T0229472

Safety Law

Occupational Safety & Health Guide Series

Series Editor:
Thomas D. Schneid
Eastern Kentucky University
Richmond, Kentucky

PUBLISHED TITLES

Motor Carrier Safety: A Guide to Regulatory Compliance
E. Scott Dunlap

Occupational Health Guide to Violence in the Workplace
Thomas D. Schneid

Physical Hazards of the Workplace, Second Edition
Barry Spurlock

Physical Security and Safety: A Field Guide for the Practitioner
Truett A. Ricks, Bobby E. Ricks, and Jeffrey Dingle

Safety Performance in a Lean Environment: A Guide to
Building Safety into a Process
Paul F. English

Security Management: A Critical Thinking Approach
Michael Land, Truett Ricks, and Bobby Ricks

Security Management for Occupational Safety
Michael Land

Workplace Safety and Health: Assessing Current Practices and
Promoting Change in the Profession
Thomas D. Schneid

Safety Law: Legal Aspects in Occupational Safety and Health
Thomas D. Schneid

FORTHCOMING TITLES

Safety and Human Resource Law for the Safety Professional
Thomas D. Schneid

Human Resources & Change Management for Safety Professionals
Thomas D. Schneid and Shelby L. Schneid

Safety Law
Legal Aspects in Occupational Safety and Health

Thomas D. Schneid

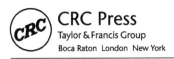

CRC Press
Taylor & Francis Group
Boca Raton London New York

CRC Press is an imprint of the
Taylor & Francis Group, an **informa** business

CRC Press
Taylor & Francis Group
6000 Broken Sound Parkway NW, Suite 300
Boca Raton, FL 33487-2742

First issued in paperback 2023

© 2018 by Taylor & Francis Group, LLC
CRC Press is an imprint of Taylor & Francis Group, an Informa business

No claim to original U.S. Government works

ISBN 13: 978-1-03-257026-6 (pbk)
ISBN 13: 978-0-8153-5496-3 (hbk)

DOI: 10.1201/9781351130998

This book contains information obtained from authentic and highly regarded sources. Reasonable efforts have been made to publish reliable data and information, but the author and publisher cannot assume responsibility for the validity of all materials or the consequences of their use. The authors and publishers have attempted to trace the copyright holders of all material reproduced in this publication and apologize to copyright holders if permission to publish in this form has not been obtained. If any copyright material has not been acknowledged please write and let us know so we may rectify in any future reprint.

Except as permitted under U.S. Copyright Law, no part of this book may be reprinted, reproduced, transmitted, or utilized in any form by any electronic, mechanical, or other means, now known or hereafter invented, including photocopying, microfilming, and recording, or in any information storage or retrieval system, without written permission from the publishers.

For permission to photocopy or use material electronically from this work, please access www.copyright.com (http://www.copyright.com/) or contact the Copyright Clearance Center, Inc. (CCC), 222 Rosewood Drive, Danvers, MA 01923, 978-750-8400. CCC is a not-for-profit organization that provides licenses and registration for a variety of users. For organizations that have been granted a photocopy license by the CCC, a separate system of payment has been arranged.

Trademark Notice: Product or corporate names may be trademarks or registered trademarks, and are used only for identification and explanation without intent to infringe.

Publisher's Note
The publisher has gone to great lengths to ensure the quality of this reprint but points out that some imperfections in the original copies may be apparent.

Visit the Taylor & Francis Web site at
http://www.taylorandfrancis.com

and the CRC Press Web site at
http://www.crcpress.com

Contents

Foreword

Law, Society and Interpretation of Rules… All of these elements are critically important to our community today, and in the future. I first met Dr. Tom Schneid in the 1980s, when OSHA was a young field, and maturing day by day. The study of Occupational Safety and Health, including the case law, is critical to improving the safety of our community as a whole. As you read Tom's latest book, understand that OSHA in and of itself does not keep us safe, YOU do as part of your chosen safety profession.

As I was taught many years ago, when I was a Special Government Employee for OSHA during my VPP work, we must observe, listen, learn, and apply our skills, knowledge, and understanding of improvement of safety and health. I have been a safety practitioner since the 1970s. My career has been in general industry, construction, and government operations. I was a federal safety officer at the Oklahoma City bombing in 1995 as well as at the World Trade Center Attacks in New York City in 2001 for over 100 days.

OSHA was formed in 1971 and has been providing guidance and support since its inception. These cases are critical to your understanding and application of OSHA. As you read this text, understand that you have the opportunity to view and apply decades of guidance and interpretation. We did not have that luxury when I started my safety career in the beginning when OSHA was in its infancy. It is important to note that OSHA standards are not the ceiling or the epitome of your program, but merely a starting point. They are Minimums, and that your programs must be constantly evolving.

In the study of OSHA law, precedent setting decisions are done differently than in Civil and Criminal cases. OSHA cases are adjudicated via an administrative process that differs. The study of these cases are critical elements to assist in your understanding of OSHA. Our desire for you is to fully immerse yourself in the study, interpretation, and application of what you will learn here.

I have had the honor of working with and for Dr. Schneid for nearly four decades and learn every day.

I applaud you for taking this next step in your career … Never stop learning … Explore new ideas….

Look for new methods. Devote yourself to being a lifelong learner.

Be safe, make a difference, and make safety your first priority.

Michael J. Fagel, PhD, CEM

Mike Fagel is an instructor in the Eastern Kentucky University Safety-Security-Emergency Management programs. He also teaches at the Illinois Institute of Technology, the National Center for Biomedical Research and Training at LSU, Northern Illinois University, and Aurora University. Fagel has authored numerous textbooks, and his latest book on Crisis Management earned textbook of the year from ASIS. His latest book on Soft Targets, Crisis Management has been adopted at several Homeland Security training programs at several universities. He can be reached at Michael.Fagel@gmail.com.

Preface

We live in a litigious and regulated society. Safety professionals are employed by corporations and other entities to not only manage inherent and created risks in the workplace in a proactive manner but also to manage the risks created through regulation and litigation. Legal and regulatory risks for corporations and individuals within the realm of safety and health have increased substantially over the past decades including, but not limited to, increased monetary penalties by the Occupational Safety and Health Administration (OSHA) and increased civil and criminal penalties under federal and state laws. Safety professionals today face a myriad of potential risks within the legal realm virtually each and every day on the job. Safety professionals must not only be knowledgeable in the methods of minimizing or eliminating risks in the workplace but also must be knowledgeable about the legal and regulatory risks and how to challenge or defend within the bounds of our judicial system.

In this text, the author has attempted to provide a broad understanding of the basic legal structure and concepts within the U.S. judicial system as well as identifying many rights and responsibilities required under the laws and regulations. Additionally, within our niche of safety and health, a specific focus has been provided to address the various legal areas which a safety professional may encounter throughout his/her career. Although the safety and health function is proactively focused, safety professionals should be prepared and anticipate legal issues including such areas as OSHA violations and citations and workers compensation claims. When these legal challenges arise, the company or organization often looks to the safety profession to take the lead and direct the defensive strategies.

Safety professionals should be aware that any type of litigation or sanction/penalty can be costly, not only in terms of money, but also in terms of job security, mental health, impact on safety and health programs, effects on employees or workforce, and in terms of numerous other negative effects. In many legal situations in which safety professionals are involved, there are no winners or losers – both combatants are bloodied and scarred. The basic concept is for safety professionals to be able to identify potential legal, governmental, or other risks or potential liabilities and formulate a proactive approach to eliminate or minimize this risk through proactively addressing the area of potential legal liability. If feasible, the safety professional should execute a "preemptive strike" to address and eliminate the risk before the risk grows and become substantially costlier.

The author reminds our readers that the law, especially in many of the areas of the law addressed in this text, is constantly changing and evolving. Although the author has made every attempt to provide the most current and accurate information, our readers are advised to research the status of the law for any specific issue and acquire competent legal counsel where necessary. Remember, ignorance of the law is never a good defense with OSHA or in a court of law! It is the author's hope that this text opens the reader's eyes and mind to the myriad of legal risks within the safety profession in order that potential legal risks can be appropriately addressed or avoided in the future.

Acknowledgements

The research and writing of a book takes a substantial amount of time. With this book, the timing was accelerated. To this end, I would like to thank my wife for her understanding that weekend work was essential to the successful completion of this text. I would also like to thank my daughters, Shelby, Madison, and Kasi for their ideas and motivation in the completion of this text.

Additionally, I would like to thank Devin Dirks, our graduate assistant, for his assistance in researching many of the cases utilized in this text as well as our many online and campus graduate students for their ideas, concepts, and inspiration in the development of this text.

And lastly, I would like to thank my parents, Robert and Rosella, for their overriding dedication to education and sacrifice they have made over the decades to ensure the success of their children and grandchildren.

Overview

Proactive v. Reactive – The primary focus of most safety professionals is to address potential risks in a proactive manner to eliminate or minimize the risk that ultimately presents the accident, injury, or illness in the workplace. In the legal realm which we will be addressing in this text, safety professionals will prepare in a reactive manner to incidents, inspections, claims, and other actions which happen after an incident, injury, or illness.

Safety professionals should be aware that there are different courts who hear cases based upon the location and other factors. There are administrative courts who address only specific issues. The highest level of courts is the federal court system that includes the U.S. Supreme Court, Courts of Appeal, and district courts. Each state has their own court systems that range from district courts to the state highest courts. Administrative courts, such as tax courts, family courts, and other "specialty" courts can be federal or state depending on the issue. The selection of the right court will depend on the issue, location, monetary amount, and other factors.

As established under the Occupational Safety and Health Act, the Occupational Safety and Health Administration (OSHA) was tasked with developing and enforcing the standards; the National Institute of Occupational Safety and Health (NIOSH) was tasked to conduct research; and the Occupational Safety and Health Review Commission (OSHRC) is the *per se* court system for the appeal of violations issues by OSHA. Although most safety professionals are familiar with OSHA and work with the OSHA standards on a daily basis, when a compliance inspection occurs and violations are found during the inspection, often monetary penalties result which the company or organization wishes to dispute. Your company or organization will look to the safety professional, as the on-site "expert," to recommend and direct the company or organization management team in determining the appropriate course of action in this the fast-paced appeal process. Safety professionals must be prepared to address the violations in a reactive manner to appropriately direct their management team in addressing or appealing the violations in a cost-effective manner.

Safety professionals should also be knowledgeable in the areas of the law, in addition to the OSH Act, which can impact them on a daily basis. Conceptually, safety does not work in a vacuum. Any number of a myriad of laws can impact the safety function on any given day. For virtually all safety professionals, individual state workers compensation laws impact virtually every work-related injury or illness that occurs in the workplace. Each state has individual laws with different requirements, monetary values, and procedures. However, in general, most states have a monetary value paid to employees who are injured on the job in the areas of time loss benefits, paid medical costs, and a monetary amount paid for permanent bodily loss. Safety professionals proactively work to prevent the injury or illness, however if/when the accident occurs and injury or illness results, the reactive nature of the state workers compensation laws become effective.

When injuries or illnesses occur to individuals who are not employees due to the alleged negligence of the company or organization, safety professionals may encounter tort actions focused on the recovery of monetary damages in state or federal civil court. Although there are several factors in determining the appropriate court and Rules of Civil Procedure that govern this type of action, safety professionals are often called upon for their expertise in testifying or assisting legal counsel in preparation for this type of legal action.

The Americans with Disabilities Act (ADA) is the most recent major legislation which can impact the safety function. Under the three-prong test within this law, individuals who possess a permanent mental or physical disability and have a record of the disability are afforded protection as well as if the company or organization treated an individual as being disabled even if the individual is not disabled. In most situations, the individual (or employee) has requested an accommodation and the employer have denied the accommodation. In these situations, the safety professional is often involved in the assessment as well as subsequent hearings before state or federal agencies.

Long story short, safety professionals must be prepared to address not only the proactive measures to safeguard their employees but also be prepared for the reactive measures that can result after an inspection or incident. Safety professionals should be aware that your company or organization will look to you, as their safety expert, to determine their appropriate course of action in these types of situations. Safety professionals must become knowledgeable in the law, especially involving the OSH Act and state workers compensation, as well as peripheral laws that can impact the safety function, such as ADA, in order to be prepared to address these situations appropriately. Knowledge of these laws, as well as other laws that impact the workplace, can offer a level of protection and forethought wherein the safety professional can identify the potential risk and turn a potentially reactive situation into a proactive elimination of such risk along with the correlating costs.

Safety professionals should be aware that the law is an ever-changing organism with court decisions being made daily at all levels of the federal, state, and administrative court systems. It is imperative that safety professionals not only understand the applicable laws but also know the methodology through which to identify, research, and understand the applicable law as it stands on any given day. Please remember that under our three-pronged system, the duty of the courts is to interpret the laws and different courts can have different opinions and which opinions or decisions are applicable to your situation.

> The law should be loved a little because it is felt to be just; feared a little because it is severe; hated a little because it is a certain degree out of sympathy with the prevalent temper of the day; and respected because it is felt to be a necessity.
>
> **Emile Fourget**

ANALYZING AND BRIEFING A COURT DECISION

Safety professionals work with and for the law on a daily basis. In the United States, laws can be made by the executive branch (i.e. executive order) or the legislative branch (i.e. new laws) and the judicial branch is to review and assess the validity and applicability of these laws. This assessment by the judicial branch of our government is often called "case law" and is the evaluation, assessment, and decisions of the courts at all levels up to and including the U.S. Supreme Court.

Safety professionals should be aware that there are state courts as well as federal courts and even specialty courts such as Family Law courts and Traffic Courts. Although the court name may vary, both the state and federal courts possess a hierarchy wherein each court decision can be appealed to a higher court by any of the parties involved in the actions. The highest court in most state judiciary systems as well as the federal judiciary system is the Supreme Court. For safety professionals who may be unfamiliar with their individual state judiciary system or the federal judiciary system, it is important to acquire a basic knowledge of the levels of the courts, namely the specialty courts, such as tax court, the district or trial courts (where most trials take place), the appellate courts, and the state top court or the U.S. Supreme Court.

When reading a court decision, safety professionals may wish to utilize the following outline:

1. Identify the court and date of the case at the top of the decision.
2. Look up any legal terms you are not familiar with.
3. Read the case in total.
4. Determine the type of case you are reading.
5. Review the case summary or headnotes.
6. Read the case again and identify the court's decision.
7. If an appellate case, identify if the decision was unanimous or a split decision.
8. Did the minority provide a dissenting opinion?
9. Re-read the case. Identify the parties, issues, and facts of the case.
10. Brief your case in writing so you will remember the issues, facts, and decision at a later date.

Safety professionals should be aware that although the courts are not supposed to make law, their decisions are in fact shaping and making new law. The decisions of the courts are often called "case law" which is the accumulation of court decisions that provide guidance and direction on current and future cases and decisions. As identified above, cases usually start at the lowest level in either the state or federal judiciary system and are appealed upward within the system to the top court but can stop at any level. The decision of the higher court usually supercedes the decision of the lower court in whole or in part.

It is important that safety professionals acquire the skill and ability to carefully analyze these court decisions in order to know the status of the law on any given day. Safety professionals can find the court's decisions at most courthouses or law libraries however databases, such as Westlaw and Lexis, provide all cases to the safety professional as near as his/her computer. Court decisions are identified by name, *Jones v. Smith*, as well as the volume and page number within the identified location of the case and the year of the decision. As an example, Jones v. Smith, 22

U.S. 25 (2011). The parties are Jones being the action against Smith. Jones would be the plaintiff and Smith would be the defendant. The case can be count in volume 22 within the U.S. Supreme Court cases at page 25. The decision was rendered by the U.S. Supreme Court in 2011.

As identified above, it is important that the safety professional first read the case in full to identify the type of case, e.g. criminal or civil, as well as acquire a flavor of the case. Safety and health professionals should identify the parties, the type of case, what are the broad issues and the identified defenses as well as the court's decision. After the initial reading of the case, safety professionals should re-read the case with an eye to the detail provided within the case. On the third reading, the safety professional should take notes and begin to assemble the structure of the case brief which the safety professional can use to refresh his/her memory of the case or for use in whatever activity is at hand.

The primary reason safety professionals should brief a case is to provide an understanding of the particular issues and decisions in the cases as well as to provide a method of remembering the cases when a large number of cases are involved in the situation. Although there are various methods of briefing a case, the following method is provided as one example. Safety professionals should find a method in which they are comfortable and utilize this method consistently in their work.

BRIEFING A CASE Methodology:

1. CASE – List the case name, the court, and the date of the case at the top of the brief.
2. ISSUE – In a clear and concise manner of no more than 1–3 sentences, completely explain the issue(s) in the case.
3. FACTS – In a clear and concise manner of no more than 1–2 paragraphs, identify all the pertinent facts of the case.
4. HOLDING OR DECISION – Clearly and concisely identify the decision of the court.
5. DISSENT OR DISSENTING OPINION – If the minority provided a dissenting opinion, provide a clear and concise explanation of the dissenting judge's position.
6. YOUR OPINION – It is important for safety professionals to identify why they agree or disagree with the decision of the court.

Most case briefs should be one page in length but no more than 2 pages. Safety professionals who exceed the one page limit may want to reassess their analysis and reduce the verbage to address only the issues, facts, and decision provided by the court. In essence, the brief is a short, concise and "to the point" document which safety professionals can use to remember the case and possess a quick review of the important aspects of the case. If additional details are needed, the safety professional should go back and review the entire case.

Below please find an example of a very basic case brief for your review and use:

Case Name: *Smith v. Jones, Inc,* 10 Anystate Court, 21 (2011)

Issues: Smith alleged she was discriminated against by her employer, Jones, Inc., in violation of the Pregnancy Discrimination Act and Title VII of the Civil Rights Act.

Facts: Smith, employed by Jones, Inc. for five years, was terminated from her employment. Jones alleges Smith was terminated for theft of company property. Smith alleges she was terminated when she informed her boss that she was pregnant.

Holding: For the Defendant, Jones, Inc. The court found that the termination of Smith for theft was appropriate and found no discrimination based on her pregnancy.

My Opinion: I disagree with the decision of the court. Jones possessed a history of terminating employees who file for any type of leave of absence. Smith was constructively terminated under the precursor of theft that was simply a company pen she forgot in her purse.

Authors

Thomas D. Schneid is the chair of the Department of Safety and Security and a tenured professor in the School of Safety, Security and Emergency Management in the College of Justice and Safety at Eastern Kentucky University. Tom has worked in the safety, human resource, and legal fields and has represented numerous corporations and individuals in OSHA and labor/employment related litigations throughout the United States. Tom has earned a BS in education, MS and CAS in safety as well as his Juris Doctor (JD in law) from West Virginia University and LLM (Graduate Labor and Employment Law) from the University of San Diego as well as post tenure PhD in Environmental Engineering and MS in International Business. Tom is a member of the bar for the U.S. Supreme Court, 6th Circuit Court of Appeals, and a number of federal districts as well as the Kentucky and West Virginia Bar.

Tom has authored and co-authored numerous texts on including Workplace Safety and Health: *Assessing Current Practices and Promoting Change in the Profession* (2014); *Corporate Safety Compliance: Law, OSHA and Ethics* (2008); *Labor and Employment Issues for Safety Professional* (2011); *Americans With Disabilities Act: A Compliance Guide* (1994); *ADA: A Manager's Guide* (1993); *Legal Liabilities for Safety and Loss Prevention Professionals* (2010); *Fire and Emergency Law Casebook* (1996); *Creative Safety Solutions* (1998); *Occupational Health Guide to Violence in the Workplace* (1999); *Legal Liabilities in Emergency Management* (2001); and *Fire Law* (1995). Tom has also co-authored several texts including *Food Safety Law* (1997), *Legal Liabilities for Safety and Loss Prevention Professionals* (1997), *Physical Hazards in the Workplace* (2001), and *Disaster Management and Preparedness* (2000) as well as over 100 articles on safety and legal topics.

Tom's current areas of academic interest include Drone Law, Licensure for the Safety Profession, and the Changing Labor Landscape in the United States.

1 Constitution of the United States and Constitutional Law

Laws are not invented; they grow out of circumstance.

Azarias

Laws should be made like clothes. They should be made to fit the people they are meant to serve.

Clarence Darrow

STUDENT LEARNING OBJECTIVES

1. Acquire an understanding of the U.S. Constitution.
2. Acquire an understanding of the Amendments to the U.S. Constitution.
3. Acquire an understanding of the Powers granted by the U.S. Constitution.
4. Acquire an understanding of the Bill of Rights.
5. Acquire an understanding of U.S. Supreme Court.

The Constitution of the United States is the root for the tree of laws that governs the United States. The U.S. Constitution, drafted in 1787 by the Founding Fathers, contains seven (7) short sections, called "Articles," and contains approximately 4,400 words. The first 10 Amendments to the Constitution, known commonly as the "Bill of Rights," was added four years later. The U.S. Constitution established the framework for the United States including the separation of powers; checks and balances; freedom of speech, religion, and the press; right to bear arms; judicial review; and due process and equal protection. All laws and virtually everything the government does must adhere to the U.S. Constitution.

Constitutional law is the interpretation of the U.S. Constitution by the courts and the application of the rights and responsibilities granted under the U.S. Constitution to a myriad of issues. Since the writing of the U.S. Constitution and the original 10 Amendments, Congress has added only 17 additional Amendments over the past 230± years. However, Constitutional law is one of the most hotly debated areas of the law due to the fact that it impacts virtually every other area of the law; the issues are usually political or impact individual values and often address the processes and powers to make or apply other laws. The U.S. Supreme Court is the ultimate authority in interpreting the U.S. Constitution.

In the area of Constitutional law, the U.S. Constitution is the top law; however, each state also has individual state constitutions that provide another layer of rights and protections. Although many state constitutions are mirrored after the U.S. Constitution, state constitutions are often more detailed and establish a parallel state government that includes legislative, executive, and judicial branches and often a state bill of rights. Constitutional law, in essence, is the courts address the conflicts and powers granted to federal and state governments under the U.S. Constitution as well as individual state constitutions.

The U.S. Constitution establishes the executive branch (i.e. the President), the legislative branch (i.e. the Congress), and the judicial branch (i.e. the courts). In this "balance of powers," the U.S. Supreme Court is often the final arbitrator in conflicts. The U.S. Supreme Court has the power to review federal as well as state legislation to determine whether the law is constitutional. The federal court system also has acquired jurisdiction over many other issues that are not constitutionally related such as civil cases arising under federal laws, cases involving citizens of different states, and cases involving crime, such as drug offenses, which violate federal laws.

Under Article I of the Constitution, Congress was granted the power to "lay and collect taxes," "borrow money," "declare war," and "raise and support Armies" as well as "to regulate Commerce with foreign nations, and among the several States, and with Indian Tribes." Through court decisions, each and every word within the Constitution granting powers to Congress have been defined and expanding the power of Congress to include commerce between states, establishing federal crimes, and numerous other powers within the scope of the Constitutional perimeters.

The U.S. Constitution specifically granted the President the ability to act as the commander in chief of the armed forces; the ability to appoint ambassadors to represent the United States in foreign countries; the ability to appoint judges in the federal courts; the ability to appoint officials within the executive branch (with the consent of the U.S. Senate); and to veto legislation which Congress may propose. Where the lines of power between Congress and the President has been the source of numerous court decisions ranging from the President's power to initiate military action to the power to collect "penalties" (or taxes).

Although the Constitution provides little guidance and explicitly grants few rights in the document to the states, the concept of *federalism,* the idea that governmental power is shared between the state and national governments, is one of the foundational concepts of our constitutional system. In essence, the states have general authority, while the federal government possesses only the power specifically enumerated in the Constitution.

For a substantial period, the Supreme Court tended to favor state's authority over federal authority, citing the commerce clause and other provisions of the Constitution as limiting federal authority. This concept, generally known as "dual sovereignty," identified that the states possess one sphere of power and the federal government possesses another sphere of power and neither side could operate in the other side's sphere of power. Over the years, the concept of dual sovereignty has lessened, and the concept of "preemption" has emerged. Under this doctrine, when the federal government enforces a law, the federal law preempts state law in any areas that potentially conflicts with federal law. However, if the federal government does not act, the state law would take precedent. However, sometimes if the federal government does not act, the state could still be barred from acting if the federal power is considered dormant.

(Preamble)

We the People of the United States, in Order to form a more perfect Union, establish Justice, insure domestic Tranquility, provide for the common defence, promote the general Welfare, and secure the Blessings of Liberty to ourselves and our Posterity, do ordain and establish this Constitution for the United States of America.

Article I (Article 1 – Legislative)

SECTION 1

All legislative Powers herein granted shall be vested in a Congress of the United States, which shall consist of a Senate and House of Representatives.

SECTION 2

1: The House of Representatives shall be composed of Members chosen every second Year by the People of the several States, and the Electors in each State shall have the Qualifications requisite for Electors of the most numerous Branch of the State Legislature.

2: No Person shall be a Representative who shall not have attained to the Age of twenty five Years, and been seven Years a Citizen of the United States, and who shall not, when elected, be an Inhabitant of that State in which he shall be chosen.

3: Representatives and direct Taxes shall be apportioned among the several States which may be included within this Union, according to their respective Numbers, which shall be determined by adding to the whole Number of free Persons, including those bound to Service for a Term of Years, and excluding Indians not taxed, three fifths of all other Persons. The actual Enumeration shall be made within three Years after the first Meeting of the Congress of the United States, and within every subsequent Term of ten Years, in such Manner as they shall by Law direct. The Number of Representatives shall not exceed one for every thirty Thousand, but each State shall have at Least one Representative; and until such enumeration shall be made, the State of New Hampshire shall be entitled to chuse three, Massachusetts eight, Rhode-Island and Providence Plantations one, Connecticut five, New-York six, New Jersey four, Pennsylvania eight, Delaware one, Maryland six, Virginia ten, North Carolina five, South Carolina five, and Georgia three.

4: When vacancies happen in the Representation from any State, the Executive Authority thereof shall issue Writs of Election to fill such Vacancies.

5: The House of Representatives shall chuse their Speaker and other Officers; and shall have the sole Power of Impeachment.

SECTION 3

1: The Senate of the United States shall be composed of two Senators from each State, chosen by the Legislature thereof, for six Years; and each Senator shall have one Vote.

2: Immediately after they shall be assembled in Consequence of the first Election, they shall be divided as equally as may be into three Classes. The Seats of the Senators of the first Class shall be vacated at the Expiration of the second Year, of the second Class at the Expiration of the fourth Year, and of the third Class at the Expiration of the sixth Year, so that one third may be chosen every second Year; and if Vacancies happen by Resignation, or otherwise, during the Recess of the Legislature of any State, the Executive thereof may make temporary Appointments until the next Meeting of the Legislature, which shall then fill such Vacancies.

3: No Person shall be a Senator who shall not have attained to the Age of thirty Years, and been nine Years a Citizen of the United States, and who shall not, when elected, be an Inhabitant of that State for which he shall be chosen.

4: The Vice President of the United States shall be President of the Senate, but shall have no Vote, unless they be equally divided.

5: The Senate shall chuse their other Officers, and also a President pro tempore, in the Absence of the Vice President, or when he shall exercise the Office of President of the United States.

6: The Senate shall have the sole Power to try all Impeachments. When sitting for that Purpose, they shall be on Oath or Affirmation. When the President of the United States is tried, the Chief Justice shall preside: And no Person shall be convicted without the Concurrence of two thirds of the Members present.

7: Judgment in Cases of impeachment shall not extend further than to removal from Office, and disqualification to hold and enjoy any Office of honor, Trust or Profit under the United States: but the Party convicted shall nevertheless be liable and subject to Indictment, Trial, Judgment and Punishment, according to Law.

SECTION 4

1: The Times, Places and Manner of holding Elections for Senators and Representatives, shall be prescribed in each State by the Legislature thereof; but the Congress may at any time by Law make or alter such Regulations, except as to the Places of chusing Senators.

2: The Congress shall assemble at least once in every Year, and such Meeting shall be on the first Monday in December, unless they shall by Law appoint a different Day.

SECTION 5

1: Each House shall be the Judge of the Elections, Returns and Qualifications of its own Members, and a Majority of each shall constitute a Quorum to do Business; but a smaller Number may adjourn from day to day, and may be authorized to compel the Attendance of absent Members, in such Manner, and under such Penalties as each House may provide.

2: Each House may determine the Rules of its Proceedings, punish its Members for disorderly Behaviour, and, with the Concurrence of two thirds, expel a Member.

3: Each House shall keep a Journal of its Proceedings, and from time to time publish the same, excepting such Parts as may in their Judgment require Secrecy; and the Yeas and Nays of the Members of either House on any question shall, at the Desire of one fifth of those Present, be entered on the Journal.

4: Neither House, during the Session of Congress, shall, without the Consent of the other, adjourn for more than three days, nor to any other Place than that in which the two Houses shall be sitting.

SECTION 6

1: The Senators and Representatives shall receive a Compensation for their Services, to be ascertained by Law, and paid out of the Treasury of the United States. They shall in all Cases, except Treason, Felony and Breach of the Peace, be privileged from Arrest during their Attendance at the Session of their respective Houses, and in going to and returning from the same; and for any Speech or Debate in either House, they shall not be questioned in any other Place.

2: No Senator or Representative shall, during the Time for which he was elected, be appointed to any civil Office under the Authority of the United States, which shall have been created, or the Emoluments whereof shall have been encreased during such time; and no Person holding any Office under the United States, shall be a Member of either House during his Continuance in Office.

SECTION 7

1: All Bills for raising Revenue shall originate in the House of Representatives; but the Senate may propose or concur with Amendments as on other Bills.

2: Every Bill which shall have passed the House of Representatives and the Senate, shall, before it become a Law, be presented to the President of the United States; If he approve he shall sign it, but if not he shall return it, with his Objections to that House in which it shall have originated, who shall enter the Objections at large on their Journal, and proceed to reconsider it. If after such Reconsideration two thirds of that House shall agree to pass the Bill, it shall be sent, together with the Objections, to the other House, by which it shall likewise be reconsidered, and if approved by two thirds of that House, it shall become a Law. But in all such Cases the Votes of both Houses shall be determined by yeas and Nays, and the Names of the Persons voting for and against the Bill shall be entered on the Journal of each House respectively. If any Bill shall not be returned by the President within ten Days (Sundays excepted) after it shall have been presented to him, the Same shall be a Law, in like Manner as if he had signed it, unless the Congress by their Adjournment prevent its Return, in which Case it shall not be a Law.

3: Every Order, Resolution, or Vote to which the Concurrence of the Senate and House of Representatives may be necessary (except on a question of Adjournment) shall be presented to the President of the United States; and before the Same shall take Effect, shall be approved by him, or being disapproved by him, shall be repassed by two thirds of the Senate and House of Representatives, according to the Rules and Limitations prescribed in the Case of a Bill.

SECTION 8

1: The Congress shall have Power To lay and collect Taxes, Duties, Imposts and Excises, to pay the Debts and provide for the common Defence and general Welfare of the United States; but all Duties, Imposts and Excises shall be uniform throughout the United States;

2: To borrow Money on the credit of the United States;

3: To regulate Commerce with foreign Nations, and among the several States, and with the Indian Tribes;

4: To establish an uniform Rule of Naturalization, and uniform Laws on the subject of Bankruptcies throughout the United States;

5: To coin Money, regulate the Value thereof, and of foreign Coin, and fix the Standard of Weights and Measures;

6: To provide for the Punishment of counterfeiting the Securities and current Coin of the United States;

7: To establish Post Offices and post Roads;

8: To promote the Progress of Science and useful Arts, by securing for limited Times to Authors and Inventors the exclusive Right to their respective Writings and Discoveries;

9: To constitute Tribunals inferior to the Supreme Court;

10: To define and punish Piracies and Felonies committed on the high Seas, and Offences against the Law of Nations;

11: To declare War, grant Letters of Marque and Reprisal, and make Rules concerning Captures on Land and Water;

12: To raise and support Armies, but no Appropriation of Money to that Use shall be for a longer Term than two Years;

13: To provide and maintain a Navy;

14: To make Rules for the Government and Regulation of the land and naval Forces;

15: To provide for calling forth the Militia to execute the Laws of the Union, suppress Insurrections and repel Invasions;

16: To provide for organizing, arming, and disciplining, the Militia, and for governing such Part of them as may be employed in the Service of the United States, reserving to the States respectively, the Appointment of the Officers, and the Authority of training the Militia according to the discipline prescribed by Congress;

17: To exercise exclusive Legislation in all Cases whatsoever, over such District (not exceeding ten Miles square) as may, by Cession of particular States, and the Acceptance of Congress, become the Seat of the Government of the United States, and to exercise like Authority over all Places purchased by the Consent of the Legislature of the State in which the Same shall be, for the Erection of Forts, Magazines, Arsenals, dock-Yards, and other needful Buildings; – And

18: To make all Laws which shall be necessary and proper for carrying into Execution the foregoing Powers, and all other Powers vested by this Constitution in the Government of the United States, or in any Department or Officer thereof.

SECTION 9

1: The Migration or Importation of such Persons as any of the States now existing shall think proper to admit, shall not be prohibited by the Congress prior to the Year one thousand eight hundred and eight, but a Tax or duty may be imposed on such Importation, not exceeding ten dollars for each Person.

2: The Privilege of the Writ of Habeas Corpus shall not be suspended, unless when in Cases of Rebellion or Invasion the public Safety may require it.

3: No Bill of Attainder or ex post facto Law shall be passed.

4: No Capitation, or other direct, Tax shall be laid, unless in Proportion to the Census or Enumeration herein before directed to be taken.

5: No Tax or Duty shall be laid on Articles exported from any State.

6: No Preference shall be given by any Regulation of Commerce or Revenue to the Ports of one State over those of another: nor shall Vessels bound to, or from, one State, be obliged to enter, clear, or pay Duties in another.

7: No Money shall be drawn from the Treasury, but in Consequence of Appropriations made by Law; and a regular Statement and Account of the Receipts and Expenditures of all public Money shall be published from time to time.

8: No Title of Nobility shall be granted by the United States: And no Person holding any Office of Profit or Trust under them, shall, without the Consent of the Congress, accept of any present, Emolument, Office, or Title, of any kind whatever, from any King, Prince, or foreign State.

SECTION 10

1: No State shall enter into any Treaty, Alliance, or Confederation; grant Letters of Marque and Reprisal; coin Money; emit Bills of Credit; make any Thing but gold and silver Coin a Tender in Payment of Debts; pass any Bill of Attainder, ex post facto Law, or Law impairing the Obligation of Contracts, or grant any Title of Nobility.

2: No State shall, without the Consent of the Congress, lay any Imposts or Duties on Imports or Exports, except what may be absolutely necessary for executing it's inspection Laws: and the net Produce of all Duties and Imposts, laid by any State on Imports or Exports, shall be for the Use of the Treasury of the United States; and all such Laws shall be subject to the Revision and Controul of the Congress.

3: No State shall, without the Consent of Congress, lay any Duty of Tonnage, keep Troops, or Ships of War in time of Peace, enter into any Agreement or Compact with another State, or with a foreign Power, or engage in War, unless actually invaded, or in such imminent Danger as will not admit of delay.

Article II (Article 2 – Executive)

SECTION 1

1: The executive Power shall be vested in a President of the United States of America. He shall hold his Office during the Term of four Years, and, together with the Vice President, chosen for the same Term, be elected, as follows

2: Each State shall appoint, in such Manner as the Legislature thereof may direct, a Number of Electors, equal to the whole Number of Senators and Representatives to which the State may be entitled in the Congress: but no Senator or Representative, or Person holding an Office of Trust or Profit under the United States, shall be appointed an Elector.

3: The Electors shall meet in their respective States, and vote by Ballot for two Persons, of whom one at least shall not be an Inhabitant of the same State with themselves. And they shall make a List of all the Persons voted for, and of the Number of Votes for each; which List they shall sign and certify, and transmit sealed to the Seat of the Government of the United States, directed to the President of the Senate. The President of the Senate shall, in the Presence of the Senate and House of Representatives, open all the Certificates, and the Votes shall then be counted. The Person having the greatest Number of Votes shall be the President, if such Number be a Majority of the whole Number of Electors appointed; and if there be more than one who have such Majority, and have an equal Number of Votes, then the House of Representatives shall immediately chuse by Ballot one of them for President; and if no Person have a Majority, then from the five highest on the List the said House shall in like Manner chuse the President. But in chusing the President, the Votes shall be taken by States, the Representation from each State having one Vote; A quorum for this Purpose shall consist of a Member or Members from two thirds of the States, and a Majority of all the States shall be necessary to a Choice. In every Case, after the Choice of the President, the Person having the greatest Number of Votes of the Electors shall be the Vice President. But if there should remain two or more who have equal Votes, the Senate shall chuse from them by Ballot the Vice President.

4: The Congress may determine the Time of chusing the Electors, and the Day on which they shall give their Votes; which Day shall be the same throughout the United States.

5: No Person except a natural born Citizen, or a Citizen of the United States, at the time of the Adoption of this Constitution, shall be eligible to the Office of President; neither shall any Person be eligible to that Office who shall not have attained to the Age of thirty five Years, and been fourteen Years a Resident within the United States.

6: In Case of the Removal of the President from Office, or of his Death, Resignation, or Inability to discharge the Powers and Duties of the said Office, the Same shall devolve on the Vice President, and the Congress may by Law provide for the Case of Removal, Death, Resignation or Inability, both of the President and Vice President, declaring what Officer shall then act as President, and such Officer shall act accordingly, until the Disability be removed, or a President shall be elected.

7: The President shall, at stated Times, receive for his Services, a Compensation, which shall neither be increased nor diminished during the Period for which he shall have been elected, and he shall not receive within that Period any other Emolument from the United States, or any of them.

8: Before he enter on the Execution of his Office, he shall take the following Oath or Affirmation: – "I do solemnly swear (or affirm) that I will faithfully execute the Office of President of the United States, and will to the best of my Ability, preserve, protect and defend the Constitution of the United States."

SECTION 2

1: The President shall be Commander in Chief of the Army and Navy of the United States, and of the Militia of the several States, when called into the actual Service of the United States; he may require the Opinion, in writing, of the principal Officer in each of the executive Departments, upon any Subject relating to the Duties of their respective Offices, and he shall have Power to grant Reprieves and Pardons for Offences against the United States, except in Cases of Impeachment.

2: He shall have Power, by and with the Advice and Consent of the Senate, to make Treaties, provided two thirds of the Senators present concur; and he shall nominate, and by and with the Advice and Consent of the Senate, shall appoint Ambassadors, other public Ministers and Consuls, Judges of the supreme Court, and all other Officers of the United States, whose Appointments are not herein otherwise provided for, and which shall be established by Law: but the Congress may by Law vest the Appointment of such inferior Officers, as they think proper, in the President alone, in the Courts of Law, or in the Heads of Departments.

3: The President shall have Power to fill up all Vacancies that may happen during the Recess of the Senate, by granting Commissions which shall expire at the End of their next Session.

SECTION 3

He shall from time to time give to the Congress Information of the State of the Union, and recommend to their Consideration such Measures as he shall judge necessary and expedient; he may, on extraordinary Occasions, convene both Houses, or either of them, and in Case of Disagreement between them, with Respect to the Time of Adjournment, he may adjourn them to such Time as he shall think proper; he shall receive Ambassadors and other public Ministers; he shall take Care that the Laws be faithfully executed, and shall Commission all the Officers of the United States.

SECTION 4

The President, Vice President and all civil Officers of the United States, shall be removed from Office on Impeachment for, and Conviction of, Treason, Bribery, or other high Crimes and Misdemeanors.

Article III (Article 3 – Judicial)

SECTION 1

The judicial Power of the United States, shall be vested in one Supreme Court, and in such inferior Courts as the Congress may from time to time ordain and establish. The Judges, both of the supreme and inferior Courts, shall hold their Offices during good Behaviour, and shall, at stated Times, receive for their Services, a Compensation, which shall not be diminished during their Continuance in Office.

SECTION 2

1: The judicial Power shall extend to all Cases, in Law and Equity, arising under this Constitution, the Laws of the United States, and Treaties made, or which shall be made, under their Authority; – to all Cases affecting Ambassadors, other public Ministers and Consuls; – to all Cases of admiralty and maritime Jurisdiction; – to Controversies to which the United States shall be a Party; – to Controversies between two or more States; – between a State and Citizens of another State; – between Citizens of different States, – between Citizens of the same State claiming Lands under Grants of different States, and between a State, or the Citizens thereof, and foreign States, Citizens or Subjects.

2: In all Cases affecting Ambassadors, other public Ministers and Consuls, and those in which a State shall be Party, the Supreme Court shall have original Jurisdiction. In all the other Cases before mentioned, the Supreme Court shall have appellate Jurisdiction, both as to Law and Fact, with such Exceptions, and under such Regulations as the Congress shall make.

3: The Trial of all Crimes, except in Cases of Impeachment, shall be by Jury; and such Trial shall be held in the State where the said Crimes shall have been committed; but when not committed within any State, the Trial shall be at such Place or Places as the Congress may by Law have directed.

SECTION 3

1: Treason against the United States, shall consist only in levying War against them, or in adhering to their Enemies, giving them Aid and Comfort. No Person shall be convicted of Treason unless on the Testimony of two Witnesses to the same overt Act, or on Confession in open Court.

2: The Congress shall have Power to declare the Punishment of Treason, but no Attainder of Treason shall work Corruption of Blood, or Forfeiture except during the Life of the Person attainted.

Article IV (Article 4 – States' Relations)

SECTION 1

Full Faith and Credit shall be given in each State to the public Acts, Records, and judicial Proceedings of every other State. And the Congress may by general Laws prescribe the Manner in which such Acts, Records and Proceedings shall be proved, and the Effect thereof.

SECTION 2

1: The Citizens of each State shall be entitled to all Privileges and Immunities of Citizens in the several States.

2: A Person charged in any State with Treason, Felony, or other Crime, who shall flee from Justice, and be found in another State, shall on Demand of the executive Authority of the State from which he fled, be delivered up, to be removed to the State having Jurisdiction of the Crime.

3: No Person held to Service or Labour in one State, under the Laws thereof, escaping into another, shall, in Consequence of any Law or Regulation therein, be discharged from such Service or Labour, but shall be delivered up on Claim of the Party to whom such Service or Labour may be due.

SECTION 3

1: New States may be admitted by the Congress into this Union; but no new State shall be formed or erected within the Jurisdiction of any other State; nor any State be formed by the Junction of two or more States, or Parts of States, without the Consent of the Legislatures of the States concerned as well as of the Congress.

2: The Congress shall have Power to dispose of and make all needful Rules and Regulations respecting the Territory or other Property belonging to the United States; and nothing in this Constitution shall be so construed as to Prejudice any Claims of the United States, or of any particular State.

SECTION 4

The United States shall guarantee to every State in this Union a Republican Form of Government, and shall protect each of them against Invasion; and on Application of the Legislature, or of the Executive (when the Legislature cannot be convened) against domestic Violence.

Article V (Article 5 – Mode of Amendment)

The Congress, whenever two thirds of both Houses shall deem it necessary, shall propose Amendments to this Constitution, or, on the Application of the Legislatures of two thirds of the several States, shall call a Convention for proposing Amendments, which, in either Case, shall be valid to all Intents and Purposes, as Part of this Constitution, when ratified by the Legislatures of three fourths of the several States, or by Conventions in three fourths thereof, as the one or the other Mode of Ratification may be proposed by the Congress; Provided that no Amendment which may be made prior to the Year One thousand eight hundred and eight shall in any Manner affect the first and fourth Clauses in the Ninth Section of the first Article; and that no State, without its Consent, shall be deprived of its equal Suffrage in the Senate.

Article VI (Article 6 – Prior Debts, National Supremacy, Oaths of Office)

1: All Debts contracted and Engagements entered into, before the Adoption of this Constitution, shall be as valid against the United States under this Constitution, as under the Confederation.

2: This Constitution, and the Laws of the United States which shall be made in Pursuance thereof; and all Treaties made, or which shall be made, under the Authority of the United States, shall be the supreme Law of the Land; and the Judges in every State shall be bound thereby, any Thing in the Constitution or Laws of any State to the Contrary notwithstanding.

3: The Senators and Representatives before mentioned, and the Members of the several State Legislatures, and all executive and judicial Officers, both of the United States and of the several States, shall be bound by Oath or Affirmation, to support this Constitution; but no religious Test shall ever be required as a Qualification to any Office or public Trust under the United States.

Article VII (Article 7 – Ratification)

The Ratification of the Conventions of nine States, shall be sufficient for the Establishment of this Constitution between the States so ratifying the Same.

The Word "the," being interlined between the seventh and eight Lines of the first Page, The Word "Thirty" being partly written on an Erazure in the fifteenth Line of the first Page. The Words "is tried" being interlined between the thirty second and thirty third Lines of the first Page and the Word "the" being interlined between the forty third and forty fourth Lines of the second Page.

done *in Convention by the Unanimous Consent of the States present the Seventeenth Day of September in the Year of our Lord one thousand seven hundred and Eighty seven and of the Independence of the United States of America the Twelfth* **In witness** *whereof We have hereunto subscribed our Names,*

Attest William Jackson Secretary

Go: Washington -Presidt. and deputy from Virginia

Delaware
    Geo: Read
    Gunning Bedford jun
    John Dickinson
    Richard Bassett
    Jaco: Broom
Maryland
    James McHenry
    Dan of St Thos. Jenifer
    Danl Carroll.
Virginia
    John Blair—
    James Madison Jr.
North Carolina
    Wm Blount
    Richd. Dobbs Spaight.
    Hu Williamson
South Carolina
    J. Rutledge
    Charles Cotesworth Pinckney

(Continued)

Charles Pinckney
Pierce Butler.
Georgia
William Few
Abr Baldwin
New Hampshire
John Langdon
Nicholas Gilman
Massachusetts
Nathaniel Gorham
Rufus King
Connecticut
Wm. Saml. Johnson
Roger Sherman
New York
Alexander Hamilton
New Jersey
Wil. Livingston
David Brearley.
Wm. Paterson.
Jona: Dayton
Pennsylvania
B Franklin
Thomas Mifflin
Robt Morris
Geo. Clymer
Thos. FitzSimons
Jared Ingersoll
James Wilson.
Gouv Morris

Note: U.S. Constitution, National Archives.

The first 10 Amendments, commonly known as the "Bill of Rights," was added by the founding fathers soon after the completion of the U.S. Constitution. These first 10 Amendments were designed to protect individual citizens from the powers granted to the newly formed federal government. The 13th, 14th, and 15th Amendments were added after the Civil War abolishing slavery, protecting and ensuring voting rights, extending due process requirements to the states, and extending equal protection. Through the Supreme Court's adoption of the approach called *selective incorporation*, the court selectively applied many of the provisions from the Amendments to the Bill of Rights and to states.

Of particular importance to safety professionals, as well as all citizens of the United States, are the rights granted under the U.S. Constitution. Every constitutional right is founded in one or more provisions of the text of the "Bill of Rights" in the Constitution. These foundational rights include the right to free speech in the First Amendment, the right to bear arms in the Second Amendment, and additional enumerated rights as identified below.

Congress OF THE United States, begun and held at the City of New-York, on Wednesday the fourth of March, one thousand seven hundred and eighty nine.

THE Conventions of a number of the States, having at the time of their adopting the Constitution, expressed a desire, in order to prevent misconstruction or abuse of its powers, that further declaratory and restrictive clauses should be added: And as extending the ground of public confidence in the Government, will best ensure the beneficent ends of its institution.

RESOLVED by the Senate and House of Representatives of the United States of America, in Congress assembled, two thirds of both Houses concurring, that the following Articles be proposed to the Legislatures of the several States, as amendments to the Constitution of the United States, all, or any of which Articles, when ratified by three fourths of the said Legislatures, to be valid to all intents and purposes, as part of the said Constitution; viz.

ARTICLES in addition to, and Amendment of the Constitution of the United States of America, proposed by Congress, and ratified by the Legislatures of the several States, pursuant to the fifth Article of the original Constitution.

(Articles I through X are known as the Bill of Rights)

-

Article the first… After the first enumeration required by the first Article of the Constitution, there shall be one Representative for every thirty thousand, until the number shall amount to one hundred, after which, the proportion shall be so regulated by Congress, that there shall be not less than one hundred Representatives, nor less than one Representative for every forty thousand persons, until the number of Representatives shall amount to two hundred, after which the proportion shall be so regulated by Congress, that there shall not be less than two hundred Representatives, nor more than one Representative for every fifty thousand persons.

-

Article the second… No law, varying the compensation for the services of the Senators and Representatives, shall take effect, until an election of Representatives shall have intervened.

Article [I] (Amendment 1 – Freedom of expression and religion)

Congress shall make no law respecting an establishment of religion, or prohibiting the free exercise thereof; or abridging the freedom of speech, or of the press; or the right of the people peaceably to assemble, and to petition the Government for a redress of grievances.

Article [II] (Amendment 2 – Bearing Arms)

A well regulated Militia, being necessary to the security of a free State, the right of the people to keep and bear Arms, shall not be infringed.

Article [III] (Amendment 3 – Quartering Soldiers)

No Soldier shall, in time of peace be quartered in any house, without the consent of the Owner, nor in time of war, but in a manner to be prescribed by law.

Article [IV] (Amendment 4 – Search and Seizure)

The right of the people to be secure in their persons, houses, papers, and effects, against unreasonable searches and seizures, shall not be violated, and no Warrants shall issue, but upon probable cause, supported by Oath or affirmation, and particularly describing the place to be searched, and the persons or things to be seized.

Article [V] (Amendment 5 – Rights of Persons)

No person shall be held to answer for a capital, or otherwise infamous crime, unless on a presentment or indictment of a Grand Jury, except in cases arising in the land or naval forces, or in the Militia, when in actual service in time of War or public danger; nor shall any person be subject for the same offence to be twice put in jeopardy of life or limb; nor shall be compelled in any criminal case to be a witness against himself, nor be deprived of life, liberty, or property, without due process of law; nor shall private property be taken for public use, without just compensation.

Article [VI] (Amendment 6 – Rights of Accused in Criminal Prosecutions)

In all criminal prosecutions, the accused shall enjoy the right to a speedy and public trial, by an impartial jury of the State and district wherein the crime shall have been committed, which district shall have been previously ascertained by law, and to be informed of the nature and cause of the accusation; to be confronted with the witnesses against him; to have compulsory process for obtaining witnesses in his favor, and to have the Assistance of Counsel for his defence.

Article [VII] (Amendment 7 – Civil Trials)

In Suits at common law, where the value in controversy shall exceed twenty dollars, the right of trial by jury shall be preserved, and no fact tried by a jury, shall be otherwise re-examined in any Court of the United States, than according to the rules of the common law.

Article [VIII] (Amendment 8 – Further Guarantees in Criminal Cases)

Excessive bail shall not be required, nor excessive fines imposed, nor cruel and unusual punishments inflicted.

Article [IX] (Amendment 9 – Unenumerated Rights)

The enumeration in the Constitution, of certain rights, shall not be construed to deny or disparage others retained by the people.

Article [X] (Amendment 10 – Reserved Powers)

The powers not delegated to the United States by the Constitution, nor prohibited by it to the States, are reserved to the States respectively, or to the people.

Attest,
John Beckley, Clerk of the
House of Representatives.
Sam. A. Otis Secretary of the Senate.

Frederick Augustus Muhlenberg Speaker of
the House of Representatives.
John Adams, Vice-President of the United
States, and President of the Senate.

(end of the Bill of Rights)

[Article XI] (Amendment 11 – Suits Against States)

The Judicial power of the United States shall not be construed to extend to any suit in law or equity, commenced or prosecuted against one of the United States by Citizens of another State, or by Citizens or Subjects of any Foreign State.

[Article XII] (Amendment 12 – Election of President)

The Electors shall meet in their respective states, and vote by ballot for President and Vice-President, one of whom, at least, shall not be an inhabitant of the same state with themselves; they shall name in their ballots the person voted for as President, and in distinct ballots the person voted for as Vice-President, and they shall make distinct lists of all persons voted for as President, and of all persons voted for as Vice-President, and of the number of votes for each, which lists they shall sign and certify, and transmit sealed to the seat of the government of the United States, directed to the President of the Senate; – The President of the Senate shall, in the presence of the Senate and House of Representatives, open all the certificates and the votes shall then be counted;—The person having the greatest number of votes for President, shall be the President, if such number be a majority of the whole number of Electors appointed; and if no person have such majority, then from the persons having the highest numbers not exceeding three on the list of those voted for as President, the House of Representatives shall choose immediately, by ballot, the President. But in choosing the President, the votes shall be taken by states, the representation from each state having one vote; a quorum for this purpose shall consist of a member or members from two-thirds of the states, and a majority of all the states shall be necessary to a choice. And if the House of Representatives shall not choose a President whenever the right of choice shall devolve upon them, before the fourth day of March next following, then the Vice-President shall act as President, as in the case of the death or other constitutional disability of the President.—The person having the greatest number of votes as Vice-President, shall be the Vice-President, if such number be a majority of the whole number of Electors appointed, and if no person have a majority, then from the two highest numbers on the list, the Senate shall choose the Vice-President; a quorum for the purpose shall consist of two-thirds of the whole number of Senators, and a majority of the whole number shall be necessary to a choice. But no person constitutionally ineligible to the office of President shall be eligible to that of Vice-President of the United States.

Article XIII (Amendment 13 – Slavery and Involuntary Servitude)

Neither slavery nor involuntary servitude, except as a punishment for crime whereof the party shall have been duly convicted, shall exist within the United States, or any place subject to their jurisdiction.

Congress shall have power to enforce this article by appropriate legislation.

Article XIV (Amendment 14 – Rights Guaranteed: Privileges and Immunities of Citizenship, Due Process, and Equal Protection)

1: All persons born or naturalized in the United States, and subject to the jurisdiction thereof, are citizens of the United States and of the State wherein they reside. No State shall make or enforce any law which shall abridge the privileges or immunities of citizens of the United States; nor shall any State deprive any person of life, liberty, or property, without due process of law; nor deny to any person within its jurisdiction the equal protection of the laws.

2: Representatives shall be apportioned among the several States according to their respective numbers, counting the whole number of persons in each State, excluding Indians not taxed. But when the right to vote at any election for the choice of electors for President and Vice President of the United States, Representatives in Congress, the Executive and Judicial officers of a State, or the members of the Legislature thereof, is denied to any of the male inhabitants of such State, being twenty-one years of age, and citizens of the United States, or in any way abridged, except for participation in rebellion, or other crime, the basis of representation therein shall be reduced in the proportion which the number of such male citizens shall bear to the whole number of male citizens twenty-one years of age in such State.

3: No person shall be a Senator or Representative in Congress, or elector of President and Vice President, or hold any office, civil or military, under the United States, or under any State, who, having previously taken an oath, as a member of Congress, or as an officer of the United States, or as a member of any State legislature, or as an executive or judicial officer of any State, to support the Constitution of the United States, shall have engaged in insurrection or rebellion against the same, or given aid or comfort to the enemies thereof. But Congress may by a vote of two-thirds of each House, remove such disability.

4: The validity of the public debt of the United States, authorized by law, including debts incurred for payment of pensions and bounties for services in suppressing insurrection or rebellion, shall not be questioned. But neither the United States nor any State shall assume or pay any debt or obligation incurred in aid of insurrection or rebellion against the United States, or any claim for the loss or emancipation of any slave; but all such debts, obligations and claims shall be held illegal and void.

5: The Congress shall have power to enforce, by appropriate legislation, the provisions of this article.

Article XV (Amendment 15 – Rights of Citizens to Vote)

The right of citizens of the United States to vote shall not be denied or abridged by the United States or by any State on account of race, color, or previous condition of servitude.

The Congress shall have power to enforce this article by appropriate legislation.

Article XVI (Amendment 16 – Income Tax)

The Congress shall have power to lay and collect taxes on incomes, from whatever source derived, without apportionment among the several States, and without regard to any census or enumeration.

[Article XVII] (Amendment 17 – Popular Election of Senators)

1: The Senate of the United States shall be composed of two Senators from each State, elected by the people thereof, for six years; and each Senator shall have one vote. The electors in each State shall have the qualifications requisite for electors of the most numerous branch of the State legislatures.

2: When vacancies happen in the representation of any State in the Senate, the executive authority of such State shall issue writs of election to fill such vacancies: Provided, That the legislature of any State may empower the executive thereof to make temporary appointments until the people fill the vacancies by election as the legislature may direct.

3: This amendment shall not be so construed as to affect the election or term of any Senator chosen before it becomes valid as part of the Constitution.

Article [XVIII] (Amendment 18 – Prohibition of Intoxicating Liquors)

1: After one year from the ratification of this article the manufacture, sale, or trans-portation of intoxicating liquors within, the importation thereof into, or the expor-tation thereof from the United States and all territory subject to the jurisdiction thereof for beverage purposes is hereby prohibited.

2: The Congress and the several States shall have concurrent power to enforce this article by appropriate legislation.

3: This article shall be inoperative unless it shall have been ratified as an amend-ment to the Constitution by the legislatures of the several States, as provided in the Constitution, within seven years from the date of the submission hereof to the States by the Congress.

Article [XIX] (Amendment 19 – Women's Suffrage Rights)

The right of citizens of the United States to vote shall not be denied or abridged by the United States or by any State on account of sex.
   Congress shall have power to enforce this article by appropriate legislation.

Article [XX] (Amendment 20 – Terms of President, Vice President, Members of Congress: Presidential Vacancy)

1: The terms of the President and Vice President shall end at noon on the 20th day of January, and the terms of Senators and Representatives at noon on the 3d day of

January, of the years in which such terms would have ended if this article had not been ratified; and the terms of their successors shall then begin.

2: The Congress shall assemble at least once in every year, and such meeting shall begin at noon on the 3d day of January, unless they shall by law appoint a different day.

3: If, at the time fixed for the beginning of the term of the President, the President elect shall have died, the Vice President elect shall become President. If a President shall not have been chosen before the time fixed for the beginning of his term, or if the President elect shall have failed to qualify, then the Vice President elect shall act as President until a President shall have qualified; and the Congress may by law provide for the case wherein neither a President elect nor a Vice President elect shall have qualified, declaring who shall then act as President, or the manner in which one who is to act shall be selected, and such person shall act accordingly until a President or Vice President shall have qualified.

4: The Congress may by law provide for the case of the death of any of the persons from whom the House of Representatives may choose a President whenever the right of choice shall have devolved upon them, and for the case of the death of any of the persons from whom the Senate may choose a Vice President whenever the right of choice shall have devolved upon them.

5: Sections 1 and 2 shall take effect on the 15th day of October following the ratification of this article.

6: This article shall be inoperative unless it shall have been ratified as an amendment to the Constitution by the legislatures of three-fourths of the several States within seven years from the date of its submission.

Article [XXI] (Amendment 21 – Repeal of Eighteenth Amendment)

1: The eighteenth article of amendment to the Constitution of the United States is hereby repealed.

2: The transportation or importation into any State, Territory, or possession of the United States for delivery or use therein of intoxicating liquors, in violation of the laws thereof, is hereby prohibited.

3: This article shall be inoperative unless it shall have been ratified as an amendment to the Constitution by conventions in the several States, as provided in the Constitution, within seven years from the date of the submission hereof to the States by the Congress.

Amendment XXII (Amendment 22 – Presidential Tenure)

1: No person shall be elected to the office of the President more than twice, and no person who has held the office of President, or acted as President, for more than two years of a term to which some other person was elected President shall be elected to the office of the President more than once. But this article shall not apply to any person holding the office of President when this article was proposed by the Congress, and shall not prevent any person who may be holding the office of President, or acting as President, during the term within which this article becomes operative from holding the office of President or acting as President during the remainder of such term.

2: This article shall be inoperative unless it shall have been ratified as an amendment to the Constitution by the legislatures of three-fourths of the several states within seven years from the date of its submission to the states by the Congress.

Amendment XXIII (Amendment 23 – Presidential Electors for the District of Columbia)

1: The District constituting the seat of government of the United States shall appoint in such manner as the Congress may direct: A number of electors of President and Vice President equal to the whole number of Senators and Representatives in Congress to which the District would be entitled if it were a state, but in no event more than the least populous state; they shall be in addition to those appointed by the states, but they shall be considered, for the purposes of the election of President and Vice President, to be electors appointed by a state; and they shall meet in the District and perform such duties as provided by the twelfth article of amendment.

2: The Congress shall have power to enforce this article by appropriate legislation.

Amendment XXIV (Amendment 24 – Abolition of the Poll Tax Qualification in Federal Elections)

1. The right of citizens of the United States to vote in any primary or other election for President or Vice President, for electors for President or Vice President, or for Senator or Representative in Congress, shall not be denied or abridged by the United States or any state by reason of failure to pay any poll tax or other tax.

2. The Congress shall have power to enforce this article by appropriate legislation.

Amendment XXV (Amendment 25 – Presidential Vacancy, Disability, and Inability)

1: In case of the removal of the President from office or of his death or resignation, the Vice President shall become President.

2: Whenever there is a vacancy in the office of the Vice President, the President shall nominate a Vice President who shall take office upon confirmation by a majority vote of both Houses of Congress.

3: Whenever the President transmits to the President pro tempore of the Senate and the Speaker of the House of Representatives his written declaration that he is unable to discharge the powers and duties of his office, and until he transmits to them a written declaration to the contrary, such powers and duties shall be discharged by the Vice President as Acting President.

4: Whenever the Vice President and a majority of either the principal officers of the executive departments or of such other body as Congress may by law provide, transmit to the President pro tempore of the Senate and the Speaker of the House of Representatives their written declaration that the President is unable to discharge the powers and duties of his office, the Vice President shall immediately assume the powers and duties of the office as Acting President.

Thereafter, when the President transmits to the President pro tempore of the Senate and the Speaker of the House of Representatives his written declaration that no inability exists, he shall resume the powers and duties of his office unless the Vice President and a majority of either the principal officers of the executive department or of such other body as Congress may by law provide, transmit within four days to the President pro tempore of the Senate and the Speaker of the House of Representatives their written declaration that the President is unable to discharge the powers and duties of his office. Thereupon Congress shall decide the issue, assembling within forty-eight hours for that purpose if not in session. If the Congress, within twenty-one days after receipt of the latter written declaration, or, if Congress is not in session, within twenty-one days after Congress is required to assemble, determines by two-thirds vote of both Houses that the President is unable to discharge the powers and duties of his office, the Vice President shall continue to discharge the same as Acting President; otherwise, the President shall resume the powers and duties of his office.

Amendment XXVI (Amendment 26 – Reduction of Voting Age Qualification)

1: The right of citizens of the United States, who are 18 years of age or older, to vote, shall not be denied or abridged by the United States or any state on account of age.

2: The Congress shall have the power to enforce this article by appropriate legislation.

Amendment XXVII (Amendment 27 – Congressional Pay Limitation)

No law varying the compensation for the services of the Senators and Representatives shall take effect until an election of Representatives shall have intervened.[*]

Safety professionals do not need to be Constitutional law experts but should have a basic grasp of the concepts and rights in order to be able to appropriately discuss and assist counsel who may be pursuing a constitutional rights defense to a violation or penalty issued by the Occupational Safety and Health Administration (OSHA) or state plan program. The above information is simply a shortened overview of some of the myriad of constitutional issues and concepts which have developed from this important document over the last 230 years. The U.S. Constitution is the foundation upon which our federal government has been established. Although sometimes vague, our judicial system interprets the language in this document to keep our laws updated with our changing society, technology, and other aspects. Although the concepts remain the same as written by our founding fathers, the interpretation has changed along with the changes in the United States.

---

[*] Id.

As noted by Edmund De S. Brunner, "Democracy is something we must always be working at. It is a process never finished, never ending. And each new height gained opens broader vistas over the sweep of history; thus it must continue to be if democracy is to continue as a working tool in the hands of free men."

Questions

1. What are the powers granted under the Bill of Rights?
2. How is the Second Amendment being interpreted today?
3. What speech is covered under the First Amendment?
4. Why are there Amendments to the U.S. Constitution and what are they?
5. What are the duties and responsibilities of the U.S. Supreme Court?

SELECTED CASE STUDY

Case modified for the purpose of this text
436 U.S. 307 (1978)
MARSHALL, SECRETARY OF LABOR, ET AL.
v
BARLOW'S, INC.
No. 76-1143.
Supreme Court of the United States.
Argued January 9, 1978.
Decided May 23, 1978.

APPEAL FROM THE UNITED STATES DISTRICT COURT FOR THE DISTRICT OF IDAHO

Solicitor General McCree argued the cause for appellants. With him on the briefs were *Deputy Solicitor General Wallace, Stuart A. Smith,* and *Michael H. Levin.*

John L. Runft argued the cause for appellee. With him on the brief was *Iver J. Longeteig.*[1]

MR. JUSTICE WHITE delivered the opinion of the Court.

Section 8 (a) of the Occupational Safety and Health Act of 1970 (OSHA or Act)[2] empowers agents of the Secretary of Labor (Secretary) to search the work area of any employment facility within the Act's jurisdiction. The purpose of the search is to inspect for safety hazards and violations of OSHA regulations. No search warrant or other process is expressly required under the Act.

On the morning of September 11, 1975, an OSHA inspector entered the customer service area of Barlow's, Inc., an electrical and plumbing installation business located in Pocatello, Idaho. The president and general manager, Ferrol G. "Bill" Barlow, was on hand; and the OSHA inspector, after showing his credentials,[3] informed Mr. Barlow that he wished to conduct a search of the working areas of the business. Mr. Barlow inquired whether any complaint had been received about his company. The inspector answered no, but that Barlow's, Inc., had simply turned up in the agency's selection process. The inspector again asked to enter the nonpublic area of the business; Mr. Barlow's response was to inquire whether the inspector had a search warrant. The inspector had none. Thereupon, Mr. Barlow refused the inspector admission to the employee area of his business. He said he was relying on his rights as guaranteed by the Fourth Amendment of the United States Constitution.

Three months later, the Secretary petitioned the United States District Court for the District of Idaho to issue an order compelling Mr. Barlow to admit the inspector.[4] The requested order was issued on December 30, 1975, and was presented to Mr. Barlow on January 5, 1976. Mr. Barlow again refused admission, and he sought his own injunctive relief against the warrantless searches assertedly permitted by OSHA. A three-judge court was convened. On December 30, 1976, it ruled in Mr. Barlow's favor. 424 F. Supp. 437. Concluding that *Camara* v. *Municipal Court,* 387 U.S. 523, 528–29 (1967), and *See* v. *Seattle,* 387 U.S. 541, 543 (1967), controlled this case, the court held that the Fourth Amendment required a warrant for the type of search involved here[5] and that the statutory authorization for warrantless inspections was unconstitutional. An injunction against searches or inspections pursuant to § 8 (a) was entered. The Secretary appealed, challenging the judgment, and we noted probable jurisdiction. 430 U.S. 964.

I

The Secretary urges that warrantless inspections to enforce OSHA are reasonable within the meaning of the Fourth Amendment. Among other things, he relies on § 8 (a) of the Act, 29 U.S.C. § 657 (a), which authorizes inspection of business premises without a warrant and which the Secretary urges represents a congressional construction of the Fourth Amendment that the courts should not reject. Regrettably, we are unable to agree.

The Warrant Clause of the Fourth Amendment protects commercial buildings as well as private homes. To hold otherwise would belie the origin of that Amendment and the American colonial experience. An important forerunner of the first 10 Amendments to the United States Constitution, the Virginia Bill of Rights, specifically opposed "general warrants, whereby an officer or messenger may be commanded to search suspected places without evidence of a fact committed."[6] The general warrant was a recurring point of contention in the Colonies immediately preceding the Revolution.[7] The particular offensiveness it engendered was acutely felt by the merchants and businessmen whose premises and products were inspected for compliance with the several parliamentary revenue measures that most irritated the colonists.[8] "[T]he Fourth Amendment's commands grew in large measure out of the colonists' experience with the writs of assistance ... [that] granted sweeping power to customs officials and other agents of the King to search at large for smuggled goods." *United States* v. *Chadwick,* 433 U.S. 1, 7–8 (1977). See also *G. M. Leasing Corp.* v. *United States,* 429 U.S. 338, 355 (1977). Against this background, it is untenable that the ban on warrantless searches was not intended to shield places of business as well as of residence.

This Court has already held that warrantless searches are generally unreasonable, and that this rule applies to commercial premises as well as homes. In *Camara* v. *Municipal Court, supra,* at 528–29, we held:

> [E]xcept in certain carefully defined classes of cases, a search of private property without proper consent is `unreasonable' unless it has been authorized by a valid search warrant.

On the same day, we also ruled:

> As we explained in *Camara,* a search of private houses is presumptively unreasonable if conducted without a warrant. The businessman, like the occupant of a residence, has a constitutional right to go about his business free from unreasonable official entries upon his private commercial property. The businessman, too, has that right placed in jeopardy if the decision to enter and inspect for violation of regulatory laws can be made and enforced by the inspector in the field without official authority evidenced by a warrant.

> *See v. Seattle, supra, at 543.*

These same cases also held that the Fourth Amendment prohibition against unreasonable searches protects against warrantless intrusions during civil as well as criminal investigations. *Ibid.* The reason is found in the "basic purpose of this Amendment ... [which] is to safeguard the privacy and security of individuals against arbitrary invasions by governmental officials." *Camara, supra,* at 528. If the government intrudes on a person's property, the privacy interest suffers whether the government's motivation is to investigate violations of criminal laws or breaches of other statutory or regulatory standards. It therefore appears that unless some recognized exception to the warrant requirement applies, *See* v. *Seattle* would require a warrant to conduct the inspection sought in this case.

The Secretary urges that an exception from the search warrant requirement has been recognized for "pervasively regulated business[es]," *United States* v. *Biswell,* 406 U.S. 311, 316 (1972), and for "closely regulated" industries "long subject to close supervision and inspection." *Colonnade Catering Corp.* v. *United States,* 397 U.S. 72, 74, 77 (1970). These cases are indeed exceptions, but they represent responses to relatively unique circumstances. Certain industries have such a history of government oversight that no reasonable expectation of privacy, see *Katz* v. *United States,* 389 U.S. 347, 351–52 (1967), could exist for a proprietor over the stock of such an enterprise. Liquor (*Colonnade*) and firearms (*Biswell*) are industries of this type; when an entrepreneur embarks upon such a business, he has voluntarily chosen to subject himself to a full arsenal of governmental regulation.

Industries such as these fall within the "certain carefully defined classes of cases," referenced in *Camara,* 387 U.S., at 528. The element that distinguishes these enterprises from ordinary businesses is a long tradition of close government supervision, of which any person who chooses to enter such a business must already be aware. "A central difference between those cases *[Colonnade* and *Biswell]* and this one is that businessmen engaged in such federally licensed and regulated enterprises accept the burdens as well as the benefits of their trade, whereas the petitioner here was not engaged in any regulated or licensed business. The businessman in a regulated industry in effect consents to the restrictions placed upon him." *Almeida-Sanchez* v. *United States,* 413 U.S. 266, 271 (1973).

The clear import of our cases is that the closely regulated industry of the type involved in *Colonnade* and *Biswell* is the exception. The Secretary would make it the rule. Invoking the Walsh-Healey Act of 1936, 41 U.S.C. § 35 *et seq.,* the Secretary attempts to support a conclusion that all businesses involved in interstate commerce have long been subjected to close supervision of employee safety and health conditions. But the degree of federal involvement in employee working circumstances has never been of the order of specificity and pervasiveness that OSHA mandates. It is quite unconvincing to argue that the imposition of minimum wages and maximum hours on employers who contracted with the Government under the Walsh-Healey Act prepared the entirety of American interstate commerce for regulation of working conditions to the minutest detail. Nor can any but the most fictional sense of voluntary consent to later searches be found in the single fact that one conducts a business affecting interstate commerce; under current practice and law, few businesses can be conducted without having some effect on interstate commerce.

The Secretary also attempts to derive support for a *Colonnade-Biswell-type* exception by drawing analogies from the field of labor law. In *Republic Aviation Corp.* v. *NLRB,* 324 U.S. 793 (1945), this Court upheld the rights of employees to solicit for a union during nonworking time where efficiency was not compromised. By opening up his property to employees, the employer had yielded so much of his private property rights as to allow those employees to exercise § 7 rights under the National Labor Relations Act. But this Court also held that the private property rights of an owner prevailed over the intrusion of nonemployee organizers, even in nonworking areas of the plant and during nonworking hours. *NLRB* v. *Babcock & Wilcox Co.,* 351 U.S. 105 (1956).

The critical fact in this case is that entry over Mr. Barlow's objection is being sought by a Government agent.[9] Employees are not being prohibited from reporting OSHA violations. What they observe in their daily functions is undoubtedly beyond the employer's reasonable expectation of privacy. The Government inspector, however, is not an employee. Without a warrant, he stands in no better position than a member of the public. What is observable by the public is observable, without a warrant, by the Government inspector as well.[10] The owner of a business has not, by the necessary utilization of employees in his operation, thrown open the areas where employees alone are permitted to the warrantless scrutiny of Government agents. That an employee is free to report, and the Government is free to use, any evidence of noncompliance with OSHA that the employee observes furnishes no justification for federal agents to enter a place of business from which the public is restricted and to conduct their own warrantless search.[11]

II

The Secretary nevertheless stoutly argues that the enforcement scheme of the Act requires warrantless searches, and that the restrictions on search discretion contained in the Act and its regulations already protect as much privacy as a warrant would. The Secretary thereby asserts the actual reasonableness of OSHA searches, whatever the general rule against warrantless searches might be. Because "reasonableness is still the ultimate standard," *Camara v. Municipal Court*, 387 U.S., at 539, the Secretary suggests that the Court decide whether a warrant is needed by arriving at a sensible balance between the administrative necessities of OSHA inspections and the incremental protection of privacy of business owners a warrant would afford. He suggests that only a decision exempting OSHA inspections from the Warrant Clause would give "full recognition to the competing public and private interests here at stake." *Ibid.*

The Secretary submits that warrantless inspections are essential to the proper enforcement of OSHA because they afford the opportunity to inspect without prior notice and hence to preserve the advantages of surprise. While the dangerous conditions outlawed by the Act include structural defects that cannot be quickly hidden or remedied, the Act also regulates a myriad of safety details that may be amenable to speedy alteration or disguise. The risk is that during the interval between an inspector's initial request to search a plant and his procuring a warrant following the owner's refusal of permission, violations of this latter type could be corrected and thus escape the inspector's notice. To the suggestion that warrants may be issued *ex parte* and executed without delay and without prior notice, thereby preserving the element of surprise, the Secretary expresses concern for the administrative strain that would be experienced by the inspection system, and by the courts, should *ex parte* warrants issued in advance become standard practice.

We are unconvinced, however, that requiring warrants to inspect will impose serious burdens on the inspection system or the courts, will prevent inspections necessary to enforce the statute, or will make them less effective. In the first place, the great majority of businessmen can be expected in normal course to consent to inspection without warrant; the Secretary has not brought to this Court's attention any widespread pattern of refusal.[12] In those cases where an owner does insist on a warrant, the Secretary argues that inspection efficiency will be impeded by the advance notice and delay. The Act's penalty provisions for giving advance notice of a search, 29 U.S.C. § 666 (f), and the Secretary's own regulations, 29 CFR § 1903.6 (1977), indicate that surprise searches are indeed contemplated. However, the Secretary has also promulgated a regulation providing that upon refusal to permit an inspector to enter the property or to complete his inspection, the inspector shall attempt to ascertain the reasons for the refusal and report to his superior, who shall "promptly take appropriate action, including compulsory process, if necessary." 29 CFR § 1903.4 (1977).[13] The regulation represents a choice to proceed by process where entry is refused; and on the basis of evidence available from present practice, the Act's effectiveness has not been crippled by providing those owners who wish to refuse an initial requested entry with a time lapse while the inspector obtains the necessary process.[14] Indeed, the kind of process sought in this case and apparently anticipated by the regulation provides notice to the business operator.[15] If this safeguard endangers the efficient administration of OSHA, the Secretary should never have adopted it, particularly when the Act does not require it. Nor is it immediately apparent why the advantages of surprise would be lost if, after being refused entry, procedures were available for the Secretary to seek an *ex parte* warrant and to reappear at the premises without further notice to the establishment being inspected.[16]

Whether the Secretary proceeds to secure a warrant or other process, with or without prior notice, his entitlement to inspect will not depend on his demonstrating probable cause to believe that conditions in violation of OSHA exist on the premises. Probable cause in the criminal law sense is not required. For purposes of an administrative search such as this, probable cause justifying the issuance of a warrant may be based not only on specific evidence of an existing violation[17] but also on showing that "reasonable legislative or administrative standards for conducting an ... inspection are satisfied with respect to a particular [establishment]." *Camara* v. *Municipal Court,* 387 U.S., at 538. A warrant showing that a specific business has been chosen for an OSHA search on the basis of a general administrative plan for the enforcement of the Act derived from neutral sources such as, for example, dispersion of employees in various types of industries across a given area, and the desired frequency of searches in any of the lesser divisions of the area, would protect an employer's Fourth Amendment rights.[18] We doubt that the consumption of enforcement energies in the obtaining of such warrants will exceed manageable proportions.

Finally, the Secretary urges that requiring a warrant for OSHA inspectors will mean that, as a practical matter, warrantless-search provisions in other regulatory statutes are also constitutionally infirm. The reasonableness of a warrantless search, however, will depend upon the specific enforcement needs and privacy guarantees of each statute. Some of the statutes cited apply only to a single industry, where regulations might already be so pervasive that a *Colonnade-Biswell* exception to the warrant requirement could apply. Some statutes already envision resort to federal-court enforcement when entry is refused, employing specific language in some cases[19] and general language in others.[20] In short, we base today's opinion on the facts and law concerned with OSHA and do not retreat from a holding appropriate to that statute because of its real or imagined effect on other, different administrative schemes.

Nor do we agree that the incremental protections afforded the employer's privacy by a warrant are so marginal that they fail to justify the administrative burdens that may be entailed. The authority to make warrantless searches devolves almost unbridled discretion upon executive and administrative officers, particularly those in the field, as to when to search and whom to search. A warrant, by contrast, would provide assurances from a neutral officer that the inspection is reasonable under the Constitution, is authorized by statute, and is pursuant to an administrative plan containing specific neutral criteria.[21] Also, a warrant would then and there advise the owner of the scope and objects of the search, beyond which limits the inspector is not expected to proceed.[22] These are important functions for a warrant to perform, functions which underlie the Court's prior decisions that the Warrant Clause applies to inspections for compliance with regulatory statutes.[23] *Camara* v. *Municipal Court,* 387 U.S. 523 (1967); *See* v. *Seattle,* 387 U.S. 541 (1967). We conclude that the concerns expressed by the Secretary do not suffice to justify warrantless inspections under OSHA or vitiate the general constitutional requirement that for a search to be reasonable a warrant must be obtained.

III

We hold that Barlow's was entitled to a declaratory judgment that the Act is unconstitutional insofar as it purports to authorize inspections without warrant or its equivalent and to an injunction enjoining the Act's enforcement to that extent.[24] The judgment of the District Court is therefore affirmed.

So ordered.

MR. JUSTICE BRENNAN took no part in the consideration or decision of this case.

MR. JUSTICE STEVENS, with whom MR. JUSTICE BLACKMUN and MR. JUSTICE REHNQUIST join, dissenting.

Congress enacted the Occupational Safety and Health Act to safeguard employees against hazards in the work areas of businesses subject to the Act. To ensure compliance, Congress authorized the Secretary of Labor to conduct routine, nonconsensual inspections. Today, the Court holds that the Fourth Amendment prohibits such inspections without a warrant. The Court also holds that the constitutionally required warrant may be issued without any showing of probable cause. I disagree with both of these holdings.

The Fourth Amendment contains two separate Clauses, each flatly prohibiting a category of governmental conduct. The first Clause states that the right to be free from unreasonable searches "shall not be violated,"[25] the second unequivocally prohibits the issuance of warrants except "upon probable cause."[26] In this case, the ultimate question is whether the category of warrantless searches authorized by the statute is "unreasonable" within the meaning of the first Clause.

In cases involving the investigation of criminal activity, the Court has held that the reasonableness of a search generally depends upon whether it was conducted pursuant to a valid warrant. See, *e. g. Coolidge v. New Hampshire,* 403 U.S. 443. There is, however, also a category of searches which are reasonable within the meaning of the first Clause even though the probable-cause requirement of the Warrant Clause cannot be satisfied. See *United States* v. *Martinez-Fuerte,* 428 U.S. 543; *Terry* v. *Ohio,* 392 U.S. 1; *South Dakota* v. *Opperman,* 428 U.S. 364; *United States* v. *Biswell,* 406 U.S. 311. The regulatory inspection program challenged in this case, in my judgment, falls within this category.

I

The warrant requirement is linked "textually ... to the probable-cause concept" in the Warrant Clause. *South Dakota* v. *Opperman, supra,* at 370 n. 5. The routine OSHA inspections are, by definition, not based on cause to believe there is a violation on the premises to be inspected. Hence, if the inspections were measured against the requirements of the Warrant Clause, they would be automatically and unequivocally unreasonable.

Because of the acknowledged importance and reasonableness of routine inspections in the enforcement of federal regulatory statutes such as OSHA, the Court recognizes that requiring full compliance with the Warrant Clause would invalidate all such inspection programs. Yet, rather than simply analyzing such programs under the "Reasonableness" Clause of the Fourth Amendment, the Court holds the OSHA program invalid under the Warrant Clause and then avoids a blanket prohibition on all routine, regulatory inspections by relying on the notion that the "probable cause" requirement in the Warrant Clause may be relaxed whenever the Court believes that the governmental need to conduct a category of "searches" outweighs the intrusion on interests protected by the Fourth Amendment.

The Court's approach disregards the plain language of the Warrant Clause and is unfaithful to the balance struck by the Framers of the Fourth Amendment – "the one procedural safeguard in the Constitution that grew directly out of the events which immediately preceded the revolutionary struggle with England."[27] This preconstitutional history includes the controversy in England over the issuance of general warrants to aid enforcement of the seditious libel laws and the colonial experience with writs of assistance issued to facilitate collection of the various import duties imposed by Parliament. The Framers' familiarity with the abuses attending the issuance of such general warrants provided the principal stimulus for the restraints on arbitrary governmental intrusions embodied in the Fourth Amendment.

> [O]ur constitutional fathers were not concerned about warrantless searches, but about overreaching warrants. It is perhaps too much to say that they feared the warrant more than the search, but it is plain enough that the warrant was the prime object of their concern. Far from looking at the warrant as a protection against unreasonable searches, they saw it as an authority for unreasonable and oppressive searches...[28]

> Since the general warrant, not the warrantless search, was the immediate evil at which the Fourth Amendment was directed, it is not surprising that the Framers placed precise limits on its issuance. The requirement that a warrant only issue on a showing of particularized probable cause was the means adopted to circumscribe the warrant power. While the subsequent course of Fourth Amendment jurisprudence in this Court emphasizes the dangers posed by warrantless searches conducted without probable cause, it is the general reasonableness standard in the first Clause, not the Warrant Clause, that the Framers adopted to limit this category of searches. It is, of course, true that the existence of a valid warrant normally satisfies the reasonableness requirement under the Fourth Amendment. But we should not dilute the requirements of the Warrant Clause in an effort to force every kind of governmental intrusion which satisfies the Fourth Amendment definition of a "search" into a judicially developed, warrant-preference scheme.

Fidelity to the original understanding of the Fourth Amendment, therefore, leads to the conclusion that the Warrant Clause has no application to routine, regulatory inspections of commercial premises. If such inspections are valid, it is because they comport with the ultimate reasonableness standard of the Fourth Amendment. If the Court were correct in its view that such inspections, if undertaken without a warrant, are unreasonable in the constitutional sense, the issuance of a "new-fangled warrant" – to use Mr. Justice Clark's characteristically expressive term – without any true showing of particularized probable cause would not be sufficient to validate them.[29]

II

Even if a warrant issued without probable cause were faithful to the Warrant Clause, I could not accept the Court's holding that the Government's inspection program is constitutionally unreasonable because it fails to require such a warrant procedure. In determining whether a warrant is a necessary safeguard in a given class of cases, "the Court has weighed the public interest against the Fourth Amendment interest of the individual ..." *United States* v. *Martinez-Fuerte,* 428 U.S., at 555. Several considerations persuade me that this balance should be struck in favor of the routine inspections authorized by Congress.

Congress has determined that regulation and supervision of safety in the workplace furthers an important public interest and that the power to conduct warrantless searches is necessary to accomplish the safety goals of the legislation. In assessing the public interest side of the Fourth Amendment balance, however, the Court today substitutes its judgment for that of Congress on the question of what inspection authority is needed to effectuate the purposes of the Act. The Court states that if surprise is truly an important ingredient of an effective, representative inspection program, it can be retained by obtaining *ex parte* warrants in advance. The Court assures the Secretary that this will not unduly burden enforcement resources because most employers will consent to inspection.

The Court's analysis does not persuade me that Congress' determination that the warrantless-inspection power as a necessary adjunct of the exercise of the regulatory power is unreasonable. It was surely not unreasonable to conclude that the rate at which employers deny entry to inspectors would increase if covered businesses, which may have safety violations on their premises, have a right to deny warrantless entry to a compliance inspector. The Court is correct that this problem could be avoided by requiring inspectors to obtain a warrant prior to every inspection visit. But the adoption of such a practice undercuts the Court's explanation of why a warrant requirement would not create undue enforcement problems. For, even if it were true that many employers would not exercise their right to demand a warrant, it would provide little solace to those charged with administration of OSHA; faced with an increase in the rate of refusals and the added costs generated by futile trips to inspection sites where entry is denied, officials may be compelled to adopt a general practice of obtaining warrants in advance. While the Court's prediction of the effect a warrant requirement would have on the behavior of covered employers may turn out to be accurate, its judgment is essentially empirical. On such an issue, I would defer to Congress' judgment regarding the importance of a warrantless-search power to the OSHA enforcement scheme.

The Court also appears uncomfortable with the notion of second-guessing Congress and the Secretary on the question of how the substantive goals of OSHA can best be achieved. Thus, the Court offers an alternative explanation for its refusal to accept the legislative judgment. We are told that, in any event, the Secretary, who is charged with enforcement of the Act, has indicated that inspections without delay are not essential to the enforcement scheme. The Court bases this conclusion on a regulation prescribing the administrative response when a compliance inspector is denied entry. It provides: "The Area Director shall immediately consult with the Assistant Regional Director and the Regional Solicitor, who shall promptly take appropriate action, including compulsory process, if necessary." 29 CFR § 1903.4 (1977). The Court views this regulation as an admission by the Secretary that no enforcement problem is generated by permitting employers to deny entry and delaying the inspection until a warrant has been obtained. I disagree. The regulation was promulgated against the background of a statutory right to immediate entry, of which covered employers are presumably aware and which Congress and the Secretary obviously thought would keep denials of entry to a minimum. In these circumstances, it was surely not unreasonable for the Secretary to adopt an orderly procedure for dealing with what he believed would be the occasional denial of entry. The regulation does not imply a judgment by the Secretary that delay caused by numerous denials of entry would be administratively acceptable.

Even if a warrant requirement does not "frustrate" the legislative purpose, the Court has no authority to impose an additional burden on the Secretary unless that burden is required to protect the employer's Fourth Amendment interests.[30] The essential function of the traditional warrant requirement is the interposition of a neutral magistrate between the citizen and the presumably zealous law enforcement officer so that there might be an objective determination of probable cause. But this purpose is not served by the newfangled inspection warrant. As the Court acknowledges, the inspector's "entitlement to inspect will not depend on his demonstrating probable cause to believe that conditions in violation of OSHA exist on the premises.... For purposes of an administrative search such as this, probable cause justifying the issuance of a warrant may be based ... on a showing that 'reasonable legislative or administrative standards for conducting an ... inspection are satisfied with respect to a particular [establishment].'" *Ante,* at 320. To obtain a warrant, the inspector need only show that "a specific business has been chosen for an OSHA search on the basis of a general administrative plan for the enforcement of the Act derived from neutral sources ..." *Ante,* at 321. Thus, the only question for the magistrate's consideration is whether the contemplated inspection deviates from an inspection schedule drawn up by higher level agency officials.

Unlike the traditional warrant, the inspection warrant provides no protection against the search itself for employers who the Government has no reason to suspect are violating OSHA regulations. The Court plainly accepts the proposition that random health and safety inspections are reasonable. It does not question Congress' determination that the public interest in workplaces free from health and safety hazards outweighs the employer's desire to conduct his business only in the presence of permittees, except in those rare instances when the Government has probable cause to suspect that the premises harbor a violation of the law.

What purposes, then, are served by the administrative warrant procedure? The inspection warrant purports to serve three functions: to inform the employer that the inspection is authorized by the statute, to advise him of the lawful limits of the inspection, and to assure him that the person demanding entry is an authorized inspector. *Camara* v. *Municipal Court,* 387 U.S. 523, 532. An examination of these functions in the OSHA context reveals that the inspection warrant adds little to the protections already afforded by the statute and pertinent regulations, and the slight additional benefit it might provide is insufficient to identify a constitutional violation or to justify overriding Congress' judgment that the power to conduct warrantless inspections is essential.

The inspection warrant is supposed to assure the employer that the inspection is in fact routine, and that the inspector has not improperly departed from the program of representative inspections established by responsible officials. But to the extent that harassment inspections would be reduced by the necessity of obtaining a warrant, the Secretary's present enforcement scheme would have precisely the same effect. The representative inspections are conducted "in accordance with criteria based upon accident experience and the number of employees exposed in particular industries." *Ante,* at 321 n. 17. If, under the present scheme, entry to covered premises is denied, the inspector can gain entry only by informing his administrative superiors of the refusal and seeking a court order requiring the employer to submit to the inspection. The inspector who would like to conduct a nonroutine search is just as likely to be deterred by the prospect of informing his superiors of his intention and of making false representations to the court when he seeks compulsory process as by the prospect of having to make bad-faith representations in an *ex parte* warrant proceeding.

The other two asserted purposes of the administrative warrant are also adequately achieved under the existing scheme. If the employer has doubts about the official status of the inspector, he is given adequate opportunity to reassure himself in this regard before permitting entry. The OSHA inspector's statutory right to enter the premises is conditioned upon the presentation of appropriate credentials. 29 U.S.C. § 657 (a) (1). These credentials state the inspector's name, identify him as an OSHA compliance officer, and contain his photograph and signature. If the employer still has doubts, he may make a toll-free call to verify the inspector's authority, *Usery* v. *Godfrey Brake & Supply Service, Inc.,* 545 F. 2d 52, 54 (CA8 1976), or simply deny entry and await the presentation of a court order.

The warrant is not needed to inform the employer of the lawful limits of an OSHA inspection. The statute expressly provides that the inspector may enter all areas in a covered business "where work is performed by an employee of an employer," 29 U.S.C. § 657 (a) (1), "to inspect and investigate during regular working hours and at other reasonable times, and within reasonable limits and in a reasonable manner ... all pertinent conditions, structures, machines, apparatus, devices, equipment, and materials therein ..." 29 U.S.C. § 657 (a)(2). See also 29 CFR § 1903 (1977). While it is true that the inspection power granted by Congress is broad, the warrant procedure required by the Court does not purport to restrict this power but simply to ensure that the employer is apprised of its scope. Since both the statute and the pertinent regulations perform this informational function, a warrant is superfluous.

Requiring the inspection warrant, therefore, adds little in the way of protection to that already provided under the existing enforcement scheme. In these circumstances, the warrant is essentially a formality. In view of the obviously enormous cost of enforcing a health and safety scheme of the dimensions of OSHA, this Court should not, in the guise of construing the Fourth Amendment, require formalities which merely place an additional strain on already overtaxed federal resources.

Congress, like this Court, has an obligation to obey the mandate of the Fourth Amendment. In the past the Court "has been particularly sensitive to the Amendment's broad standard of 'reasonableness' where ... authorizing statutes permitted the challenged searches." *Almeida-Sanchez* v. *United States,* 413 U.S. 266,

290 (WHITE, J., dissenting). In *United States* v. *Martinez-Fuerte,* 428 U.S. 543, for example, respondents challenged the routine stopping of vehicles to check for aliens at permanent checkpoints located away from the border. The checkpoints were established pursuant to statutory authority and their location and operation were governed by administrative criteria. The Court rejected respondents' argument that the constitutional reasonableness of the location and operation of the fixed checkpoints should be reviewed in a *Camara* warrant proceeding. The Court observed that the reassuring purposes of the inspection warrant were adequately served by the visible manifestations of authority exhibited at the fixed checkpoints.

Moreover, although the location and method of operation of the fixed checkpoints were deemed critical to the constitutional reasonableness of the challenged stops, the Court did not require Border Patrol officials to obtain a warrant based on a showing that the checkpoints were located and operated in accordance with administrative standards. Indeed, the Court observed that "[t]he choice of checkpoint locations must be left largely to the discretion of Border Patrol officials, to be exercised in accordance with statutes and regulations that may be applicable ... [and] [m]any incidents of checkpoint operation also must be committed to the discretion of such officials." 428 U.S., at 559–60, n. 13. The Court had no difficulty assuming that those officials responsible for allocating limited enforcement resources would be "unlikely to locate a checkpoint where it bears arbitrarily or oppressively on motorists as a class." *Id.,* at 559.

The Court's recognition of Congress' role in balancing the public interest advanced by various regulatory statutes and the private interest in being free from arbitrary governmental intrusion has not been limited to situations in which, for example, Congress is exercising its special power to exclude aliens. Until today, we have not rejected a congressional judgment concerning the reasonableness of a category of regulatory inspections of commercial premises.[31] While businesses are unquestionably entitled to Fourth Amendment protection, we have "recognized that a business, by its special nature and voluntary existence, may open itself to intrusions that would not be permissible in a purely private context." *G. M. Leasing Corp.* v. *United States,* 429 U.S. 338, 353. Thus, in *Colonnade Catering Corp.* v. *United States,* 397 U.S. 72, the Court recognized the reasonableness of a statutory authorization to inspect the premises of a caterer dealing in alcoholic beverages, noting that "Congress has broad power to design such powers of inspection under the liquor laws as it deems necessary to meet the evils at hand." *Id.,* at 76. And in *United States* v. *Biswell,* 406 U.S. 311, the Court sustained the authority to conduct warrantless searches of firearm dealers under the Gun Control Act of 1968 primarily on the basis of the reasonableness of the congressional evaluation of the interests at stake.[32]

The Court, however, concludes that the deference accorded Congress in *Biswell* and *Colonnade* should be limited to situations where the evils addressed by the regulatory statute are peculiar to a specific industry and that industry is one which has long been subject to Government regulation. The Court reasons that only in those situations can it be said that a person who engages in business will be aware of and consent to routine, regulatory inspections. I cannot agree that the respect due the congressional judgment should be so narrowly confined.

In the first place, the longevity of a regulatory program does not, in my judgment, have any bearing on the reasonableness of routine inspections necessary to achieve adequate enforcement of that program. Congress' conception of what constitute urgent federal interests need not remain static. The recent vintage of public and congressional awareness of the dangers posed by health and safety hazards in the workplace is not a basis for according less respect to the considered judgment of Congress. Indeed, in *Biswell,* the Court upheld an inspection program authorized by a regulatory statute enacted in 1968. The Court there noted that "[f]ederal regulation of the interstate traffic in firearms is not as deeply rooted in history as is governmental control of the liquor industry, but close scrutiny of this traffic is undeniably" an urgent federal interest. 406 U.S., at 315. Thus, the critical fact is the congressional determination that federal regulation would further significant public interests, not the date that determination was made.

In the second place, I see no basis for the Court's conclusion that a congressional determination that a category of regulatory inspections is reasonable need only be respected when Congress is legislating on an industry-by-industry basis. The pertinent inquiry is not whether the inspection program is authorized by a regulatory statute directed at a single industry, but whether Congress has limited the exercise of the inspection power to those commercial premises where the evils at which the statute is directed are to be found. Thus, in *Biswell,* if Congress had authorized inspections of all commercial premises as a means of restricting the illegal traffic in firearms, the Court would have found the inspection program unreasonable; the power to inspect was upheld because it was tailored to the subject matter of Congress' proper exercise of regulatory power. Similarly, OSHA is directed at health and safety hazards in the workplace, and the inspection power granted the Secretary extends only to those areas where such hazards are likely to be found.

Finally, the Court would distinguish the respect accorded Congress' judgment in *Colonnade* and *Biswell* on the ground that businesses engaged in the liquor and firearms industry "accept the burdens as well as the benefits of their trade ..." *Ante,* at 313. In the Court's view, such businesses consent to the restrictions placed upon them, while it would be fiction to conclude that a businessman subject to OSHA consented to routine safety inspections. In fact, however, consent is fictional in both contexts. Here, as well as in *Biswell,* businesses are required to be aware of and comply with regulations governing their business activities. In both situations, the validity of the regulations depends not upon the consent of those regulated, but on the existence of a federal statute embodying a congressional determination that the public interest in the health of the Nation's work force or the limitation of illegal firearms traffic outweighs the businessman's interest in preventing a Government inspector from viewing those areas of his premises which relate to the subject matter of the regulation.

The case before us involves an attempt to conduct a warrantless search of the working area of an electrical and plumbing contractor. The statute authorizes such an inspection during reasonable hours. The inspection is limited to those areas over which Congress has exercised its proper legislative authority.[33] The area is also one to which employees have regular access without any suggestion that the work performed or the equipment used has any special claim to confidentiality.[34] Congress has determined that industrial safety is an urgent federal interest requiring regulation and supervision, and further, that warrantless inspections are necessary to accomplish the safety goals of the legislation. While one may question the wisdom of pervasive governmental oversight of industrial life, I decline to question Congress' judgment that the inspection power is a necessary enforcement device in achieving the goals of a valid exercise of regulatory power.[35]

I respectfully dissent.

NOTES

1. *Warren Spannaus,* Attorney General of Minnesota, *Richard B. Allyn,* Solicitor General, and *Steven M. Gunn* and *Richard A. Lockridge,* Special Assistant Attorneys General, filed a brief for 11 States as *amici curiae* urging reversal, joined by the Attorneys General for their respective States as follows: *Frank J. Kelley* of Michigan, *William F. Hyland* of New Jersey, *Toney Anaya* of New Mexico, *Rufus Edmisten* of North Carolina, *Robert P. Kane* of Pennsylvania, *Daniel R. McLeod* of South Carolina, *M. Jerome Diamond* of Vermont, *Anthony F. Troy* of Virginia, and *V. Frank Mendicino* of Wyoming. Briefs of *amici curiae* urging reversal were filed by *J. Albert Woll* and *Laurence Gold* for the American Federation of Labor and Congress of Industrial Organizations; and by *Michael R. Sherwood* for the Sierra Club et al.

   Briefs of *amici curiae* urging affirmance were filed by *Wayne L. Kidwell,* Attorney General of Idaho, and *Guy G. Hurlbutt,* Chief Deputy Attorney General, *Robert B. Hansen,* Attorney General of Utah, and *Michael L. Deamer,* Deputy Attorney General, for the States of Idaho and Utah; by *Allen A. Lauterbach* for the American Farm Bureau Federation; by *Robert T. Thompson, Lawrence Kraus,* and *Stanley T. Kaleczyc* for the Chamber of Commerce of the United States; by *Anthony J. Obadal, Steven R. Semler, Stephen C. Yohay, Leonard J. Theberge, Edward H. Dowd,* and *James Watt* for the Mountain States Legal Foundation; by *James D. McKevitt* for the National Federation of Independent Business; and by *Ronald A. Zumbrun, John H. Findley, Albert Ferri, Jr.,* and *W. Hugh O'Riordan* for the Pacific Legal Foundation.

   Briefs of *amici curiae* were filed by *Robert E. Rader, Jr.,* for the American Conservative Union; and by *David Goldberger, Barbara O'Toole, McNeill Stokes, Ira J. Smotherman, Jr.,* and *David Rudenstine* for the Roger Baldwin Foundation, Inc., of the American Civil Liberties Union, Illinois Division.

2. "In order to carry out the purposes of this chapter, the Secretary, upon presenting appropriate credentials to the owner, operator, or agent in charge, is authorized—

   (1) to enter without delay and at reasonable times any factory, plant, establishment, construction site, or other area, workplace or environment where work is performed by an employee of an employer; and
   (2) to inspect and investigate during regular working hours and at other reasonable times, and within reasonable limits and in a reasonable manner, any such place of employment and all pertinent conditions, structures, machines, apparatus, devices, equipment, and materials therein, and to question privately any such employer, owner, operator, agent, or employee.

   84 Stat. 1598, 29 U.S.C. § 657 (a)

3. This is required by the Act. See n. 1, *supra.*
4. A regulation of the Secretary, 29 CFR § 1903.4 (1977), requires an inspector to seek compulsory process if an employer refuses a requested search. See *infra,* at 317, and n. 12.
5. No *res judicata* bar arose against Mr. Barlow from the December 30, 1975, order authorizing a search, because the earlier decision reserved the constitutional issue. See 424 F. Supp. 437.

6. H. Commager, Documents of American History 104 (8th ed. 1968).
7. See, e.g., Dickerson, Writs of Assistance as a Cause of the Revolution in The Era of the American Revolution 40 (R. Morris ed. 1939).
8. The Stamp Act of 1765, the Townshend Revenue Act of 1767, and the tea tax of 1773 are notable examples. See Commager, *supra,* n. 5, at 53, 63. For commentary, see 1 S. Morison, H. Commager, & W. Leuchtenburg, The Growth of the American Republic 143, 149, 159 (1969).
9. The Government has asked that Mr. Barlow be ordered to show cause why he should not be held in contempt for refusing to honor the inspection order, and its position is that the OSHA inspector is now entitled to enter at once, over Mr. Barlow's objection.
10. Cf. *Air Pollution Variance Bd.* v. *Western Alfalfa Corp.,* 416 U.S. 861 (1974).
11. The automobile-search cases cited by the Secretary are even less helpful to his position than the labor cases. The fact that automobiles occupy a special category in Fourth Amendment case law is by now beyond doubt due, among other factors, to the quick mobility of a car, the registration requirements of both the car and the driver, and the more available opportunity for plain-view observations of a car's contents. *Cady* v. *Dombrowski,* 413 U.S. 433, 441–442 (1973); see also *Chambers* v. *Maroney,* 399 U.S. 42, 48–51 (1970). Even so, probable cause has not been abandoned as a requirement for stopping and searching an automobile.
12. We recognize that today's holding itself might have an impact on whether owners choose to resist requested searches; we can only await the development of evidence not present on this record to determine how serious an impediment to effective enforcement this might be.
13. It is true, as the Secretary asserts, that § 8 (a) of the Act, 29 U.S.C. § 657 (a), purports to authorize inspections without warrant; but it is also true that it does not forbid the Secretary from proceeding to inspect only by warrant or other process. The Secretary has broad authority to prescribe such rules and regulations as he may deem necessary to carry out his responsibilities under this chapter, "including rules and regulations dealing with the inspection of an employer's establishment." § 8 (g) (2), 29 U.S.C. § 657 (g) (2). The regulations with respect to inspections are contained in 29 CFR Part 1903 (1977). Section 1903.4, referred to in the text, provides as follows:

> Upon a refusal to permit a Compliance Safety and Health Officer, in the exercise of his official duties, to enter without delay and at reasonable times any place of employment or any place therein, to inspect, to review records, or to question any employer, owner, operator, agent, or employee, in accordance with § 1903.3, or to permit a representative of employees to accompany the Compliance Safety and Health Officer during the physical inspection of any workplace in accordance with § 1903.8, the Compliance Safety and Health Officer shall terminate the inspection or confine the inspection to other areas, conditions, structures, machines, apparatus, devices, equipment, materials, records, or interviews concerning which no objection is raised. The Compliance Safety and Health Officer shall endeavor to ascertain the reason for such refusal, and he shall immediately report the refusal and the reason therefor to the Area Director. The Area Director shall immediately consult with the Assistant Regional Director and the Regional Solicitor, who shall promptly take appropriate action, including compulsory process, if necessary.

When his representative was refused admission by Mr. Barlow, the Secretary proceeded in federal court to enforce his right to enter and inspect, as conferred by 29 U.S.C. § 657.
14. A change in the language of the Compliance Operations Manual for OSHA inspectors supports the inference that, whatever the Act's administrators might have thought at the start, it was eventually concluded that enforcement efficiency would not be jeopardized by permitting employers to refuse entry, at least until the inspector obtained compulsory process. The 1972 Manual included a section specifically directed to obtaining "warrants," and one provision of that section dealt with *ex parte* warrants:

> In cases where a refusal of entry is to be expected from the past performance of the employer, or where the employer has given some indication prior to the commencement of the investigation of his intention to bar entry or limit or interfere with the investigation, a warrant should be obtained before the inspection is attempted. Cases of this nature should also be referred through the Area Director to the appropriate Regional Solicitor and the Regional Administrator alerted.

Dept. of Labor, OSHA Compliance Operations Manual V-7 (Jan. 1972)

The latest available manual, incorporating changes as of November 1977, deletes this provision, leaving only the details for obtaining "compulsory process" *after* an employer has refused entry. Dept. of Labor, OSHA Field Operations Manual, Vol. V, pp. V-4-V-5. In its present form, the Secretary's regulation appears to permit establishment owners to insist on "process"; and hence their refusal to permit entry would fall short of criminal conduct within the meaning of 18 U.S.C. §§ 111 and 1114 (1976 ed.), which make it a crime forcibly to impede, intimidate, or interfere with federal officials, including OSHA inspectors, while engaged in or on account of the performance of their official duties.

15. The proceeding was instituted by filing an "Application for Affirmative Order to Grant Entry and for an Order to show cause why such affirmative order should not issue." The District Court issued the order to show cause, the matter was argued, and an order then issued authorizing the inspection and enjoining interference by Barlow's. The following is the order issued by the District Court:

> IT IS HEREBY ORDERED, ADJUDGED AND DECREED that the United States of America, United States Department of Labor, Occupational Safety and Health Administration, through its duly designated representative or representatives, are entitled to entry upon the premises known as Barlow's Inc., 225 West Pine, Pocatello, Idaho, and may go upon said business premises to conduct an inspection and investigation as provided for in Section 8 of the Occupational Safety and Health Act of 1970 (29 U.S.C. 651, *et seq.*), as part of an inspection program designed to assure compliance with that Act; that the inspection and investigation shall be conducted during regular working hours or at other reasonable times, within reasonable limits and in a reasonable manner, all as set forth in the regulations pertaining to such inspections promulgated by the Secretary of Labor, at 29 C. F. R., Part 1903; that appropriate credentials as representatives of the Occupational Safety and Health Administration, United States Department of Labor, shall be presented to the Barlow's Inc. representative upon said premises and the inspection and investigation shall be commenced as soon as practicable after the issuance of this Order and shall be completed within reasonable promptness; that the inspection and investigation shall extend to the establishment or other area, workplace, or environment where work is performed by employees of the employer, Barlow's Inc., and to all pertinent conditions, structures, machines, apparatus, devices, equipment, materials, and all other things therein (including but not limited to records, files, papers, processes, controls, and facilities) bearing upon whether Barlow's Inc. is furnishing to its employees employment and a place of employment that are free from recognized hazards that are causing or are likely to cause death or serious physical harm to its employees, and whether Barlow's Inc. is complying with the Occupational Safety and Health Standards promulgated under the Occupational Safety and Health Act and the rules, regulations, and orders issued pursuant to that Act; that representatives of the Occupational Safety and Health Administration may, at the option of Barlow's Inc., be accompanied by one or more employees of Barlow's Inc., pursuant to Section 8 (e) of that Act; that Barlow's Inc., its agents, representatives, officers, and employees are hereby enjoined and restrained from in anyway whatsoever interfering with the inspection and investigation authorized by this Order and, further, Barlow's Inc. is hereby ordered and directed to, within five working days from the date of this Order, furnish a copy of this Order to its officers and managers, and, in addition, to post a copy of this Order at its employee's bulletin board located upon the business premises; and Barlow's Inc. is hereby ordered and directed to comply in all respects with this order and allow the inspection and investigation to take place without delay and forthwith.

16. Insofar as the Secretary's statutory authority is concerned, a regulation expressly providing that the Secretary could proceed *ex parte* to seek a warrant or its equivalent would appear to be as much within the Secretary's power as the regulation currently in force and calling for "compulsory process."

17. Section 8 (f) (1), 29 U.S.C. § 657 (f) (1), provides that employees or their representatives may give written notice to the Secretary of what they believe to be violations of safety or health standards and may request an inspection. If the Secretary then determines that "there are reasonable grounds to believe that such violation or danger exists, he shall make a special inspection in accordance with the provisions of this section as soon as practicable." The statute thus purports to authorize a warrantless inspection in these circumstances.

18. The Secretary, Brief for Petitioner 9 n. 7, states that the Barlow inspection was not based on an employee complaint but was a "general schedule" investigation. "Such general inspections," he explains, "now called Regional Programmed Inspections, are carried out in accordance with criteria based upon accident experience and the number of employees exposed in particular industries. U. S. Department of Labor, Occupational Safety and Health Administration, Field Operations Manual, *supra,*1 CCH Employment Safety and Health Guide 4327.2 (1976)."

19. The Federal Metal and Nonmetallic Mine Safety Act provides: "Whenever an operator ... refuses to permit the inspection or investigation of any mine which is subject to this chapter ... a civil action for preventive relief, including an application for a permanent or temporary injunction, restraining order, or other order, may be instituted by the Secretary in the district court of the United States for the district ..." 30 U.S.C. § 733 (a). "The Secretary may institute a civil action for relief, including a permanent or temporary injunction, restraining order, or any other appropriate order in the district court ... whenever such operator or his agent ... refuses to permit the inspection of the mine ... Each court shall have jurisdiction to provide such relief as may be appropriate." 30 U.S.C. § 818. Another example is the Clean Air Act, which grants federal district courts jurisdiction "to require compliance" with the Administrator of the Environmental Protection Agency's attempt to inspect under 42 U.S.C. § 7414 (1976 ed., Supp. I), when the Administrator has commenced "a civil action" for injunctive relief or to recover a penalty. 42 U.S.C. § 7413 (b) (4) (1976 ed., Supp. I).

20. Exemplary language is contained in the Animal Welfare Act of 1970 which provides for inspections by the Secretary of Agriculture; federal district courts are vested with jurisdiction "specifically to enforce, and to prevent and restrain violations of this chapter, and shall have jurisdiction in all other kinds of cases arising under this chapter." 7 U.S.C. § 2146 (c) (1976 ed.). Similar provisions are included in other agricultural inspection Acts; see, e.g., 21 U.S.C. § 674 (meat product inspection); 21 U.S.C. § 1050 (egg product inspection). The Internal Revenue Code, whose excise tax provisions requiring inspections of businesses are cited by the Secretary, provides: "The district courts ... shall have such jurisdiction to make and issue in civil actions, writs and orders of injunction ... and such other orders and processes, and to render such ... decrees as may be necessary or appropriate for the enforcement of the internal revenue laws." 26 U.S.C. § 7402 (a). For gasoline inspections, federal district courts are granted jurisdiction to restrain violations and enforce standards (one of which, 49 U.S.C. § 1677, requires gas transporters to permit entry or inspection). The owner is to be afforded the opportunity for notice and response in most cases, but "failure to give such notice and afford such opportunity shall not preclude the granting of appropriate relief [by the district court]." 49 U.S.C. § 1679 (a).

21. The application for the inspection order filed by the Secretary in this case represented that "the desired inspection and investigation are contemplated as a part of an inspection program designed to assure compliance with the Act and are authorized by Section

8 (a) of the Act." The program was not described, however, or any facts presented that would indicate why an inspection of Barlow's establishment was within the program. The order that issued concluded generally that the inspection authorized was "part of an inspection program designed to assure compliance with the Act."

22. Section 8 (a) of the Act, as set forth in 29 U.S.C. § 657 (a), provides that "[i]n order to carry out the purposes of this chapter" the Secretary may enter any establishment, area, work place or environment "where work is performed by an employee of an employer" and "inspect and investigate" any such place of employment and all "pertinent conditions, structures, machines, apparatus, devices, equipment, and materials therein, and ... question privately any such employer, owner, operator, agent, or employee." Inspections are to be carried out "during regular working hours and at other reasonable times, and within reasonable limits and in a reasonable manner." The Secretary's regulations echo the statutory language in these respects. 29 CFR § 1903.3 (1977). They also provide that inspectors are to explain the nature and purpose of the inspection and to "indicate generally the scope of the inspection." 29 CFR § 1903.7 (a) (1977). Environmental samples and photographs are authorized, 29 CFR § 1903.7 (b) (1977), and inspections are to be performed so as "to preclude unreasonable disruption of the operations of the employer's establishment." 29 CFR § 1903.7 (d) (1977). The order that issued in this case reflected much of the foregoing statutory and regulatory language.

23. Delineating the scope of a search with some care is particularly important where documents are involved. Section 8 (c) of the Act, 29 U.S.C. § 657 (c), provides that an employer must "make, keep and preserve, and make available to the Secretary [of Labor] or to the Secretary of Health, Education and Welfare" such records regarding his activities relating to OSHA as the Secretary of Labor may prescribe by regulation as necessary or appropriate for enforcement of the statute or for developing information regarding the causes and prevention of occupational accidents and illnesses. Regulations requiring employers to maintain records of and to make periodic reports on "work-related deaths, injuries and illnesses" are also contemplated, as are rules requiring accurate records of employee exposures to potential toxic materials and harmful physical agents.

   In describing the scope of the warrantless inspection authorized by the statute, § 8 (a) does not expressly include any *records* among those items or things that may be examined, and § 8 (c) merely provides that the employer is to "make available" his pertinent records and to make periodic reports.

   The Secretary's regulation, 29 CFR § 1903.3 (1977), however, expressly includes among the inspector's powers the authority "to review records required by the Act and regulations published in this chapter, and other records which are directly related to the purpose of the inspection." Further, § 1903.7 requires inspectors to indicate generally "the records specified in § 1903.3 which they wish to review" but "such designations of records shall not preclude access to additional records specified in § 1903.3." It is the Secretary's position, which we reject, that an inspection of documents of this scope may be effected without a warrant.

   The order that issued in this case included among the objects and things to be inspected "all other things therein (including but not limited to records, files, papers, processes, controls and facilities) bearing upon whether Barlow's, Inc. is furnishing to its employees employment and a place of employment that are free from recognized hazards that are causing or are likely to cause death or serious physical harm to its employees, and whether Barlow's, Inc. is complying with ..." the OSHA regulations.

24. The injunction entered by the District Court, however, should not be understood to forbid the Secretary from exercising the inspection authority conferred by § 8 pursuant to regulations and judicial process that satisfy the Fourth Amendment. The District Court did not address the issue whether the order for inspection that was issued in this case was the functional equivalent of a warrant, and the Secretary has limited his

submission in this case to the constitutionality of a warrantless search of the Barlow establishment authorized by § 8 (a). He has expressly declined to rely on 29 CFR § 1903.4 (1977) and upon the order obtained in this case. Tr. of Oral Arg. 19. Of course, if the process obtained here, or obtained in other cases under revised regulations, would satisfy the Fourth Amendment, there would be no occasion for enjoining the inspections authorized by § 8 (a).

25. "The right of the people to be secure in their persons, houses, papers, and effects, against unreasonable searches and seizures, shall not be violated...."

26. "[A]nd no Warrants shall issue, but upon probable cause, supported by Oath or affirmation, and particularly describing the place to be searched, and the persons or things to be seized."

27. J. Landynski, Search and Seizure and the Supreme Court 19 (1966).

28. T. Taylor, Two Studies in Constitutional Interpretation 41 (1969).

29. *See* v. *Seattle,* 387 U. S. 541, 547 (Clark, J., dissenting).

30. When it passed OSHA, Congress was cognizant of the fact that in light of the enormity of the enforcement task "the number of inspections which it would be desirable to have made will undoubtedly for an unforeseeable period, exceed the capacity of the inspection force ..." Senate Committee on Labor and Public Welfare, Legislative History of the Occupational Safety and Health Act of 1970, 92d Cong., 1st Sess., 152 (Comm. Print 1971).

31. The Court's rejection of a legislative judgment regarding the reasonableness of the OSHA inspection program is especially puzzling in light of recent decisions finding law enforcement practices constitutionally reasonable, even though those practices involved significantly more individual discretion than the OSHA program. See, *e. g., Terry* v. *Ohio, 392 U. S. 1; Adams* v. *Williams,* 407 U. S. 143; *Cady* v. *Dombrowski,* 413 U. S. 433; *South Dakota* v. *Opperman,* 428 U. S. 364.

32. The Court held:

> In the context of a regulatory inspection system of business premises that is carefully limited in time, place, and scope, the legality of the search depends ... on the authority of a valid statute.
> ...
> We have little difficulty in concluding that where, as here, regulatory inspections further urgent federal interest, and the possibilities of abuse and the threat to privacy are not of impressive dimensions, the inspection may proceed without a warrant where specifically authorized by statute.
>
> 406 U. S., at 315, 317

33. What the Court actually decided in *Camara* v. *Municipal Court,* 387 U. S. 523, and *See* v. *Seattle,* 387 U. S. 541, does not require the result it reaches today. *Camara* involved a residence, rather than a business establishment; although the Fourth Amendment extends its protection to commercial buildings, the central importance of protecting residential privacy is manifest. The building involved in *See* was, of course, a commercial establishment, but a holding that a locked warehouse may not be entered pursuant to a general authorization to "enter all buildings and premises, except the interior of dwellings, as often as may be necessary," 387 U. S., at 541, need not be extended to cover more carefully delineated grants of authority. My view that the *See* holding should be narrowly confined is influenced by my favorable opinion of the dissent written by Mr. Justice Clark and joined by Justices Harlan and STEWART. As *Colonnade* and *Biswell* demonstrate, however, the doctrine of *stare decisis* does not compel the Court to extend those cases to govern today's holding.

34. The Act and pertinent regulation provide protection for any trade secrets of the employer. 29 U.S.C. §§ 664–665; 29 CFR § 1903.9 (1977).

35. The decision today renders presumptively invalid numerous inspection provisions in federal regulatory statutes. *E. g.,* 30 U.S.C. § 813 (Federal Coal Mine Health and Safety Act of 1969); 30 U.S.C. §§ 723, 724 (Federal Metal and Nonmetallic Mine Safety Act); 21 U.S.C. § 603 (inspection of meat and food products). That some of these provisions apply only to a single industry, as noted above, does not alter this fact. And the fact that some "envision resort to federal-court enforcement when entry is refused" is also irrelevant since the OSHA inspection program invalidated here requires compulsory process when a compliance inspector has been denied entry. *Ante,* at 321.

2 Federal Court System

Morality cannot be legislated, but behavior can be regulated. Judicial decrees may not change the heart, but they can restrain the heartless.

Martin Luther King, Jr.

Society fails to recognize that the tension between the police and the judiciary has always been fundamental to our constitutional system. It is intentional and healthy and constitutes the real difference between a free society and a police state.

Nicholas Katzenbach

STUDENT LEARNING OBJECTIVES

1. Acquire an understanding of the Structure of the Federal Court System.
2. Acquire an understanding of the Jurisdiction of the Federal Courts.
3. Acquire an understanding of Civil Procedure.
4. Acquire an understanding of Criminal Procedure.
5. Acquire an understanding of the Judicial Process.

As identified in Chapter 1, the federal courts were established through Article III of the U.S. Constitution. The judiciary branch, one of the three separate and distinct branches that include the executive (i.e. the President) and legislative branches (i.e. Congress), is often called the protector of the Constitution because their court decisions protect the rights and liberties guaranteed by the Constitution. The federal courts, through their fair and impartial judgments, interpret and apply the law to resolve disputes between parties. As delineated by the founding fathers, the federal courts do not enact laws (this power belongs to the legislative branch) and does not enforce laws (this power belongs to the executive branch). It only interprets the Constitution and resolves disputes through fair, impartial, and independent judgments.

The founding fathers considered an independent federal judiciary to be essential in order to ensure fairness and equal justice for all citizens. In the Constitution, the founding fathers promoted the independent judiciary in two major ways: (1) Article III identified that federal judges would be appointed for life and could only be removed from the bench through impeachment and conviction by Congress for "Treason, Bribery, or other High Crimes and Misdemeanors"; and (2) a judge's compensation "shall not be diminished during their Continuance in Office."* This means, in essence, that neither the President nor Congress can reduce the salary

---

* Article III of the U.S. Constitution.

or remove a federal judge from the bench (exceptional cases: treason, bribery, or a major crime). These protections permit federal judges to be independent to decide cases free from political influences and current passions.

Under the Constitution, Congress (legislative branch) was granted the power to create federal courts other than the Supreme Court and to determine the jurisdiction of these federal courts. It is Congress, not the federal courts, which control the types of cases that can be addressed in the federal courts. Congress has three basic responsibilities that determine how the federal courts operate including the following: (1) how many judges there will be and where they will be located; (2) confirmation of federal judges; and (3) approval of federal courts' budgets and appropriations of monies for the federal courts to operate.

The executive branch also plays a vital role in the federal courts under the Constitution. The President appoints judicial nominees who can, with the consent of the Senate, become federal judges. In addition to the executive branch's power to appoint new federal judges, several executive branch agencies, such as the U.S. Marshals Service, work with the judiciary branch. (Note: The Department of Justice, which is responsible for prosecuting federal crimes and representing the government in civil litigation, carries the heaviest caseload in the federal court system.)

Congress also created specialized courts under Article I of the Constitution for efficiency as well as to ensure impartiality and removal of political influences. These specialty courts and federal administrative agencies adjudicate disputes and benefit programs involving specific federal laws. These nonjudiciary courts, such as the U.S. Tax Court and U.S. Court of Appeals for the Armed Forces, can decide cases and their decisions are often appealable to the federal courts created under Article III.

Within the structure and hierarchy of the federal court system, the specialty courts and tribunals, such as the Court of Appeals for Veterans Claims, are at the initial level of the court system. Decisions from these Article I specialty courts and tribunals are often appealable to the federal district courts. For safety professionals, the Occupational Safety and Health Review Commission is considered an Article I court or tribunal. Decisions from the Occupational Safety and Health Review Commission can be appealed to the federal district court in the District of Columbia or in the local federal district court.

The U.S. district courts, often referred to as the federal "trial courts," are usually the entry level for the federal court system. The federal district courts are strategically located throughout the states (94 federal judicial districts), as well as in the District of Columbia, Puerto Rica, Guam, the U.S. Virgin Islands, and the Northern Mariana Islands. Each state has at least one federal trial court, and each district includes a U.S. bankruptcy court as part of the federal district court structure. There are two special federal courts which are provided nationwide jurisdiction over certain types of cases. The Court of International Trade hears cases involving international trade and customs disputes. The U.S. Court of Federal Claims has jurisdiction over claims for money damages against the United States, federal contract disputes, unlawful taking of private property by the federal government and other claims against the U.S. government.

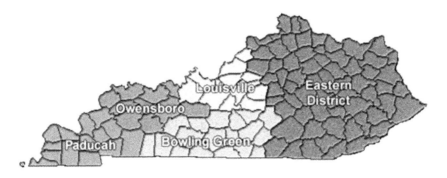

FIGURE 2.1   Counties in federal court districts in Kentucky.

Example: Federal District Courts for the Eastern and Western Districts of Kentucky (Figure 2.1).

The Appellate Courts, often referred to as "Courts of Appeal," are strategically placed in 12 regional circuits throughout the United States and 1 federal circuit court of appeals. The 94 district courts are organized into the 12 regional circuits to hear challenges from the decisions of the district courts within the appellate court's jurisdiction. Additionally, the Court of Appeals possesses nationwide jurisdiction to hear appeals in specialty cases, such as patent law and cases from the Court of International Trade and Court of Federal Claims (Figure 2.2).

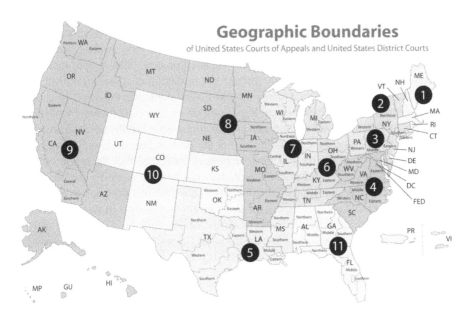

FIGURE 2.2   Federal Circuit Courts of Appeal Regions.

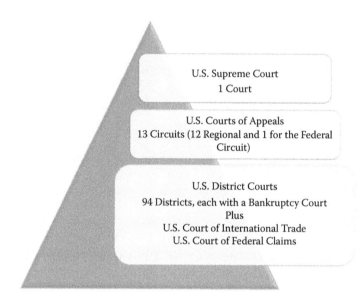

FIGURE 2.3   Federal court system.

The U.S. Supreme Court, located in Washington D.C., consists of a Chief Justice and eight associate justices. Within certain guidelines established by Congress and at its discretion, the Supreme Court hears a small number of cases from the Appellate Courts each year. Supreme Court cases are often selected from appellate court cases where different circuits have different decisions for the same or similar issues, often called a "split" in the circuits, or the circuits have addressed important questions or issues involving the Constitution or other federal law (Figure 2.3).

In order that a case can be heard by a federal court, certain conditions must be met before the federal court can acquire jurisdiction over the case. First, as identified in the Constitution, federal courts can exercise only judicial powers. "This means that federal judges may interpret the law only through the resolution of actual legal disputes, referred to in Article III of the Constitution as Cases and Controversies."[*] In short, the court cannot answer a hypothetical legal question or correct a problem by its own initiative. Second, there must be an actual case or controversy and the person bring the lawsuit, or plaintiff, must have "standing" to ask the court to hear the case. "Standing" means the person bringing the suit must have been legally harmed or aggrieved by another, referred to as the defendant. Third, the case being brought by the plaintiff must present a category of dispute "that the law in question was designed to address, and it must be a complaint that the court has the power to remedy."[†] In short, the court must have the authority to hear the case under the Constitution or federal law. Lastly, the case must present an ongoing issue for the courts to resolve. If there is no ongoing issue, the case is considered "moot" or no issue is present for the court to address.

---

[*] *Understanding The Federal Courts*, Administrative Office of the U.S. Courts, Page 6.
[†] Id.

The federal courts can only hear certain types of cases as established by the Constitution or Congress. Federal question jurisdiction "arises in cases that involve the U.S. government, the U.S. Constitution or federal law, or controversies between states or between U.S. and foreign governments."[*] Examples of federal question jurisdiction include claims for Social Security benefits and criminal prosecution for a federal crime. Federal jurisdiction can also be found where there is a "diversity of citizenship" meaning the parties are from different states or a U.S. citizen and a citizen of a foreign country. It should be noted that in cases where "diversity of citizenship" is utilized, the case must involve more than $75,000.00 in potential damages to be filed in federal court. Claims below $75,000.00, even where "diversity of citizenship" exists, must be filed in state court.

Congress determined that all bankruptcy cases must be heard in federal court, usually in U.S. Bankruptcy Court (i.e. bankruptcy cases may NOT be filed in state court). The primary purpose of the law of bankruptcy is to provide an honest debtor a "fresh start" in life by relieving debts, to repay creditors in a fair and orderly manner, to reorganize a failing business by restructuring debt, or to provide a method through which liquidation of assets of a failing organization is used to pay the debt. In bankruptcy proceedings, businesses or individuals identify that they can no longer pay their creditors. The business or individual requests that the court provide court-supervised liquidation of their assets or ask the court to reorganize their financial assets and develop a plan through which making payment of their credits the amount owed to them. There are several categories of bankruptcy cases which can be brought before the U.S. Bankruptcy Court including the following:

Chapter 7 – Liquidation of Assets – Designed to sell most of the debtor's property to repay debts owed to the creditor. The Bankruptcy Court often appoints a trustee to take over debtor's property. Debtor is often permitted to keep a limited amount of the property as specified by law. Property is sold and proceeds distributed to the creditors in accordance with the bankruptcy laws.

Chapter 9 – Municipality – Designed for debt adjustment for cities, towns, counties, public agencies, and other instrumentalities of the state.

Chapter 11 – Reorganization – Designed to provide an operating business the ability to resolve financial problems through reorganization. The business is often permitted to continue in operation, and a trustee is appointed to oversee the operating business.

Chapter 12 – Family Farm – Designed to offer relief similar to Chapter 13 for family farms only.

Chapter 13 – Debt Adjustment – Designed to permit the debtor to keep the property; however, the debtor must repay the creditors in installments taken from future earnings. Usually, the debtor is required to submit a plan for approval by the court. Often a trustee is appointed, and the debtor pays the trustee and the trustee pays the creditors.

Chapter 15 – Cross-Border Insolvencies – Designed to address debt relief in foreign cases.

---

[*] Id.

In summation, the U.S. Constitution established the U.S. Supreme Court, and Congress established the appellate and district federal courts. The federal courts are responsible for all bankruptcy cases. For a case to be heard before the federal courts, specific requirements must be met including diversity of citizenship, federal crime controversies between states and related jurisdictional requirements, as well as a minimum of $75,000.00 in damages for civil cases. Federal civil and criminal cases usually start at the trial or district levels with appeals to the Court of appeals and to the Supreme Court. However, the Supreme Court usually hears a small number of cases and usually make decisions where there is a split in the circuit courts. The Supreme Court is the "final arbitrator" of all cases within our judicial system.

Questions

1. What is the purpose of the federal court system?
2. How many and where are the federal district courts in your state located?
3. What is the makeup of the U.S. Supreme Court and where is it located?
4. Please explain the judicial hierarchy of the federal court system.
5. What is the difference between the Rules of Criminal and Rules of Civil Procedure?

FEDERAL JUDICIAL CASELOAD STATISTICS 2016

> In accordance with 28 U.S.C. § 604(a)(2), each year, the Administrative Office of the United States Courts is required to provide a report of statistical information on the caseload of the federal courts for the 12-month period ending March 31.

This report presents data on the work of the appellate, district, and bankruptcy courts and on the probation and pretrial services systems. Below is a summary of key findings provided for the year ending March 31, 2016.

- In the U.S. courts of appeals, filings held steady, dropped by 1 percent.
- The bankruptcy appellate panels reported a 20 percent reduction in filings.
- Filings in the U.S. Court of Appeals for the Federal Circuit grew 6 percent.
- In the U.S. district courts, filings of civil cases decreased by 2.5 percent, while filings for defendants charged with crimes fell less than 1 percent.
- The U.S. bankruptcy courts received 9 percent fewer petitions.
- The number of persons under supervision by the federal probation system on March 31, 2015 was 3 percent higher than the total reported one year earlier.
- The number of pretrial services cases activated in the past 12 months dropped by 3 percent.

U.S. COURTS OF APPEALS

Filings in the 12 regional courts of appeals remained relatively stable. Civil appeals, administrative agency decisions appeals, and bankruptcy appeals had declines in filings. Increases occurred in filings of criminal appeals and of original proceedings and miscellaneous applications.

Civil appeals dropped by 2,157 filings (down by 7 percent) to 28,066.

- Prisoner petitions decreased by 7 percent.
- Civil appeals not filed by prisoners declined by 8 percent.
- Criminal appeals increased by 15 percent to 12,275. This growth resulted from a 45 percent rise in appeals by persons convicted of drug offenses, most of them seeking reductions in their sentences following the implementation of the United States Sentencing Commission's Amendment 782, which adjusted by two levels the Drug Quantity Table used for sentencing pursuant to 18 U.S.C. §3582(c).
- Seventy-nine percent of criminal appeals involved four offense categories: drugs, immigration, firearms and explosives, and property offenses (including fraud).
- Administrative agency appeals fell by 4 percent to 6,866, largely because of a 7 percent reduction in appeals of decisions by the Board of Immigration Appeals (BIA).
- BIA appeals accounted for 81 percent of administrative agency appeals and constituted the largest category of administrative agency appeals filed in each circuit except the D.C. Circuit.
- Original proceedings and miscellaneous applications went up by 5 percent to 5,634.
- Sixty-seven percent of filings in the original proceedings and miscellaneous applications category involved second or successive motions for writs of habeas corpus, 21 percent involved writs of mandamus, and 10 percent were miscellaneous cases.
- Of the 583 miscellaneous applications reported, class actions accounted for 56 percent of the total.

Bankruptcy appeals decreased by 5 percent to 808 (Table 2.1).

Terminations of appeals decreased by 2 percent to 53,673. Pending appeals remained relatively unchanged, falling less than 1 percent to 40,922.

BANKRUPTCY APPELLATE PANELS

The bankruptcy appellate panels (BAPs) reported that filings decreased by 20 percent to 649 (down by 166 appeals). Filings fell in all five circuits with BAPs. The BAPs are units of the federal courts of appeals, and each BAP must be established by a circuit council.

Filings dropped by 125 appeals (down by 22 percent) in the Ninth Circuit, by 18 appeals (down by 32 percent) in the Eight Circuit, by 8 appeals (down by 12 percent) in the Tenth Circuit, by 8 appeals (down by 11 percent) in the First Circuit, and by 7 appeals (down by 11 percent) in the Sixth Circuit.

TABLE 2.1
Appeals Court Filings Percent Change Over Time

	Since 2007	Since 2012	Since 2015
Total filings	−11.57	−5.25	−1.10
Criminal appeals	−12.91	−5.90	15.21
Civil appeals	−9.12	−8.78	−7.14
U.S. prisoner petitions	−14.98	−13.06	−16.34
Other U.S. civil	−8.46	−5.99	−5.44
Private prisoner petitions	−12.98	−9.88	−1.73
Other private civil	−3.47	−6.87	−8.12
Bankruptcy appeals	3.46	11.91	−5.28
Administrative agency appeals	−38.62	−16.15	−3.80
Original proceedings and miscellaneous applications[a]	51.25	44.39	4.78

[a] Beginning in March 2014, data include miscellaneous cases not included previously.

U.S. COURT OF APPEALS FOR THE FEDERAL CIRCUIT

Filings in the U.S. Court of Appeals for the Federal Circuit grew by 6 percent to 1,736.

- Appeals arising from the U.S. Patent and Trademark Office had the largest numeric increase, a rise of 229 appeals to 546 (up by 72 percent).
- Appeals of decisions by the U.S. district courts had the largest numeric decrease, a drop of 33 appeals to 559 (down by 6 percent) (Table 2.2).

Terminations of appeals increased by 135 appeals to 1,604 (up by 9 percent). The pending caseload rose by 132 appeals to 1,293 (up by 11 percent).

U.S. DISTRICT COURTS

Combined filings for civil cases and criminal defendants in the U.S. district courts decreased by 7, 350 (down by 2 percent) to 354,339. Terminations held steady, rising by 2,627 (up by less than 1 percent) to 350,455. The total for pending cases and defendants remained fairly stable, growing by 3,285 (up by less than 1 percent) to 441,846.

TABLE 2.2
Federal Circuit Dilings Percent Change Over Time

	Since 2007	Since 2012	Since 2015
Total filings	3	28	6
U.S. District court appeals	24	18	−6
U.S. Patent and trademark office appeals	825	296	72
U.S. Merit systems protection board appeals	−46	−11	−10

CIVIL FILINGS

Civil filings in the U.S. district courts fell by 2.5 percent (down by 7,056 cases) to 274,552.

Diversity of citizenship filings (i.e. cases between citizens of different states) declined by 5 percent to 82,990.

- Diversity of citizenship filings involving personal injury/product liability decreased by 5 percent to 38,652.
- Driving this overall decline was a reduction of more than 3,500 multidistrict litigation cases involving personal injury/product liability in the Southern District of West Virginia. During the previous year, the same district had received more than 21,000 such cases alleging injuries from pelvic repair system products.
- Federal question filings remained relatively stable, decreased by less than 1 percent to 149,509.
- Personal injury/product liability cases dropped by 40 percent to 40,139 (down by 987 cases) in response to lower filings of asbestos cases (down by 464 cases) and other product liability cases (down by 426 cases).
- Contract filings declined by 17 percent to 4,058 as insurance cases fell by 34 percent (down by 574 cases).
- Intellectual property rights filings fell by 4 percent to 13,257, mainly due to a 17 percent reduction in trademark cases (down by 644 cases).
- Filings of cases with the United States as defendant decreased by 2 percent to 36,641.
- Social Security filings went down by 7 percent to 17,931 as supplemental security income cases dropped by 11 percent.
- Filings with the United States as plaintiff fell by 15 percent to 5,401.
- Forfeiture and penalty cases dropped by 34 percent (down by 592 cases), largely in response to declines in other forfeiture and penalty suits (down by 345 cases) and cases addressing the drug-related seizure of property (down by 246 cases).
- Cases involving defaulted student loans decreased by 16 percent to 1,212 (Table 2.3).
- Civil case terminations increased by 2 percent to 270,515.
- The Southern District of West Virginia terminated more than 8,400 multidistrict litigation cases related to pelvic repair system products.
- Pending civil cases grew by 1 percent to 344,715.

TABLE 2.3
Civil Case Filings Percent Change Over Time

	Since 2007	Since 2012	Since 2015
Total filings	6.6	−1.4	−2.5
Federal question cases	5.6	4.5	−0.4
Diversity of citizenship cases	−10.3	−13.2	−5.4
U.S. defendant cases	4.7	0.9	−1.9
U.S. plaintiff cases	−41.1	−47.6	−14.6

CRIMINAL FILINGS

Filings for criminal defendants (including transfers) in the U.S. district courts remained stable, falling less than 1 percent (down by 294 defendants) to 79,787.

Filings involving drug offenses, which accounted for 32 percent of total defendant filings, increased by 3 percent to 25,454.

- Defendants charged with marijuana offenses dropped by 7 percent to 5,347.
- Defendants charged with crimes involving drugs other than marijuana rose by 6 percent to 20,000.
- Defendants charged with immigration offenses, which constituted 26 percent of all criminal defendant filings, declined by less than 1 percent to 21,016.
- Eighty percent of immigration defendant filings occurred in the five southwestern border districts.
- Filings decreased by 27 and 3 percent in the Southern District of California and Western District of Texas, respectively.
- Filings grew by 12, 11, and 3 percent in the Southern District of Texas, District of New Mexico, and District of Arizona, respectively.
- Filings associated with property offenses, which amounted to 15 percent of all defendant filings, fell by 9 percent to 11,697.
- Fraud defendants declined by 7 percent to 8,392.

Defendant filings for firearms and explosives crimes climbed by13 percent to 8, 466. Defendants accused of sex offenses rose by 4 percent to 3,430. Defendants charged with general offenses (i.e. public-order crimes such as money laundering) increased by 2 percent to 1,897.

Traffic offense filings decreased by 21 percent to 2,423 (this total does not include defendants charged with traffic crimes in petty offense cases disposed of by magistrate judges). Defendants charged with justice system offenses (i.e. crimes related to judicial proceedings, such as obstruction of justice or failure to appear) fell by 8 percent to 804 (Table 2.4).

Terminations for criminal defendants dropped by 5 percent to 79,940. As terminations slightly exceeded filings, the number for defendants pending declined by 1 percent to 97,131.

TABLE 2.4
Criminal Defendant Filings (Excluding Transfers) Percent Change Over Time

	Since 2007	Since 2012	Since 2015
Total defendants filed	−8.5	−19.5	−0.4
Immigration defendants	23.8	−20.9	−0.7
Property defendants	−25.7	−28.8	−9.3
Sex offense defendants	59.1	−1.4	3.8
Drug defendants	−15.7	−19.8	2.6
Firearms and explosives defendants	−11.7	−3.9	12.6

U.S. BANKRUPTCY COURTS

Filings of bankruptcy petitions fell by 9 percent to 833,515 (down 77,571 petitions). Of the 90 bankruptcy courts, 84 reported declines in filings.

- The largest percentage decrease was a 20 percent reduction in the Southern District of Florida.
- Percentage increases were reported by the District of Alaska (up by 6 percent), Northern District of Alabama (up by 4 percent), Southern District of Mississippi (up by 3 percent), Middle District of Alabama (up by 2 percent), Southern District of Alabama (up by 2 percent), and Western District of Virginia (up by 1 percent).

Fewer petitions were filed under chapters 7 and 13 of the bankruptcy code. More petitions were filed under chapters 11 and 12.

- Chapter 7 filings dropped by 12 percent to 523,394.
- Chapter 13 filings fell by 1 percent to 302,193
- Chapter 11 filings rose by 5 percent to 7,380.
- Chapter 12 filings increased by 25 percent to 440.

Petitions filed by debtors with predominantly business debts declined by 5 percent to 24,797. Debtors with predominantly nonbusiness (i.e. consumer) debts filed 808,718 petitions, 9 percent fewer than the previous year. Consumer cases accounted for 97 percent of all petitions (Table 2.5).

Terminations of bankruptcy cases fell by 10 percent to 947,587. Because terminations exceeded filings, the number of cases pending on March 31, 2016 dropped by 9 percent from the previous year's total to 1,208,606.

Bankruptcy filings have fluctuated since the Bankruptcy Abuse Prevention and Consumer Protection Act (BAPCPA) took effect in October 2005. The courts received 695,575 petitions in 12 months ending March 31, 2007. Thereafter, filings increased every year until 2011 where 1,571,183 petitions were filed. In each of the last five years, filings have declined. Total filings for 2016 are 47 percent below the post-BAPCPA peak reached in 2011, but 20 percent above the 2007 filing level.

TABLE 2.5
Bankruptcy Court Filings Percent Change Over Time

	Since 2007	Since 2012	Since 2015
Total filings	−54	−47	−9
Chapter 7	−64	−53	−12
Chapter 11	14	−44	5
Chapter 13	−15	−31	−2

ADVERSARY PROCEEDINGS

Adversary proceedings are separate civil lawsuits that arise in bankruptcy cases, including actions to object to or revoke discharges, to obtain injunctions or other equitable relief, and to determine the dischargeable debt. Adversary proceedings may be associated with consumer bankruptcy cases, but most arise in cases filed under chapter 11. They generally reflect the level of chapter 11 bankruptcy petitions filed two years earlier.

During 12 months ending March 31, 2016, filings of adversary proceedings decreased by 6 percent to 32,227. Fifty-nine of the 90 bankruptcy courts experienced declines in filings during this reporting period. These reductions were attributed to the overall drop in bankruptcy filings.

Terminations of adversary proceedings dropped by 8 percent to 35,910. Pending adversary proceedings fell by 8 percent to 44,687.

POST-CONVICTION SUPERVISION

The number of persons under post-conviction supervision as of March 31, 2016, rose by 3 percent from the prior year to 138,074 (up by 4,622 persons). Persons serving terms of supervised release on that date following release from a correctional institution increased by 5 percent to 118,099.

- Eighty-six percent of persons under post-conviction supervision on March 31, 2016 were serving terms of supervised release, increased from 84 percent one year earlier.
- Fourteen percent of persons under post-conviction supervision were under supervision following the imposition of sentences of probation, and 1 percent were on parole.

Cases remaining open on March 31, 2016 that involved probation imposed by district and magistrate judges decreased by 3 percent from the previous year's total to 18,643.

Persons on parole, special parole, military parole, and mandatory release on the last day of the reporting period declined by 11 percent to 1,186.

The number of persons received for post-conviction supervision was 67,911, an increase of 9 percent from the previous year (Table 2.6).

Closings of post-conviction supervision cases (excluding transfers and deaths) rose 2 by percent to 54,646 (up by 1,097 cases).

TABLE 2.6
Persons under Post-conviction Supervision Percent Change Over Time

	Since 2007	Since 2012	Since 2015
Total under supervision	20.1	4.3	3.5
Serving terms of supervised release	35.0	9.4	4.9
On probation	−24.2	−17.1	−3.4
On parole	−57.1	−30.8	−11.0

In addition to their supervision duties, probation officers conduct investigations and prepare comprehensive reports to aid judges in sentencing convicted defendants. The officers' presentence reports contain detailed background information on defendants and discuss issues related to the advisory sentencing guidelines.

- In 2016, probation officers wrote 65,021 presentence reports, a 3 percent decrease from the previous year.
- Ninety-two percent of the presentence reports addressed offenses for which the U.S. Sentencing Commission has promulgated sentencing guidelines.

PRETRIAL SERVICES

The number of cases opened in the pretrial services system equaled 93,005, a decrease of 3 percent from 2015.

- A total of 644 pretrial diversion cases were activated, a drop of 18 percent from the previous year.
- Defendants received for pretrial services supervision fell by 2 percent to 24,301.
- Defendants received for pretrial diversion supervision dropped by 14 percent to 929 (Table 2.7).
- A total of 91,676 pretrial services cases were closed, a reduction of 8 percent.
- Pretrial services officers prepare reports for judges to help in determining whether to order the release or detention of defendants. They also provide information judges use in establishing appropriate conditions for released defendants.
- Pretrial services officers interviewed 51,717 defendants (up by 5 percent) and prepared 90,050 pretrial services reports (down by 3 percent).
- For persons under pretrial supervision, officers monitored their compliance with release conditions set by the courts, made referrals for support services that offer alternatives to detention (such as substance abuse treatment), and informed the courts and U.S. attorneys of apparent violations of release conditions.
- Defendants with release conditions dropped by 1 percent to 26,583.

TABLE 2.7
Pretrial Services Filings Percent Change Over Time

	Since 2007	Since 2012	Since 2015
Total cases activated	−2.1	−16.7	−3.3
Pretrial services cases activated	−1.1	−16.6	−3.1
Pretrial diversion cases activated	−59.0	−30.5	−18.1
Released on supervision	−25.9	−19.1	−1.9
Pretrial supervision	−25.4	−18.6	−1.3
Diversion supervision	−37.7	−30.1	−14.5

Questions

1. Where is your local federal district court located?
2. What Appellate Circuit are you located in?
3. How long does a federal judge serve in this capacity?
4. Where is the U.S. Supreme Court located?
5. Identify one (1) specialty court in the federal court system.

3 The Court Process and Procedures

Laws are sand, customs are rock. Laws can be evaded and punishment escaped, but an openly transgressed custom brings sure punishment.

Mark Twain

The execution of the laws is more important than the making of them.

Thomas Jefferson

STUDENT LEARNING OBJECTIVES

1. Analyze and assess federal court procedures.
2. Analyze the adversarial process utilized by the courts.
3. Assess and analyze the difference between civil and criminal processes.
4. Analyze the steps in a trial proceeding.

Although the Constitution provides individuals their day in court, the process of litigation is adversarial, and it relies on the parties to present the facts of their dispute to a neutral judge or jury. When an individual or a company brings the legal action, they are usually referred to as the "plaintiff" at the trial level. The individual or company in which the action is against is usually referred to as the "defendant." Each party is required to collect their own evidence and prepare their presentation to the court. Generally, the parties pay their own court costs, attorney fees, expert fees, and other related costs whether they win or lose. In criminal cases, the government pays the costs for the investigation and prosecution and the court, when appropriate, provides an attorney to the defendant at no cost if he/she is not able to afford an attorney. In civil cases, the parties usually pay for their own costs; however, plaintiffs who cannot pay the court fees may seek permission from the court to waive the court costs only.

The courts have well-defined rules, including the federal Rules of Evidence, federal Rules of Civil Procedure, Rules of Criminal Procedure, appellate rules, and others that govern all types of cases in the trial and appellate courts. These rules are often technical and are designed to promote a level playing field and minimize expense and delay. Strict adherence to these rules is required and actions can be dismissed for failure to follow the rules.

Civil and criminal actions have significantly different "burden of proof." Please remember that civil actions are usually concerned about money, while criminal actions involve the taking of freedom from an individual. Thus, the burden of proof is far greater in criminal actions than civil actions. In criminal cases, the government (or prosecution) must prove each and every element of the crime "beyond a reasonable doubt." The defendant is not required to testify, and the defendant is not required to prove his/her innocence. In a civil case, the burden of proof is by the "preponderance of the evidence" and a majority rule of the jury. Thus, the burden of proof is far greater in a criminal trial than a civil trial.

In federal court, a civil case usually involves a dispute between 2 or more parties, and the court has jurisdiction over the specific dispute. A civil action starts with the plaintiff filing a "complaint" document with the court and "serving" a copy of the complaint to the defendants. The "complaint" document described the plaintiff's injury or the damages allegedly caused by the defendant(s), explains how the defendant allegedly caused the damages, addresses why this specific federal court has jurisdiction over this matter, and asks the court to grant monetary or other relief (such as stopping a particular action).

In addition to being an adversarial process, civil cases often take a substantial amount of time, even years, to get to trial. Criminal cases, due to the "Speedy Trial Act,"* take precedence over civil cases. After the plaintiff files the complaint and serves the complaint on the defendant, the parties may conduct "discovery." In essence, discovery can include, but is not limited to, depositions, witness lists, and copies of documents. The general purpose of discovery is for the parties to prepare for trial by requiring the parties to assemble their evidence and prepare their witnesses. Additionally, the parties may also file "motions" or requests to the court seeking rulings from the court regarding the discovery of evidence, procedures to be followed, and other issues.

As identified above, one common practice in discovery is the use of a deposition. Depositions can be used by either party in a dispute. A deposition is usually held outside of the courtroom at an attorney's office or conference room, with a court reporter present and transcribing each and every word said during the deposition. The witness is usually under oath, and the attorneys take turns asking the witness questions that the witness is required to answer. Upon completion, the court reporter transcribes each and every work and produces a written document called a "transcript" of the deposition.

Given the expansive caseload for most judges as well as the expense and delay of having a trial, judges often "twist the arm" of the parties in hopes that the parties will reach an agreement before trial. As the evidence is gathered by both parties, the plaintiff and the defendant can acquire a clearer picture as to the strength or weakness of their case. Although the parties often settle the matter outside of trial with court approval, alternate dispute resolution, such as mediation and arbitration, is often encouraged by the court.

---

* Title I of the Speedy Trial Act of 1974, 88 Stat. 2080, as amended August 2, 1979, 93 Stat. 328, is set forth in 18 U.S.C. §§ 3161–3174. The Act establishes time limits for completing the various stages of a federal criminal prosecution. The information or indictment must be filed within 30 days from the date of arrest or service of the summons. 18 U.S.C. § 3161(b). **Trial must commence within 70 days from the date the information or indictment** was filed, or from the date the defendant appears before an officer of the court in which the charge is pending, whichever is later. 18 U.S.C. § 3161(c)(1). (Emphasis added)

ELEMENTS OF A TRIAL

- Jury Selection (if applicable).
- Opening Statements by the Parties.
- Direct and Cross-Examination of the Witnesses.
- Closing Statements by the Parties.
- Jury Deliberation and Verdict.

In the event that a civil case is not settled, the judge will schedule a trial with the parties. In most civil actions, either side may request a trial by jury. If the parties waive their right to a trial by jury, the case will be heard and determined only by the judge (known as a bench trial). After selection of a jury, the procedures of a civil trial usually include opening statements by each of the parties, the calling of witnesses and cross-examination by the opposing party, closing statements by both parties, and deliberation by the jury before a decision is rendered. Witnesses at trial are required to be disclosed to the opposition and testify under oath and under the supervision of the judge. The judge determines which information can be presented and the attorneys can object to the question(s) asked by opposing counsel. The judge will rule off each and every objection either by sustaining the objection (the witness does not answer the question) or by overruling the objection (the question stands and the witness must answer).

After all witnesses and evidences are presented and each party is provided time for their closing arguments, the jury is usually instructed by the Judge as to their responsibilities and tasks and the jury is moved to a private area for deliberations. In a civil trial, the jury is usually asked to determine, by the "preponderance of the evidence," which side prevailed and the scope of any damages. In a bench trial, the judge decides who prevailed and the damages or relief to be granted to the winning party. Either party has the right to appeal the decision to the appropriate appellate court.

It should be noted that a large percentage of civil cases are settled or dismissed prior to trial. Given the fact that each side bears their own costs, the cost of the litigation itself may be a deciding factor in pursuing alternate dispute resolution or settlement. Additionally, the time involved from complaint to a decision by the judge or jury may involve several years. For safety professionals, being pro-active in preventing or minimizing risks that could evolve into a civil action is paramount. Although the sole remedy for workplace injuries and illnesses is often individual state workers compensation, injury to others, contract disputes, and other potential sources of civil litigation should be identified and addressed in a proactive manner.

In summation, safety professionals should be aware of the processes and procedures in a civil trial to be able to adequately assess and provide guidance to their management teams as to the risks and costs involved in any civil action. As can be seen from the numerous television commercials, billboards, and other advertisements by law firms, we live in a litigious society and prudent safety professionals should be knowledgeable, prepared, and ready for the inevitable complaint to be served upon their company or organization.

Questions

1. What is the difference between a civil and criminal trial?
2. What is "discovery" in a civil action?
3. What is the difference in the "burden of proof" between a civil and criminal action?
4. What is a bench trial?
5. What is a deposition?

CURRENT RULES OF PRACTICE & PROCEDURE

*Below are links to the national federal rules and forms in effect, as well as local rules (which are required to be **consistent with the national rules**) **prescribed by district** courts and courts of appeal.*

RULES OF APPELLATE PROCEDURE

The Federal Rules of Appellate Procedure (eff. December 1, 2016) govern procedure in the U.S. courts of appeals. The Supreme Court first adopted the Rules of Appellate Procedure by order dated December 4, 1967, transmitted to Congress on January 15, 1968, and effective July 1, 1968. The Appellate Rules and accompanying forms were last amended in 2016.

RULES OF BANKRUPTCY PROCEDURE

The Federal Rules of Bankruptcy Procedure (eff. December 1, 2016) govern procedures for bankruptcy proceedings. For many years, such proceedings were governed by the General Orders and Forms in Bankruptcy promulgated by the Supreme Court. By order dated April 24, 1973, effective October 1, 1973, the Supreme Court prescribed, pursuant to 28 U.S.C. § 2075, the Bankruptcy Rules and Official Bankruptcy Forms, which abrogated previous rules and forms. Over the years, the Bankruptcy Rules and Official Forms have been amended many times, most recently in 2016.

> Interim Bankruptcy Rule 1007-I
>
> The National Guard and Reservists Debt Relief Act of 2008, Pub. L. No. 110–438, as amended by Public Law No.114-107, provides a temporary exclusion from the bankruptcy means test for certain reservists and members of the National Guard. At the request of the Judicial Conference's Advisory Committee on Bankruptcy Rules, Interim Rule 1007-I was transmitted to the courts for adoption as a local rule to implement the temporary exclusion.

RULES OF CIVIL PROCEDURE

The Federal Rules of Civil Procedure (eff. December 1, 2016) govern civil proceedings in the U.S. district courts. Their purpose is "to secure the just, speedy, and inexpensive determination of every action and proceeding." Fed. R. Civ. P. 1. The rules were first adopted by order of the Supreme Court on December 20, 1937, transmitted to Congress on January 3, 1938, and effective September 16, 1938. The Civil Rules were last amended in 2016.

RULES OF CRIMINAL PROCEDURE

The Federal Rules of Criminal Procedure (eff. December 16, 2016) govern criminal proceedings and prosecutions in the U.S. district courts, the courts of appeals, and the Supreme Court. Their purpose is to "provide for the just determination of every criminal proceeding, to secure simplicity in procedure and fairness in administration, and to eliminate unjustifiable expense and delay." Fed. R. Crim. P. 2. The original rules were adopted by order of the Supreme Court on December 26, 1944, transmitted to Congress on January 3, 1945, and effective March 21, 1946. The rules have since been amended numerous times, most recently in 2016.

RULES OF EVIDENCE

The Federal Rules of Evidence (eff. December 1, 2016) govern the admission or exclusion of evidence in most proceedings in the U.S. courts. The Supreme Court submitted proposed Federal Rules of Evidence to Congress on February 5, 1973, but Congress exercised its power under the Rules Enabling Act to suspend their implementation. The Federal Rules of Evidence became federal law on January 2, 1975, when President Ford signed the Act to Establish Rules of Evidence for Certain Courts and Proceedings, Pub. L. No. 93-595. As enacted, the Evidence Rules included amendments by Congress to the rules originally proposed by the Supreme Court. The most recent amendments to the Federal Rules of Evidence were adopted in 2014.

RULES GOVERNING SECTION 2254 AND SECTION 2255 PROCEEDINGS

Generally, the Rules Governing Section 2254 Cases in the U.S. district courts govern habeas corpus petitions filed in a U.S. district court pursuant to 28 U.S.C. § 2254 by a person in custody challenging his or her current or future custody under a state-court judgment on the grounds that such custody violates the Constitution or laws or treaties of the United States. The Rules Governing Section 2255 Proceedings for the U.S. district courts govern motions to vacate, set aside or correct a sentence filed pursuant to 28 U.S.C. § 2255. Such motions must be filed in the sentencing court by a person in custody attacking the sentence imposed on the ground that the sentence was imposed in violation of the Constitution or laws of the United States, that the court was without jurisdiction to impose such sentence, or that the sentence was in excess of the maximum authorized by law, or is otherwise subject to collateral attack.

The Supreme Court submitted proposed rules and forms governing proceedings under Section 2254 and Section 2255 to Congress on April 26, 1976, but Congress exercised its power under the Rules Enabling Act to suspend their implementation. The Rules Governing Section 2254 and Section 2255 Proceedings, as amended by Congress, became federal law on September 28, 1976, and made applicable to petitions filed under Section 2254 and motions filed under section 2255 on or after February 1, 1977. Pub. L. No. 94-426. The rules were last amended in 2009.

RULES OF THE FOREIGN INTELLIGENCE SURVEILLANCE COURT

The Rules of Procedure for the Foreign Intelligence Surveillance Court were promulgated pursuant to 50 U.S.C. § 1803(g). They govern all proceedings in the Foreign Intelligence Surveillance Court and were last amended in 2010.

LOCAL COURT RULES

U.S. district courts and courts of appeals often prescribe local rules governing practice and procedure. Such rules must be consistent with both Acts of Congress and the Federal Rules of Practice and Procedure, and may only be prescribed after notice and an opportunity for public comment. A court's authority to prescribe local rules is governed by both statute and the Federal Rules of Practice and Procedure. See 28 U.S.C. §§ 2071(a)–(b); Fed. R. App. P. 47; Fed. R. Bankr. P. 9029; Fed. R. Civ. P. 83; Fed. R. Crim. P. 57.

Section 205 of the E-Government Act of 2002, Pub. L. No. 107-347, requires that federal courts post local rules on their websites. Visit the Court Locator for a listing of all federal court websites.

FORMS ACCOMPANYING THE FEDERAL RULES OF PROCEDURE AND EVIDENCE

- Appellate Rules Forms
- Bankruptcy Forms
- National Court Forms[*]

Supp. 1096

United States District Court,
S.D. Georgia,
Brunswick Division.
Darris F. LEE and Linda Lee, Plaintiffs

v.

Johnny SIKES and Marvis W. Driggers, Defendants.
Civ. A. No. CV293-109.
October 4, 1994.

Prison inmate who was attacked by boar hog while working at assigned duties in prison's hog farm operation brought civil rights suit against warden and supervisor of operation. On defense motion for partial summary judgment, the District Court, Alaimo, J., held that: (1) inmate failed to show "deliberate indifference" by supervisor

---

[*] Federal Rules of Court at www.uscourts.gov.

of operation or prison warden, and thus failed to establish Eighth Amendment violation, and (2) inmate was protected by Eighth Amendment, which provides explicit protection to prisoners against cruel and unusual punishment, and could not bring separate, independent claim for same behavior by prison officials based on substantive due process.

Motion granted.

ORDER

District Judge.

Plaintiff, Darris F. Lee ("Lee"), formerly an inmate at Rogers Correctional Institution, was attacked by a boar hog while working at his assigned duties in the prison's hog farm operation. He now brings this federal question action against Johnny Sikes, Warden at Rogers C.I., and Marvis Walter Driggers, Jr., the supervisor of the hog farm operation.

Lee alleges that Defendants deprived him of his rights, privileges and immunities under the Fifth, Eighth and Fourteenth Amendments in violation of 42 U.S.C. § 1983. Specifically, Lee claims (1) an Eighth Amendment violation for wanton and total disregard for his safety by failing to provide proper facilities, training and protective equipment (a workplace safety claim), (2) an Eighth Amendment violation for failure to provide adequate medical care, and (3) a Fourteenth Amendment violation based on the same conduct. Lee also alleges state law claims including negligent employment, failure to train and supervise, and failure to warn of unsafe conditions. His wife, Linda Lee, claims loss of consortium.

Before the Court is Defendants' motion for summary judgment pursuant to Rule 56 of the Federal Rules of Civil Procedure. Defendants' motion is actually one for partial summary judgment, for it only addresses two of Lee's federal claims. The motion does not address Lee's Eighth Amendment claim for failure to provide adequate medical care or his state law claims. For the reasons stated below, Defendants' motion is GRANTED as to Lee's Eighth Amendment workplace safety claim and his Fourteenth Amendment claim.

FACTS

On May 20, 1991, Darris Lee was sentenced to five years in prison after pleading guilty to three counts of burglary and one count of attempted burglary. Lee initially went to Coastal Correctional Institution, Garden City, Georgia, but was eventually assigned to Rogers Correctional Institution, Reidsville, Georgia.

When Lee arrived at Reidsville, he went through a classification and testing process. He was eventually assigned to the hog barn work detail. Lee's initial duties included cleaning and feeding the hogs. After a few weeks, Lee began working in the breeding barn.

While working in the breeding barn, Lee was attacked by a boar hog. Lee claims that the hog escaped after he properly placed the hog in the breeding pen. The parties stipulate that Lee's injuries included a 10–12 centimeter laceration behind his right knee. Plaintiffs allege that Lee suffered additional injuries to his back, head and shoulders.

The parties agree that Lee was given emergency medical treatment at Georgia State Prison, but Plaintiffs contend Lee was not given proper follow up medical care and was released on parole while still undergoing treatment for his injuries.

Defendants have moved for summary judgment on the grounds that (1) Defendants did not act with deliberate indifference as required for Lee's Eighth Amendment claim and (2) there was no deprivation of a protected interest as required for Lee's Fourteenth Amendment claim.

DISCUSSION

I. SUMMARY JUDGMENT

Summary judgment requires the movant to establish the absence of genuine issues of material fact, such that the movant is entitled to judgment as a matter of law. Fed.R.Civ.P. 56(c); *Adickes v. S.H. Kress & Co.*, 398 U.S. 144, 153, 90 S.Ct. 1598, 1606, 26 L.Ed.2d 142 (1970). Summary judgment is also proper "against a party who fails to make a showing sufficient to establish the existence of an element essential to that party's case, and on which that party will bear the burden of proof at trial." *Celotex Corp. v. Catrett*, 477 U.S. 317, 322, 106 S.Ct. 2548, 2552, 91 L.Ed.2d 265 (1986). The non-moving party to a summary judgment motion need make this showing only after the moving party has satisfied its burden. *Clark v. Coats & Clark, Inc.*, 929 F.2d 604, 608 (11th Cir.1991). The court should consider the*1099* pleadings, depositions and affidavits in the case before reaching its decision, Fed.R.Civ.P. 56(c), and all reasonable inferences will be made in favor of the non-movant. *Adickes*, 398 U.S. at 158–59, 90 S.Ct. at 1608–10.

II. FEDERAL CLAIMS

A. § 1983 Liability

Section 1983 provides a civil action for persons claiming violations of their rights secured by the Constitution and laws of the United States. As stated above, Lee alleges § 1983 claims based primarily upon violations of the Eighth and Fourteenth Amendments.

B. Eighth Amendment Violation for Failure to Provide for the Safety of Darris Lee while in Defendants' Custody

Lee claims that Defendants subjected him to cruel and unusual punishment in violation of the Eighth Amendment by failing to provide him with "proper facilities, training, or protective equipment to work with the breeding hogs." (Plaintiffs' Amended Complaint at ¶ 13.) Lee further alleges that Defendants assigned him to "work directly with the hogs which were known to have vicious tendencies" in wanton and total disregard for his safety. (Plaintiff's Amended Complaint at ¶ 11.)

1. Deliberate Indifference

Prison work assignments are considered conditions of confinement subject to scrutiny under the Eighth Amendment. *Choate v. Lockhart*, 7 F.3d 1370, 1373 (8th Cir.1993). To establish an Eighth Amendment violation based on prison workplace safety, a plaintiff must show deliberate indifference. *Id.; see also Estelle v. Gamble,* 429 U.S. 97, 97 S.Ct. 285, 50 L.Ed.2d 251 (1976) (deliberate indifference required for Eighth Amendment claim for inadequate medical care); *Wilson v. Seiter,* 501 U.S. 294, 111 S.Ct. 2321, 115 L.Ed.2d 271 (1991) (deliberate indifference required for Eighth Amendment claim challenging living conditions).

3Defendants argue that summary judgment is proper because there is no genuine issue of material fact as to deliberate indifference. The Court agrees. While the hog farm operation at Reidsville may not be a perfect example of workplace safety, Defendants' conduct simply does not rise to the level of deliberate indifference.

Lee offers the following evidence of deliberate indifference to prisoner safety: Defendant, Marvis Driggers, the supervisor of inmates at the hog barn, testified that he has no input as to which inmates are assigned to the hog barn. He cannot refuse any inmates, but must work with anyone assigned to him. The inmates are not trained upon their arrival, but "kind of [fall] into the routine and learn as they go." (Marvis Driggers' dep. at 25.) The inmates are randomly assigned jobs within the hog barn operation, regardless of their background. In fact, Driggers testified that he knows nothing about the inmates' backgrounds. An arriving inmate simply assumes the responsibilities of the inmate whom he is replacing. The turnover of inmates at the hog farm is quite high. The average length of stay is three months.

The prison does have a one-page list of "Hog Unit Safety Rules and Regulations" which includes the following warning: "Herder boards should always be used when moving boars and sows. Never turn your back on a boar." Lee was not given any equipment to use when moving the hogs. Lee never saw the safety rules and neither did his supervisor, Defendant, Marvis Driggers. Having never seen the rules, Driggers could not enforce them. Driggers testified that he thought the inmates were briefed before being assigned to the hog unit. Lee was unsupervised the day a hog escaped from the breeding pen and attacked him. Driggers testified that, in the past, hogs have escaped from the various pens. The boar hogs at Rogers C.I. are quite large. They weigh between 250 and 450 pounds.

The parties have not cited and the Court has been unable to locate any Eleventh Circuit cases discussing what constitutes deliberate indifference in the workplace safety context. The Eighth Circuit, however, has dealt with this specific issue on several occasions. In deciding what constitutes deliberate indifference, mere negligence or inadvertence is insufficient. *Choate v. Lockhart,* 7 F.3d 1370, 1374 (8th Cir.1993) (citing *Wilson v. Seiter,* 501 U.S. 294, 305, 111 S.Ct. 2321, 2327, 115 L.Ed.2d 271 (1991)). Rather, in the work assignment or workplace safety context, prison officials are deliberately indifferent when they "knowingly compel convicts to perform physical labor which is beyond their strength, or which constitutes a danger to their lives or health, or which is unduly painful." *Ray v. Mabry,* 556 F.2d 881, 882 (8th Cir.1977).

A particular Eighth Circuit decision is instructive in this regard. *See Warren v. State of Mo.,* 995 F.2d 130 (8th Cir.1993). In *Warren,* an inmate suffered a broken wrist when a board kicked back from the table saw he was operating in the prison's furniture factory. The inmate brought an action under § 1983 alleging that the defendants violated his Eighth Amendment rights by failing to equip the saw with "anti-kickback fingers" despite knowledge of similar prior injuries. *Id.* at 130. The court held that "even assuming that one or more defendants had knowledge of the allegedly similar prior accidents ... this showing falls far short of creating a genuine issue of deliberate indifference to a serious issue of workplace safety." *Id.* at 131.

Likewise, even assuming that Defendants, Sikes and Driggers, knew that boar hogs were dangerous or knew that protective equipment should be used, such a showing falls short of creating a genuine issue of deliberate indifference to workplace safety. In attempting to establish a question of fact as to deliberate indifference, Lee relies almost entirely on the one-page list of "Hog Unit Safety Rules and Regulations" and Defendant, Driggers', corresponding ignorance of these rules. The Court notes, however, that in order to be *deliberately* indifferent to safety rules, Defendants would, at least, have to be aware of them. At most, Lee's evidence shows that Defendants were negligent in assigning Lee to the hog barn without proper training and equipment to cope with dangerous animals. As stated above, however, mere negligence is not enough to constitute a Constitutional violation. *Wilson,* 501 U.S. at 305, 111 S.Ct. at 2327.Accordingly, Defendants' motion for summary judgment is GRANTED as to Lee's Eighth Amendment workplace safety claim.

2. Pervasive Risk of Harm

Defendants argue that summary judgment is proper because Lee failed to show a "pervasive risk of harm." *Bellamy v. McMickens,* 692 F.Supp. 205, 211 (S.D.N.Y.1988). Lee apparently accepted Defendants' line of reasoning and sought to establish a "pervasive risk of harm" by proffering the "Hog Farm Safety Rules and Regulations." The Court notes, however, that Lee is not required to establish a "pervasive risk of harm."

In arguing that Lee must establish a pervasive risk of harm, Defendants rely entirely on analogizing this "hog attack" case to "prison attack" cases. In "prison attack" cases, inmates sue prison officials for failing to protect them from attack or sexual assault by other inmates. In this context, plaintiffs can show the required deliberate indifference by showing that prison officials ignored a "pervasive risk of harm." *LaMarca v. Turner,* 662 F.Supp. 647, 711 (S.D.Fla.1987) (§ 1983 class action against former prison superintendent for ignoring problem of gang rapes and related assaults in Glades Correctional Institution, Belle Glade, Florida). A pervasive risk of harm, however, cannot ordinarily be shown by a single incident. *O'Neal v. Evans,* 496 F.Supp. 867, 870 (S.D.Ga.1980). Defendants claim that since one "prison attack" is not enough to establish a pervasive **1101* risk of harm, one "hog attack" is likewise inadequate.

The Court **GRANTS** Defendants' motion for summary judgment as to Lee's Eight Amendment claim based on workplace safety and Lee's Fourteenth Amendment claims. All remaining claims will proceed, as they were not challenged by Defendants' motion.

SO ORDERED.

4 State Courts

The purpose of law is to prevent the strong always having their way.

Ovid

There are not enough jails, not enough policemen, not enough law courts, to enforce a law not supported by the people.

Hubert H. Humphrey

STUDENT LEARNING OBJECTIVES

1. Analyze and assess the jurisdictional boundaries between federal and state courts.
2. Analyze and understand the state judiciary systems.
3. Assess and understand the parallel between state plan programs and state judiciary systems.
4. Analyze and assess the similarities and differences between state and federal judiciary systems.

From a structure prospective, most state judicial systems mirror the federal system with a trial level, appellate level, and a high court with specialty courts usually incorporated into the trail level. Again, as with the federal level, each state has a unique constitution and specific state laws. However, judges in most states are elected or appointed to a term of years (or can be for life or a combination of methods) in comparison with a presidential nomination, confirmation by the senate and lifetime appointment as is utilized on the federal level. Although there is no uniform state court system among the 50 states, state courts often have similar names for their courts and most state courts have subject matter jurisdiction rather than exclusive jurisdiction over an issue or subject.

In most state court systems, the trial or state district court handles criminal cases in their jurisdiction, civil cases within their jurisdiction (often including contract disputes), tort cases (such as personal injury), family law (including marriage, divorce, adoption, etc.), and traffic related cases. In larger state district courts, separate family courts, traffic courts, and small claims courts are often established at the trial or district court level due to the volume of cases. At the district or trial court level, most cases are jury trials.

At the circuit level in many state courts, contract and tort actions are usually above an established dollar amount and criminal cases usually are at the felony level or criminal appeals from the district level. Circuit courts often handle cases involving real estate, domestic relations, and juvenile cases. However, again due to the volume of cases, specific juvenile courts or family courts have been established.

Appeals from the circuit level courts are usually referred to the Court of Appeals or appellate level for the individual state. The courts at this level usually hear criminal appeals (often with a limit as to the sentence), civil appeals, and appeals from administrative agencies (such as a decision by the state's equivalent of the Occupational Safety and Health Review Commission [OSHRC]) based upon the party's right to appeal. Other appeals, such as an appeal of a misdemeanor, is often provided by permission of the court. Additionally, in some states, cases may be directed by state law to start at the appellate level.

Every state judiciary system has a top level court or supreme court which is the final arbitrator of all cases. Although some cases, such as death penalty cases, can be appealed further to the federal court system, most state law cases end at the state's highest court. The top court often hears appeals on felony cases, workers' compensation appeals, and interlocutory appeals in felony cases as a right of a party. Other civil, criminal, and administrative cases can be heard by the court with their permission. The state's highest court usually has exclusive jurisdiction over death penalty cases and, in many states, has jurisdiction of cases involving the state bar involving attorney and judge disciplinary actions. Often the highest court will permit certified questions and provide advisory opinions.

What Court Do I Go To?

Federal OSHA = Federal Judiciary Court System
State Plan States = State Judiciary Court Systems

Where the specific powers of the federal judiciary are proscribed in the U.S. Constitution, the text of the U.S. Constitution provides little guidance as to state authority and explicitly grants few powers to the states. However, in the early years under the concept of *federalism*, governmental power is shared by the state and federal governments within our constitutional system. The federal government can only exercise the powers specifically granted to them under the U.S. Constitution. Each state possesses general police power and the power to do other governmental work. In concept, the states possess general authority, while the federal government possesses authority over those areas identified in the U.S. Constitution. After the civil war, the federalism concept was replaced with the concept of *dual authority or sovereignty,* where the federal and state each possesses their own sphere of authority and the state could not enter the federal sphere and vice versa. Today, the distinction of the authority of the state and federal governments is controlled by the doctrine of *preemption*. In general, under this doctrine, where the federal government acts, state law or state actions are preempted. If the federal government does not act, state law can be utilized. This is an important concept for safety professionals given the fact that the preemption doctrine has been used in cases challenging a state's right to bring criminal charges when Occupational Safety and Health Administration (OSHA) assumed jurisdiction over a case.

For safety professionals in a "state plan" state, any appeal outside of the individual state's administrative appeals procedures would be to a court within the state judiciary system. Some states have developed an appeal process that incorporates an administrative level paralleling the OSHRC on the federal level. Other states possess an appeal process to other levels within the state plan program system with an appeal to a specific court within the state's circuit court system. It is imperative that safety professionals possess a firm grasp of the state plan's appeal process as well as state court system.

State Plan States

OSHA Coverage

The Occupational Safety and Health (OSH) Act covers most private sector employers and their workers, in addition to some state and local government employers and their workers in the 50 states and certain territories and jurisdictions under federal authority. Those jurisdictions include the District of Columbia, Puerto Rico, the Virgin Islands, American Samoa, Guam, Northern Mariana Islands, Wake Island, Johnston Island, and the Outer Continental Shelf Lands as defined in the *Outer Continental Shelf Lands Act*.

Private Sector Workers

OSHA covers most private sector employers and workers in all 50 states, the District of Columbia, and the other U.S. jurisdictions—either directly through OSHA or through an OSHA-approved state plan. State plans are OSHA-approved job safety and health programs operated by individual states rather than federal OSHA. Section 18 of the OSH Act encourages states to develop and operate their own job safety and health programs and precludes state enforcement of OSHA standards unless the state has an OSHA-approved state plan.

OSHA approves and monitors all state plans and provides as much as 50 percent of the funding for each program. State-run safety and health programs must be at least as effective (ALAE) as the federal OSHA program. OSHA provides coverage to certain workers specifically excluded from a state plan (for example, those in some states who work in maritime industries or on military bases). To find the contact information of the OSHA or state plan office nearest to you, call 1-800-321-OSHA or go to www.osha.gov.

The following 22 states or territories have OSHA-approved state plans that cover both private and state and local government workers:

- Alaska
- Arizona
- California
- Hawaii
- Indiana
- Iowa
- Kentucky
- Maryland
- Michigan

- Minnesota
- Nevada
- New Mexico
- North Carolina
- Oregon
- Puerto Rico
- South Carolina
- Tennessee
- Utah
- Vermont
- Virginia
- Washington
- Wyoming

State and Local Government Workers

Workers at state and local government agencies are not covered by OSHA but have OSH Act protections if they work in states that have an OSHA-approved state plan. OSHA rules also permit states and territories to develop plans that cover state and local government workers only. In these cases, private sector workers and employers remain under federal OSHA jurisdiction.

Five additional states and one U.S. territory (Virgin Islands) have OSHA-approved state plans that cover state and local government workers only:

- Connecticut
- Illinois
- Maine
- New Jersey
- New York
- Virgin Islands

Safety professionals with multiple operations must acquire a clear understanding of the federal OSHA appeal process as well as the individual state's "state plan" appeal process. Given the fact that many state appeal process incorporate the state judiciary system within the process, knowledge of the appropriate court is also imperative. Multiple operations in different states may require the safety professional to acquire a thorough knowledge of several appeal processes as well as judiciary systems. Additionally, it is important that safety professionals acquire a grasp of the individual state's system in order to be able to prepare and present other issues, such as a workers' compensation appeal, within their scope of duty.

Questions

1. Identify at least two differences between federal and state courts.
2. What is the jurisdiction of a state district court?

3. What is the difference between OSHA and state plan states?
4. What is the state court system where your operations are located?
5. Can a citation issued in a state plan state be appealed to a federal court? Why or why not?

COMPARING FEDERAL & STATE COURTS

The U.S. Constitution is the supreme law of the land in the United States. It creates a federal system of government in which power is shared between the federal government and the state governments. Due to federalism, both the federal government and each of the state governments have their own court systems. Discover the differences in structure, judicial selection, and cases heard in both systems (Tables 4.1–4.3).

TABLE 4.1
Court Structure

The Federal Court System	The State Court System
Article III of the Constitution invests the judicial power of the United States in the federal court system. Article III, Section 1 specifically creates the U.S. Supreme Court and gives Congress the authority to create the lower federal courts.	The Constitution and laws of each state establish the state courts. A court of last resort, often known as a Supreme Court, is usually the highest court. Some states also have an intermediate Court of Appeals. Below these appeals courts are the state trial courts. Some are referred to as Circuit or District Courts.
Congress has used this power to establish the 13 U.S. Courts of Appeals, the 94 U.S. District Courts, the U.S. Court of Claims, and the U.S. Court of International Trade. U.S. Bankruptcy Courts handle bankruptcy cases. Magistrate Judges handle some District Court matters.	States also usually have courts that handle specific legal matters, e.g. probate court (wills and estates); juvenile court; family court; etc.
Parties dissatisfied with a decision of a U.S. District Court, the U.S. Court of Claims, and/or the U.S. Court of International Trade may appeal to a U.S. Court of Appeals.	Parties dissatisfied with the decision of the trial court may take their case to the intermediate Court of Appeals.
A party may ask the U.S. Supreme Court to review a decision of the U.S. Court of Appeals, but the Supreme Court usually is under no obligation to do so. The U.S. Supreme Court is the final arbiter of federal constitutional questions.	Parties have the option to ask the highest state court to hear the case.
	Only certain cases are eligible for review by the U.S. Supreme Court.

TABLE 4.2
Selection of Judges

The Federal Court System	The State Court System
The Constitution states that federal judges are to be nominated by the President and confirmed by the Senate. They hold office during good behavior, typically, for life. Through Congressional impeachment proceedings, federal judges may be removed from office for misbehavior.	State court judges are selected in a variety of ways, including • Election, • Appointment for a given number of years, • Appointment for life, and • Combinations of these methods, e.g. appointment followed by election.

TABLE 4.3
Types of Cases Heard

The Federal Court System	The State Court System
Cases that deal with the constitutionality of a law; Cases involving the laws and treaties of the U.S.; Cases involving ambassadors and public ministers; Disputes between two or more states; Admiralty law; Bankruptcy; and Habeas corpus issues.	Most criminal cases, probate (involving wills and estates) Most contract cases, tort cases (personal injuries), family law (marriages, divorces, adoptions), etc. State courts are the final arbiters of state laws and constitutions. Their interpretation of federal law or the U.S. Constitution may be appealed to the U.S. Supreme Court. The Supreme Court may choose to hear or not to hear such cases.

UNITED STATES DISTRICT COURT

WESTERN DISTRICT OF KENTUCKY AT LOUISVILLE
CIVIL ACTION NO. 3:01CV-171-H

HOSSAIN SANEII, et al.	PLAINTIFFS
V.	
WILLIAM T. ROBARDS, et al.	DEFENDANTS

MEMORANDUM OPINION

This Court now considers a number of motions, all of which address whether the Arbitration Award dated December 26, 2002, and the Supplement to the Arbitration Award (collectively the "Award") dated February 19, 2003, should be confirmed, vacated, or modified. On May 24, 2001, this Court compelled arbitration of all issues in this case, including fraudulent inducement of the contract. *See Saneii v. Robards*, 187 F.Supp.2d 710 (W.D. Ky. 2001). The Court also entered an Amended Order holding the case in abeyance until the arbitrator had reached a decision on all issues. After the arbitrator decided all issues against Plaintiffs, these motions followed.

Citing a Kentucky Court of Appeals decision, *Marks v. Bean,* 57 S.W.3d 303 (Ky. App. 2001), Plaintiffs ask the Court to vacate the arbitration award because the arbitrator was without jurisdiction to hear the claim of fraudulent inducement. The *Marks* court held that claims of fraudulent inducement were for the court, not an arbitrator, to decide. The Court of Appeals decided *Marks after* this Court had compelled arbitration but before the arbitrator began his proceedings. Naturally, Defendants' primary objective is that the Court confirm the arbitration award in their favor and dismiss all Plaintiffs' claims.

For the reasons explained below, the Court concludes that the Award must be vacated because, under Kentucky law, the arbitrator indeed exceeded his authority by deciding the fraudulent inducement issue.

I

At the heart of the current dispute is Plaintiffs' assertion that this Court was wrong to send this entire case to arbitration. This is beyond further argument, Plaintiffs say, in the light of *Marks v. Bean.* As an initial matter, therefore, the Court should probably determine whether the new Kentucky law and policy enunciated in *Marks* could decide the outcome of this case.

In *Marks,* the Kentucky Court of Appeals held that under Kentucky law an arbitration agreement does not bind a party to arbitrate a claim of fraudulent inducement to contract. A party to the contract is entitled to have a court hear such a claim. In reaching this conclusion and rejecting the majority of other state and federal courts' views, the Court of Appeals concluded that the state's strong policy against fraud supported and, indeed, required such a result.*

The facts of the *Marks* case are very similar to ours. The plaintiffs purchased a home from the defendants and alleged that the defendants fraudulently induced them into the contract to purchase the home by misrepresenting and concealing defects in the brick veneer. *Marks,* 57 S.W.3d at 304. The complaint alleged that the representations on the disclosure form were false and fraudulent and that the defendants were aware of the condition of the brick and consciously sought to conceal it from the plaintiffs. *Id.* The Sales and Purchasing Contract in *Marks* contained a binding arbitration clause very similar to the one here. It is the same as that used generally by the Kentucky Real Estate Commission. *Id.* at 305. The plaintiffs argued that the arbitration clause was not enforceable pursuant to the savings clause in K.R.S. 417.050, which excludes from arbitration "such grounds as exist as law for the revocation of any contract." *Id.* The trial court agreed and held that "[t]he existence of fraud is a factual question to be determined by the trier of fact ... the Court finds that the arbitration clause in the parties' sale contract is not enforceable." *Id.* The Kentucky Court of Appeals agreed.

---

* The majority view is represented most prominently by *Prima Paint Corp. v. Flood & Conklin Mfg. Co.,* 388 U.S. 395 (1967). It is worth noting, however, that the three-justice dissent written by Justice Black strongly supports the Court of Appeals' policy. *Id.* at 407–25.

The appellate court recognized that, despite the analogous language in the FAA and the KUAA, Kentucky courts would not adopt the majority view. The court instead determined that because the FAA interpretation "disproportionately elevates the policy favoring arbitration over the strong public policy against fraud.... When the making of the agreement itself is put in issue, as is the result of a claim of fraud in the inducement, that issue is more properly determined by those trained in the law." *Id.* at 307.* The court held that despite the arbitration agreement, the fraud in the inducement issue would go to the court and not the arbitrator.

The Court's reading of *Marks* leaves no doubt that current Kentucky law requires vacating the prior arbitration decision as to the issue of fraudulent inducement. However, serious questions remain as to whether this Court should apply Kentucky law and, if so, whether this Court can consider *Marks* in the current procedural context.

II

The FAA, where applicable, preempts all state law. The Court can apply *Marks* only if the FAA does not govern these circumstances. Therefore, the Court must consider whether this contract for the sale of residential real estate is "a transaction involving interstate commerce" within the meaning of § 2 of the FAA. 9 U.S.C.A. § 2. The reach of "involving commerce" in § 2, is as broad as Congress' exercise of its full commerce power. *See Allied-Bruce Terminix Co., Inc. v. Dobson,* 513 U.S. 265, 273–74 (1995).

The primary purpose of the FAA is to ensure the uniform enforcement of arbitration agreements. *Id.* at 270; *see also Volt Information Sciences, Inc. v. Bd. of Trustees of Leland Stanford Junior Univ.,* 489 U.S. 468 (1989). "The effect of the Arbitration Act is thus to create a body of substantive federal law on arbitration governing any agreement that is within the Act's coverage." *Foster v. Turley,* 808 F.2d 38 (10th Cir. 1986). Thus, the FAA creates uniformity by applying to all cases involving interstate commerce.

Notwithstanding its congenial effects on interstate commerce, the sale of residential real estate is inherently intrastate. Contracts strictly for the sale of residential real estate focus entirely on a commodity – the land – which is firmly planted in one particular state. The citizenship of immediate parties (the buyer and the seller) or their movements to or from that state are incidental to the real estate transaction. Those movements are not part of the transaction itself. All of the legal relationships concerning the land are bound by state law principles. Single residential real estate transactions of this type have no substantial or direct connection to interstate commerce.† For all these reasons, logic suggests that such transactions are not among those considered as involving interstate commerce.

---

* The court also noted that issues involving breach or violation of the agreement, which are primarily issues of fact, can be left to the expertise of those trained in the respective fields of arbitration.
† This is seemingly the case even if the buyer obtained financing from a bank, which happened to participate in interstate commerce. This tangential effect is not enough to bring a sale of a home within interstate commerce and the FAA.

> To characterize a residential real estate as involving interstate commerce under
> these circumstances would actually promote a lack of uniformity in the law,
> which is exactly contrary to one of the FAA's stated purpose. If the FAA applied
> to out-of-state purchasers of Kentucky real estate, different rules would apply
> in that considerable volume of transactions concerning property here. Applying
> Kentucky law to all Kentucky real estate transactions creates a more uniform
> and, therefore, a more equitable body of law.

Two district courts in the Sixth Circuit have reached the same conclusion that a real
estate contract does not involve interstate commerce for purposes of the FAA. *See
Cecala v. Moore*, 982 F.Supp. 609 (N.D.Ill.1997); *see also SI V, LLC v. FMC Corp.*,
223 F.Supp.2d 1059 (N.D.Ca. 2002). While these cases are of limited analytic value,[§]
they reinforce a common understanding that a residential real estate contract, even
one involving parties of different states, does not involve interstate commerce.

On the other hand, more complex transactions related to land may involve interstate commerce. For instance, in *Allied*-Bruce, the United States Supreme Court
found that a termite extermination contract between an Alabama homeowner and a
local Terminix franchise did involve interstate commerce. 513 U.S. at 269. The Court
came to this conclusion by applying the broad interpretation of § 2 of the FAA. *Id.*
The Court's analysis was that Terminix was a commercial entity, the parties were
from multi-states, and the termite-treating and house repairing materials used by
the defendants came from outside Alabama. *Id.* at 281. More importantly, the Court
articulated and emphasized the purposes behind the FAA and why a broad interpretation of "a contract evidencing a transaction involving commerce" was necessary
in order to be consistent with those purposes. *Id.* These circumstances are entirely
different than those here.

Other courts have also held that contracts for the construction of various commercial buildings, and even the construction of sewers, involved interstate commerce for
purposes of the FAA. *See Monte v. Southern Delaware County Authority*, 321 F.2d
870 (3rd Cir.1963); *Sears Roebuck and Co. v. Glenwal Co.*, 325 F.Supp. 86 (S.D.N.Y.
1970); *Fite and Warmath Construction Co., Inc. v. MYS Corp.*, 559 S.W.2d 729 (Ky.
1977). Although these cases concerned facilities which are located in one state and
remained in one state, like the house in the current case, the scope of these contracts
was much broader because of the interstate, commercial aspect of the transactions.
None of these cases involves a straightforward residential real estate transaction.

Bearing in mind the historical intrastate nature of residential property transactions, as well as the Supreme Court's analysis of purposes of the FAA, the Court
concludes that a residential real estate sales contract does not evidence or involve
interstate commerce. This is true despite the broad reach of "interstate commerce,"
as articulated by the United States Supreme Court in *Allied-Bruce*. 513 U.S. at 265.
The Court will apply Kentucky law, or *Marks*, to the fraudulent inducement claim.

III

Irrespective of the application of *Marks v. Bean* to our general circumstances,
Defendant raises a number of arguments why this Court should not consider the
issue. They argue (1) that Plaintiff has filed an improper motion; (2) that, in any

event, Plaintiff should have appealed to the Sixth Circuit or moved for a stay of the arbitration; and (3) that Plaintiff has waived its right to challenge the arbitration. All of these arguments contain the common theme that Plaintiffs should have raised *Marks v. Brown* prior to proceeding with arbitration. While this argument has a certain appeal, the Court cannot find any reason for not now deciding these issues correctly under Kentucky law. The Court will consider each argument in turn.

A

First, Defendants assert that because Plaintiffs did not move either to vacate the arbitration award under K.R.S. 417.160, or to modify the award under K.R.S. 417.170, the Court must now confirm the award under K.R.S. 417.150.[*] Plaintiffs' subsequent responses, [†] however, have clarified their request that the Court vacate the arbitration award because the arbitrator exceeded his authority and jurisdiction.[‡] Regardless, a pleading error of this type would not bar this Court's exercise of subject matter jurisdiction. In *Green v. Ameritech Corp.*, 200 F.3d 967, 973–74 (6th Cir. 2000), the Sixth Circuit held that a similar "pleading error did not bar the district court's exercise of subject matter jurisdiction." *Id.* The Court concludes that the form of pleading does not invalidate Plaintiffs' request to vacate.

B

Defendants next argue that, regardless of the foregoing analysis, Plaintiffs cannot raise the issue of arbitrator jurisdiction at this late date. They assert that Plaintiffs should have appealed directly to the Sixth Circuit from this Court's order compelling arbitration. The Court disagrees.

The Kentucky statute covering arbitration appeals, K.R.S. 417.220, specifically does not include court orders compelling arbitration. *See Fayette County Farm Bureau Federation v. Martin*, 758 S.W.2d 713 (Ky.App. 1988). "We must presume that they meant to exclude anything not listed and we cannot, by interpretation, 'legislate' in what they purposefully left out." *Id.* Therefore, under Kentucky law, Plaintiffs could not appeal the Order compelling arbitration until this Court entered some final judgment resulting from the arbitration, i.e. confirming or vacating this award. *Id.* at 714. This Court merely held the federal case in abeyance, so that the order compelling arbitration was not final on its own terms.

---

[*] K.R.S. 417.150 states that "[u]pon application of a party, the court *shall* confirm an award unless, within the time limits hereinafter imposed, grounds are urged for vacating or modifying or correcting the award, in which case the court shall proceed as provided in K.R.S. 417.160 and 417.170." (emphasis added)

[†] In both Plaintiffs' "Reply Memorandum in Further Support of Motion to Void Arbitration Award," on June 17, 2003, and the "Response in Opposition to Defendants' Renewed Motion for Confirmation of the Arbitration Award and to Dismiss Complaint," on June 23, 2003, the Plaintiffs clarified under what statutory provision they were asking the Court to vacate or void the arbitrator's award.

[‡] K.R.S. 417.160(c) states that one ground for the Court to vacate an arbitration award is if the arbitrators exceed their powers.

The fact that Plaintiffs could not directly appeal this order obviates Defendants' argument that by not bringing up the *Marks* case earlier, Plaintiffs wasted Defendants' time and money in the arbitration. "That a party will be exposed to the inconvenience and cost of litigation does not alone justify immediate review of an otherwise nonfinal order." *See National Gypsum Co. v. Corns,* Ky., 736 S.W.2d 325 (1987). Defendants' argument that either Plaintiffs should have appealed the arbitration compulsion sooner, or that appeal was the proper procedural mechanism, are both wrong.

Defendants also assert that Plaintiffs should have used other mechanisms, such as a motion to stay arbitration or motion to reconsider, to raise the *Marks* case sooner. Plaintiffs did not do so, Defendants argue, because they wanted first to see the result, in case favorable, before asserting the arbitrator's lack of authority. Perhaps this is true. However, one need not seek a stay of arbitration in order to preserve its objection to jurisdiction. *See Kaplan v. First Options of Chicago, Inc.,* 19 F.3d 1503, 1510 (3rd Cir.1994).

The *Kaplan* case is similar to ours in that one party argued that the other could not challenge the arbitrator's lack of jurisdiction because that party did not raise the issue earlier. It is different because it did not begin in a civil court. Instead, the parties went directly into arbitration and appellants contested jurisdiction within the arbitration, over a period of many years and including a motion to dismiss to the arbitrators. *Id.* at 1508. The court said that the fact that the appellants disputed the arbitrator's jurisdiction, while still arguing the merits before the arbitrators, was not a waiver of its subsequent jurisdictional objections. *Id.*

Kaplan stands for the proposition that it is not necessary to ask for a stay of arbitration in order to later object to the arbitrator's jurisdiction. Its logic is even more applicable here because Plaintiffs *formally* objected to the jurisdiction of the arbitrator on the issue of fraudulent inducement. Plaintiffs brought this civil action and then proceeded to unsuccessfully argue that fraudulent inducement belonged in court, not in arbitration. To now say that Plaintiffs needed to argue again, once they were ordered to arbitration and it had begun, that the arbitration should be stayed because of this *very same issue of fraudulent inducement*, places an unfair burden on Plaintiffs.

C

Finally, Defendants say that Plaintiffs waived their objection that the arbitrator exceeded his authority by not raising this argument to the arbitrator himself. Defendants assert that, instead of pointing out *Marks* to this Court or to the arbitrator, Plaintiffs waited until the end of the arbitration in order to see if the outcome was favorable. This argument is founded on a theory similar to that which the Court has just rejected.

To be sure, lawyers who practice in federal court have an obligation to assist the judges to keep within the boundaries fixed by the laws. *See BEM I, L.L.C. v. Anthropologie, Inc.,* 301 F.3d 548 (7th Cir. 2002). They also have a duty to raise jurisdictional issues. *Id.* at 551–52. However, in this case, Plaintiffs did argue that the arbitrator lacked jurisdiction to decide issues of fraudulent inducement. The Court cannot now say Plaintiffs are at fault for not reasserting the issue after the Court decided it.

True, one can find numerous cases in which a party is deemed to have waived its right to object to the arbitrator's jurisdiction or authority. However, each of those cases is distinguishable in a fundamental way from the current case. In *Mays v. Lanier Worldwide Inc.*, 115 F.Supp.2d 1330 (M.D.Ala. 2000), for instance, the district court found that plaintiff's failure to challenge arbitrability in a timely fashion, and subsequent participation in the arbitration proceedings, resulted in a waiver of the right to object. *Id.* at 1340. However, there are significant differences between *Mays* and the instant case. In *Mays*, the plaintiff actually brought the arbitration, actively participated in every phase and only after losing objected to the arbitrator's jurisdiction. *Id.* The district court found that because the plaintiff did not seek a stay in federal court, but rather vigorously prosecuted his claims in the arbitration proceedings, he could not seek a second chance in court. *Id.* at 1343.

In *Bender v. Smith Barney, Harris Upham & Co., Inc.*, 901 F.Supp.863, 869–70 (D.N.J. 1994), the court held that the plaintiff waived her right to object to the panel's jurisdiction over her claim because she failed to address the objection to the arbitrators in the first instance. The plaintiff initially brought the case to federal court but was ordered to arbitration. *Bender*, 901 F.Supp. at 869–70. The plaintiff never contested arbitration and never argued that the arbitrator was without jurisdiction. *Id.* The plaintiff only asserted lack of jurisdiction when the defendant moved to confirm the award. *Id.* In this respect *Bender* differs significantly from our case.

At all points of the litigation prior to this Court ordering arbitration, Plaintiffs have given all the necessary indications that they were against arbitrating the issue of fraudulent inducement. Failing to raise *Marks* prior to arbitration or failing to raise jurisdictional issues with the arbitrator, after a federal court had rejected those arguments, is not cause for waiver. Plaintiffs contested the arbitrator's jurisdiction over fraudulent inducement. By doing so, they have preserved their right to contest confirmation of the award.

IV

Whether an arbitrator has exceeded his authority is a question of law reviewed de novo. See MidMichigan Reg'l Med. Ctr.-Clare v. Professional Employees Div. of Local 79, Serv. Employee Int'l Union, 183 F.3d 497, 501 (6th Cir.1999); see also Green v. Ameritech Corp., 200 F.3d 967, 974 (6th Cir. 2000). Defendants argue that Plaintiffs are asking the Court to reconsider its own decision, rather than actually challenging the arbitration award. They say that the Court should confirm the arbitration award and require Plaintiffs to challenge, on appeal to the Sixth Circuit, the appropriateness of this Court referring all issues to arbitration.

Were this Court to do so, the Sixth Circuit would then look at this issue of whether the award should have been confirmed *de novo* and whether the arbitrator exceeded his power *de novo. Id.; See also Glennon v. Dean Witter Reynolds, Inc.*, 83 F.3d 132, 135 (6th Cir. 1996). The Sixth Circuit would look at *all* of Kentucky's current law, including *Marks*, in its *de novo* review. It would necessarily conclude that this Court incorrectly anticipated Kentucky law. The Sixth Circuit would likely then remand the issue of fraudulent inducement to this Court. This Court would follow *Marks*.

Such a lengthy process is unnecessary. The arbitration did not actually begin until September 24, 2002 – well after *Marks* became Kentucky law on July 20, 2001.[*] Although *Marks* was not the law when the arbitration was compelled, it was the law when the arbitration actually began. This Court can and should evaluate the arbitrator's jurisdiction according to *Marks*.

The Court will enter an order consistent with this Memorandum Opinion.

JOHN G. HEYBURN II
CHIEF JUDGE, U.S. DISTRICT COURT

cc: Counsel of Record

UNITED STATES DISTRICT COURT

WESTERN DISTRICT OF KENTUCKY AT LOUISVILLE

CIVIL ACTION NO. 3:01CV-171-H

HOSSAIN SANEII, et al.	PLAINTIFFS
V.	
WILLIAM T. ROBARDS, et al.	DEFENDANTS

ORDER

Various motions are pending which question whether the arbitration award should be affirmed or vacated. Being otherwise sufficiently advised,

IT IS HEREBY ORDERED that the arbitration order is SUSTAINED as to its finding that it did not breach the contract and is VACATED as to its finding that Defendants did not fraudulently induce Plaintiffs to enter the contract.

IT IS FURTHER ORDERED that the Court shall decide the issue of whether Plaintiffs were fraudulently induced to enter the contract.

The Court will set a pretrial conference in the near future.

This _____ day of October, 2003.

JOHN G. HEYBURN II
CHIEF JUDGE, U.S. DISTRICT COURT

cc: Counsel of Record

----

[*] The Court is not deciding whether *Marks* applies retroactively to cases decided before its issuance. The Court does not have to reach this because the actual arbitration did not begin to after the *Marks* holding.

5 Criminal Law

Dishonesty is a forsaking of permanent for temporary advantage.

Christian Bovee

Money dishonestly acquired is never worth its cost, while a good conscience never costs as much as it is worth.

J.P. Senn

STUDENT LEARNING OBJECTIVES

1. Acquire an understanding of criminal law.
2. Analyze and identify the elements of specific crimes.
3. Acquire an understanding of the burden of proof in criminal cases.
4. Acquire an understanding of potential criminal liability under the Occupational Safety and Health (OSH) Act.

Crimes and punishment – Removing an individual's freedom due to a crime against society. Criminal law is the broad body of laws, at both the federal and state levels, which address conduct and crimes prohibited by society and are generally designed to protect society. Blackstone defines "crime" as "an act committed or omitted in violation of public law, either forbidding or commanding it."[*] In essence, criminal law addresses certain prohibited acts, behaviors, and/or omissions; the violation of specific laws designed to protect society; and the punishment for the offender for violation of the law. In the United States, there are a variety of sources within the complex matrix of laws and statutes at the federal and state levels, which have their beginnings in the laws of England and have evolved over the decades with changes in our society, technology, and events.

In every society, people developed systems and laws through which to protect lives and property. Criminal laws were developed based upon the rules established by the king or by religious organizations. Criminal law in the United States was primarily based upon the laws previously developed in England. Many of the criminal laws we have today have their origins with the "common law" of early England and have been adapted into statutory laws by state legislatures over the years.

Today, when a legislative body determines specific conduct within our society should be forbidden, members of the legislative body draft a bill describing in specific detail the prohibited conduct. Both at the federal and state levels, if the bill is introduced, voted on, and passed by the House of Representatives, the Senate would then vote on the bill. If the bill is passed by vote in the Senate, the bill would move

---

[*] 4 Blackstone, Commentaries 15.

to the President at the federal level or governor at the state level. If the President or governor signs the bill, the bill become law on a specified date. If the President or governor does not sign or vetoes the bill, the legislative branch has an opportunity to override the veto with a sufficient number of votes.

The primary police power lies with the states. This means that the individual states have the power to enact and enforce laws to protect the safety and welfare of the individuals within the state boundaries. The federal government, in essence, possesses no police powers. However, under the U.S. Constitution, the federal government can exercise similar broadly interpreted powers to the states as specified in Article I, Section 8. Political subdivisions, such as cities and counties, also have limited authority to make and enforce rules and regulations.

Federal, state, and local governments are prohibited by the U.S. Constitution from enforcing "ex post facto" laws or enforcement of a crime prior to the enactment of the specific law. In essence, an individual cannot be charged with a crime retrospectively after a law has been enacted. Laws can only be enforced after then have been fully enacted.

Criminal laws are usually classified as either felonies, misdemeanors, or treason. In general, states usually distinguish the classifications based upon possible punishment or length of the sentence or jail time. Felonies are crimes punishable by death or substantial imprisonment. Misdemeanors are lessor crimes with punishment other than death or imprisonment or not designated as a felony by statute. Treason is the only crime specifically addressed in the U.S. Constitution and is provided a higher designation than a felony. According to the U.S. Constitution, "Treason against the United States shall consist only in levying war against them, or in adhering to their enemies, giving them aid and comfort."[*] Treason is a crime against the United States itself and is seldom applicable.

Under criminal law, the burden of proof for each and every element of the crime is greater than a civil action. Criminal law requires the state to prove the guilt of the accused individual or entity "beyond a reasonable doubt." The state would have the burden of proving each and every element of the crime beyond a reasonable doubt. If the state cannot prove one or more elements beyond a reasonable doubt, the accused individual or entity cannot be convicted of the crime in which charged.[†]

Safety professionals should be aware of the distinction among criminal law, tort law (civil), and contract law (civil). An action or inaction may result in be both a civil action for damages as well as criminal action against society. For example, Person X is punched by Person Y causing substantial bodily harm. Person X can pursue a civil action for damages such as medical costs, while the state could pursue assault and battery and prosecute Person Y for the same action in criminal court. Contract actions can also be both civil and criminal actions. A contract action is often one party against another party for damages due to a breach of the agreement in civil court. However, if the contract itself or required action under the contract violate statutory or case law, criminal action can be brought by the state against the

---

[*] U.S. Constitution, Article III, Section 3.

[†] Note: There are exceptions where the defendant possesses the burden of proof – affirmative defenses and the insanity defense.

contracting party. Safety professionals should be aware that the Occupational Safety and Health Act does provide for not only monetary penalties but also criminal sanctions and careful review of other injury and contract situations should be carefully analyzed for potential criminal liability.

In most crimes, the prosecutor must prove that the accused person charged committed the prohibited act or failed to act when the accused possessed a duty to act. Commonly known as *actus reus*, this principle requires the actual or affirmative physical act or verbal act to be performed. A person cannot be convicted for possessing thoughts or even evil intent without the physical or verbal act or an affirmative duty to act. Additionally, the prosecutor must prove that the act must be accompanied by the criminal intent of the accused. This is often referred to as *means rea*. Negligence or/or reckless conduct is equivalent to criminal intent. Lastly, the prosecutor must prove that the unlawful act or omission must be integrated with or related to the crime that it is proximately caused or contributed to the crime. This is referred to as *causation*. Thus, the burden is placed upon the state to prove not only the elements of the specific crime but also that the accused acted or failed to act (with a duty), the individual possessed the criminal intent, and that the physical act and state of mind were present at the time of the crime.

Safety professionals should be aware that the criminal law is substantially different than civil law, and the requirements are substantially higher due to the potential of loss of freedom. Although there have been relatively few safety related cases referred to the U.S. Department of Justice for prosecution at the federal level and a few in state plan states, circumstances of potential criminal acts do exist in the safety world. Safety professionals should be aware of the areas of potential criminal liability (often involving fatality situations) and ensure that appropriate proactive and reactive measures are taken to avoid risks in this area.

Crimes tend to be categorized according to the offense. With many of these early laws from England, there are crimes against persons, sex related crimes, crimes against property, crimes involving theft, crimes involving forgery and fraud, and "white collar" and corporate crimes. Additionally, statutory law has created laws including crimes involving morality and decency, crimes against public peace, crimes against public justice, crimes involving juveniles, and crimes involving drugs. Safety professionals should acquire a general knowledge of these laws in order to be able to identify and take appropriate action where applicable.

Crimes against persons include homicide (murder and manslaughter), aiding or soliciting suicide, assault, battery, extortion, wanton endangerment, false imprisonment, and kidnapping. In general, homicide is defined as the killing of a human being by another human being. Within the category of homicide are the crimes of murder and manslaughter. In common law, murder is defined as the "unlawful killing of a human being by another human being with malice aforethought."* Most states have incorporated a number of degrees within the crime of murder, namely first degree and second degree murder. In most states, the distinguishing factor between first and second degree murder is premeditation and/or deliberation. In some states, a homicide in the commission of a felony constitutes murder under felony-murder statutes.

---

* Black's Law Dictionary.

Manslaughter is defined as the "unlawful killing of a human being, without malice, expressed or implied. Such may be either voluntarily, upon a sudden heat, or involuntarily, but in the commission of some unlawful act."* In most states, manslaughter includes the following: "(a) it is committed recklessly; (b) a homicide which would otherwise be murder committed under the influence of extreme mental or emotional disturbance for which there is a reasonable explanation or excuse."† Extreme mental or emotional disturbance would include "heat of passion," negligent manslaughter and related defenses.

Manslaughter is often delineated by states into the crimes of involuntary manslaughter and voluntary manslaughter. Safety professionals should be aware that the few criminal cases that have been brought for workplace fatalities often fall within these category of crimes. The distinction between involuntary and voluntary manslaughter is often the "absence of intention to kill or to commit any unlawful act which might reasonably produce death or great bodily harm...."‡ Involuntary manslaughter involves a person committing an unlawful act (not a felony) involving great bodily harm or "committing a lawful act without proper precaution or requisite skill, unguardedly or undesignedly kills another." Voluntary manslaughter involves "manslaughter committed voluntarily upon a sudden heat of passion."§ In essence, voluntary manslaughter involves circumstances where a person was killed; however, the circumstances fall short of willful or deliberate intent to kill or the circumstances involve facts which are close justifiable homicide.

Miranda Rights – "You have the right to remain silent. If you do **say** anything, what you **say** can be used against you in a court of law. You have the right to consult with a lawyer and have that lawyer present during any questioning. If you cannot afford a lawyer, one will be appointed for you if you so desire."

Heat of passion defense is defined as "a state of violent and uncontrollable rage engendered by a blow or certain other provocation given.... Passion or anger suddenly aroused at the time by some immediate and reasonable provocation."¶ In most states, the heat of passion defense, if successful, can reduce a homicide from the level of murder to the level of manslaughter.

Although suicide is not considered a homicide because there is no killing by another, an individual may be prosecuted for criminal homicide if the individual causes that person to commit suicide. Additionally, in some states, an individual may be charged with the offense of aiding or soliciting suicide even if the suicide is not considered a crime. For safety professionals, suicides do happen on the job. Appropriate investigation by governmental authorities can determine if others are involved and if a crime has been committed.

For safety professionals, the crime of assault and battery is often common within the workforce primarily through their outside activities. Under common law, assault and battery are separate crimes; however, many states have combined and added degrees of assault and battery. Assault is defined as "an unlawful offer or attempt

---

* Id.
† Model Penal Code, Section 210.3.
‡ Black's Law Dictionary.
§ Model Penal Code, Section 3(1)(b).
¶ Black's Law Dictionary.

to injure another, with apparent present ability to effectuate the attempt under circumstances creating a fear of imminent peril."* In essence, one employee threatens
another employee with bodily harm. Battery is defined as "the unlawful touching of
the person of another by the aggressor, or by some substance put in motion by him."
Battery is the actual touching of the individual. Thus, together assault is the fear of
harm without touching and battery is the actual touching.

Kidnapping is defined at common law as "the forcible abduction or stealing or
carrying away of a person from own country to another."† Under most state laws, the
intent to send the victim out of the country does not constitute a necessary element
of the offense. Under the Model Penal Code, "a person is guilty of kidnapping if he
unlawfully removes another from his place of residence or business, or a substantial
distance from the vicinity where he is found, or he unlawfully confines another for
a substantial period in a place of isolation."‡ Kidnapping on a federal level addresses
child-stealing, kidnapping for ransom, and simple kidnapping.§ Kidnapping is designated as a felony of the first degree.¶

Other common crimes under state laws include mayhem (usually under state
assault statutes), extortion (obtaining property of another through threat of violence),
and wanton endangerment (reckless or malicious behavior).

Although safety professionals are seldom directly involved within the criminal
justice system, safety professionals should be aware of the laws as well as the protections if circumstances should arise. Workplace fatalities can often be investigated
for possible referral for criminal prosecution and prudent safety professionals should
ensure legal counsel is actively involved to protect individuals as well as the corporation. As it will be noted later in this text, the Occupational Safety and Health
Act does provide for criminal referrals to the U.S. Department of Justice for crimes
within the scope of their jurisdiction.

Although safety professionals seldom are directly impacted by nonconsensual
crimes involving sex, it is important to have general knowledge. The most serious
crime in this category is rape. Rape is defined as "the act of unlawful carnal knowledge by a man of a woman, forcibly and against her will."** Under most state statutes,
there are categories of forcible rape (by force or threat) and statutory rape (age or
mental incapacity). Other crimes in this category include sodomy (carnal copulation
by human beings with each other or animals), sexual assault, sexual abuse, lewdness
(open and public indecency) and corruption of a minor, solicitation, and voyeurism.

Crimes against property is the top category of crimes in the United States that
usually involve theft. Under common law, the categories included the crimes of larceny, embezzlement, extortion, and robbery. Under most state statutes today, the
common law categories have been combined and modified to include such categories
as "receiving stolen goods," "unauthorized use of an automobile," "theft of services,"

---

* Id
† Id.
‡ Model Penal Code Section 212.1.
§ Also referred to as the Lindbergh Act.
¶ Note: If the kidnapper releases the person unharmed and in a safe place, the crime can be reduced to
  kidnapping in the second degree.
** Black's Law Dictionary

and "obtaining property by false pretenses." Under common law, robbery is defined as "the felonious taking of money or goods of value from the person of another or in his presence against his will, by force or putting him in fear."* Larceny is defined as "the felonious taking of the property of another without his or her consent and against his or her will with the intent to convert it to the use of the taker or another."† Embezzlement, although not recognized under common law, was developed and implemented into law to broaden to elements of larceny. Embezzlement is defined as "willfully to take, or convert to one's own use, another's money or property, of which the wrongdoer acquired possession lawfully, by reason of some office or employment or position of trust."‡ Another crime created by statute is the obtaining of property by false pretenses. The difference between embezzlement and false pretenses is that the wrongdoer obtains title and possession of the property by means of deception.

In the category of forgery and fraud, safety professionals should take special note. Forgery, under common law, is defined as "the false making or materially altering, with the intent to defraud, of any writing, which, if genuine, more apparently be a legal efficacy or the foundation of legal liability."§ Given the significant enhancements in technology and documents, many states have broadened their statutes and use different terminology to specifically address what documents are subject to forgery and what conduct is prohibited. Many states have developed specific statutes to include credit card forgery, possession of forged documents, fraudulent destruction of documents, removal or concealment of certain documents, and tampering with records. Additionally, many states have enacted statutes addressing false advertisement or false statements in advertising. Bribery, at common law, involves only the bribing of public officials. Today, many states have broaden this crime to include agents and employees of commercial enterprises as well as public officials. Safety professionals should be aware that fraud-related statutes are different and varied among states. Some states have specific laws regarding bribery of officials in sports events, defrauding creditors, and other statutes.

Although generically referred to as "white collar" crimes, these crimes usually involve illegal behavior within corporations or sophisticated enterprises. Safety professionals should be aware that although federal agencies usually investigate matters involving white collar crimes, individual states have enacted statutes which can be more stringent than federal statutes. Within this category is the Racketeering Influence and Corrupt Organizations Act (referred to as "RICO") which was designed to address organized crime. However, the broad language utilized in this statute has permitted prosecution far beyond the traditional organized crime or mafia cases. Money laundering is the illegal concealment of money from illegal sources which is disguised as income to make it appear legitimate. These statute was designed to address monies acquire through the sale of illegal controlled substances, weapons, and related illegal items and often require financial institutions to report certain

---

* Id.
† Id.
‡ Id.
§ Id.

transactions and prohibit individual involvement where the company or organization are aware that the monies are coming from illegal activities.

Of particular importance to safety professionals is the enforcement of environmental crime statutes by both federal and state agencies. Some of these statutes include the Occupational Safety and Health Act (and state plans), Fair Labor Standards Act (FLSA), Clean Air Act, Clean Water Act, Safe Drinking Water Act, Toxic Substance Control Act, and Resource Conservation and Recovery Act (RCRA). In general, these statutes impose two general standards for imposing criminal liability on corporations, namely the following: (1) *respondeat superior* ("The master is liable for the wrongful acts of his servant") liability; and (2) specific language in the statute imposing liability on the corporation.

In the category of protecting the public order, law addressing disorderly conduct, vagrancy public drunkenness, harassment, disrupting public meetings, and cruelty of animals are often included as crimes under state statutes. In the category of crimes against public justice, safety professionals should be aware of the crime of perjury (making false statements under oath), obstruction of justice, escape from legal custody, failure to aid law enforcement, making false reports to enforcement authorities, and tampering with witnesses and tampering with evidence.

With drugs being prevalent in our society, there is a substantial probability that safety professionals will encounter drugs in the workplace. In an effort to create uniformity in the enforcement of state laws addressing illicit drugs, most states have adopted the provisions of the Uniform Controlled Substance Act which prohibited activities in detail and provide authority in an agency established by the individual states. To ensure consistency with the federal laws, the Uniform Controlled Substance Act follows the federal Controlled Substance Act and includes a specific list of all controlled substances in five schedules and includes guidelines to determine the appropriate category. The Uniform Controlled Substance Act and state statutes require persons who engage in, or intend to engage in, the manufacture, distribution, or dispensing of controlled substances to be registered with the state. All states prohibit the trafficking, possession, dispensing, obtaining by fraud, manufacture, and advertising of controlled substances. Penalties generally correlate with the category, amount, and other factors.

Of particular importance to safety professions, the OSH Act has not only monetary penalties but also criminal sanctions. Although the Occupational Safety and Health Administration (OSHA) does not prosecute criminal violations themselves, OSHA can refer criminal cases to the U.S. Department of Justice for prosecution. State plan states also possess authority to enforce criminal sanctions. Safety professionals should be aware of the issue of preemption where federal OSHA would preempt the use of state criminal codes in state plan states.

In summation, safety professionals should have a general knowledge of various criminal laws which may be applicable to their workplace. Of particular importance are the criminal laws potentially applicable to circumstances and situations involving the safety, health, and environmental functions. Prudent safety professionals may wish to discuss potential liabilities with appropriate legal counsel and be prepared to invoke constitutional rights and protections as well as other protections and defenses if applicable under the circumstances. Safety professionals should be aware of the

significant differences between criminal and civil law as well as the investigative
methods utilized when the situation is being investigated as a criminal matter.

Questions

1. Who has the burden of proof in a criminal trial and why?
2. What is the difference between an assault and a battery?
3. What is forgery?
4. What is preemption?
5. What is the difference between murder and manslaughter?

SELECTED CASE STUDY

Case modified for the purpose of this text
PEOPLE v. O'NEIL
194 Ill. App.3d 79 (1990); 550 N.E.2d 1090
*THE PEOPLE OF THE STATE OF ILLINOIS, Plaintiff-Appellee, v. STEVEN
O'NEIL et al., Defendants-Appellants.*
Appellate Court of Illinois — First District (5th Division).
Opinion filed January 19, 1990.

Reversed and remanded.
JUSTICE LORENZ delivered the opinion of the court:
Following a joint bench trial, individual defendants Steven O'Neil, Charles
Kirschbaum, and Daniel Rodriguez, agents of Film Recovery Systems, Inc. (Film
Recovery), were convicted of murder (Ill. Rev. Stat. 1981, ch. 38, par. 9-1(a)(2)) in the
death of Stefan Golab, a Film Recovery employee, from cyanide poisoning stemming
from conditions in Film Recovery's plant in Elk Grove Village, Illinois. Corporate
defendants Film Recovery and its sister corporation Metallic Marketing Systems,
Inc. (Metallic Marketing), were convicted of involuntary manslaughter (Ill. Rev.
Stat. 1981, ch. 38, par. 9-3(a)) in the same death. O'Neil, Kirschbaum, Rodriguez,
Film Recovery, and Metallic Marketing were also convicted of 14 counts of reckless
conduct (Ill. Rev. Stat. 1981, ch. 38, par. 12-5(a)) involving 14 other Film Recovery
employees.[1]

We note here that Gerald Pett and Michael T. Mackay were indicted with the other
individual defendants for murder and reckless conduct. B.R. Mackay & Sons, Inc.,
owned by Mackay, was indicted with the other corporate defendants for involuntary
manslaughter. Pett was tried for murder and reckless conduct but was acquitted of all
charges. Mackay and B.R. Mackay & Sons, Inc., could not be extradited from Utah
and were not tried.

Individual defendants O'Neil, Kirschbaum, and Rodriguez each received sentences of 25 years' imprisonment for murder and 14 concurrent 364-day imprisonment terms for reckless conduct. O'Neil and Kirschbaum were also each fined
$10,000 with respect to the murder convictions and $14,000 with respect to the

convictions for reckless conduct. Corporate defendants Film Recovery and Metallic Marketing were each fined $10,000 with respect to the convictions for involuntary manslaughter and $14,000 with respect to the convictions for reckless conduct.

On appeal, defendants urge that their convictions must be reversed and the cause remanded for retrial because the judgments rendered were inconsistent. Defendants also contend that the evidence presented at trial was insufficient to support the convictions.

We conclude that the judgments rendered are legally inconsistent. Therefore, we now reverse those convictions as to both the individual and corporate defendants and remand the matter for retrial. We summarize below those facts, as they appear in the record, which are pertinent to our disposition.

In 1982, Film Recovery occupied premises at 1855 and 1875 Greenleaf Avenue in Elk Grove Village. Film Recovery was there engaged in the business of extracting, for resale, silver from used X-ray and photographic film. Metallic Marketing operated out of the same premises on Greenleaf Avenue and owned 50% of the stock of Film Recovery. The recovery process was performed at Film Recovery's plant located at the 1855 address and involved "chipping" the film product and soaking the granulated pieces in large, open, bubbling vats containing a solution of water and sodium cyanide. The cyanide solution caused silver contained in the film to be released. A continuous flow system pumped the silver-laden solution into polyurethane tanks which contained electrically charged stainless steel plates to which the separated silver adhered. The plates were removed from the tanks to another room where the accumulated silver was scraped off. The remaining solution was pumped out of the tanks and the granulated film, devoid of silver, shovelled out.

On the morning of February 10, 1983, shortly after he disconnected a pump on one of the tanks and began to stir the contents of the tank with a rake, Stefan Golab became dizzy and faint. He left the production area to go rest in the lunchroom area of the plant. Plant workers present on that day testified Golab's body had trembled and he had foamed at the mouth. Golab eventually lost consciousness and was taken outside of the plant. Paramedics summoned to the plant were unable to revive him. Golab was pronounced dead upon arrival at Alexian Brothers Hospital.

The Cook County medical examiner performed an autopsy on Golab the following day. Although the medical examiner initially indicated Golab could have died from cardiac arrest, he reserved final determination of death pending examination of results of toxicological laboratory tests on Golab's blood and other body specimens. After receiving the toxicological report, the medical examiner determined Golab died from acute cyanide poisoning through the inhalation of cyanide fumes in the plant air.

Defendants were subsequently indicted by a Cook County grand jury. The grand jury charged defendants O'Neil, Kirschbaum, Rodriguez, Pett, and Mackay with murder, stating that, as individuals and as officers and high managerial agents of Film Recovery, they had, on February 10, 1983, knowingly created a strong probability of Golab's death. Generally, the indictment stated the individual defendants failed to disclose to Golab that he was working with substances containing cyanide and failed to advise him about, train him to anticipate, and provide adequate equipment to protect him from attendant dangers involved. The grand jury charged Film Recovery and Metallic Marketing with involuntary manslaughter stating that, through the reckless acts of their officers, directors, agents, and others, all acting within the scope of their employment, the corporate entities had, on February 10, 1983, unintentionally killed Golab.[2] Finally, the grand jury charged both individual and corporate defendants with reckless conduct as to 20 other Film Recovery employees based on the same conduct alleged in the murder indictment, but expanding the time of that conduct to "on or about March 1982 through March 1983."

Proceedings commenced in the circuit court in January 1985 and continued through the conclusion of trial in June of that year. In the course of the 24-day trial, evidence from 59 witnesses was presented, either directly or through stipulation of the parties. That testimony is contained in over 2,300 pages of trial transcript. The parties also presented numerous exhibits including photographs, corporate documents and correspondence, as well as physical evidence.

On June 14, 1985, the trial judge pronounced his judgment of defendants' guilt. The trial judge found that "the mind and mental state of a corporation is the mind and mental state of the directors, officers and high managerial personnel because they act on behalf of the corporation for both the benefit of the corporation and for themselves." Further, "if the corporation's officers, directors and high managerial personnel act within the scope of their corporate responsibilities and employment for their benefit and for the benefit of the profits of the corporation, the corporation must be held liable for what occurred in the work place."

Defendants filed timely notices of appeal, the matters were consolidated for review, and arguments were had before this court in July 1987. One of defendants' principal contentions was that the Federal Occupational Safety and Health Act of 1970 (OSH Act) (29 U.S.C. § 651 *et seq.*(1982)) preempted State criminal prosecutions against individual and corporate defendants for conditions in an industrial workplace. That identical issue was the subject of a then pending appeal before the Illinois Supreme Court in *People v. Chicago Magnet Wire Corp.* (1989), 126 Ill.2d 356, 534 N.E.2d 962. Accordingly, we postponed disposition in this case until the supreme court decided *Chicago Magnet Wire.* Following the determination in *Chicago Magnet Wire* that such prosecutions were not preempted under OSH Act, we invited the parties to file new briefs and scheduled further oral argument on the remaining issues.

OPINION

Defendants raise two contentions with respect to the consistency of the judgments rendered at trial. Each contention rests, ultimately, on the observation that the offense of murder requires a mental state different from that required for the offenses of involuntary manslaughter and reckless conduct.

In their first contention, defendants argue that the judgments for murder and reckless conduct against individual defendants O'Neil, Kirschbaum, and Rodriguez are inconsistent because, while the offense of murder requires a knowing and intentional act (see Ill. Rev. Stat. 1981, ch. 38, pars. 4–5, 9-1(a)), reckless conduct does not (see Ill. Rev. Stat. 1981, ch. 38, pars. 4–6, 12-5(a)). Defendants argue both convictions, however, arose from the same acts of the individual defendants. Defendants reason

O'Neil, Kirschbaum, and Rodriguez could not be responsible for intentional and unintentional conduct at the same time and, therefore, the judgments for murder and reckless conduct against them are inconsistent.

Defendants rely on the same logic to support the contention that the murder convictions against individual defendants O'Neil, Kirschbaum, and Rodriguez are inconsistent with the convictions for involuntary manslaughter against the corporate defendants. To arrive at that conclusion, however, defendants first note that the corporate defendants could be culpable only through the acts and omissions of the individual defendants. Defendants observe that the mind and mental state of a corporation are the collective mind and mental state of its board of directors or high managerial agents. (See Ill. Rev. Stat. 1981, ch. 38, par. 5-4(a)(2).) Further noting that involuntary manslaughter is based on unintended and reckless conduct (see Ill. Rev. Stat. 1981, ch. 38, pars. 4–6, 9-3(a)), defendants reason the convictions against the corporate entities for that offense are inconsistent with the individual defendants' convictions for murder because both offenses were based on the same conduct: the acts of the individual defendants.

We find it helpful to set out the pertinent statutory language of the offenses for which the defendants were convicted. The Criminal Code of 1961 defines "murder" as follows:

> A person who kills an individual without lawful justification commits murder if, in performing the acts which cause the death: He knows that such acts create a strong probability of death or great bodily harm to that individual[.] (Emphasis added.) (Ill. Rev. Stat. 1981, ch. 38, par. 9-1(a)(2).)

"Involuntary manslaughter" is defined as:

> A person who unintentionally kills an individual without lawful justification commits involuntary manslaughter if his acts whether lawful or unlawful which cause the death are such as are likely to cause death or great bodily harm to some individual, and he performs them recklessly[.] (Emphasis added.) (Ill. Rev. Stat. 1981, ch. 38, par. 9-3(a).)

"Reckless conduct" is defined as:

> A person who causes bodily harm to or endangers the bodily safety of an individual by any means, commits reckless conduct if he performs recklessly the acts which cause the harm or endanger safety, whether they otherwise are lawful or unlawful. (Emphasis added.) Ill. Rev. Stat. 1981, ch. 38, par. 12-5(a).

The supreme court, in *People v. Spears* (1986), 112 Ill.2d 396, 493 N.E.2d 1030, and *People v. Hoffer* (1985), 106 Ill.2d 186, 478 N.E.2d 335, has addressed issues with respect to consistency of verdicts rendered for the above offenses in light of the mental states required to sustain each.

In *Hoffer,* defendant Donald Hoffer was indicted on three counts of murder in the shooting death of Harold (Ed) Peters. In a trial before a jury, the State presented evidence that Hoffer shot Peters with a shotgun after a heated exchange of words outside Hoffer's home. Hoffer testified that he thought Peters was reaching for a gun at the time of the shooting. Hoffer stated the shotgun discharged as he lowered it with one hand and reached with his other hand to grab the gunstock.

Pursuant to Illinois Pattern Jury Instructions, the trial judge instructed the jury that the offense of murder included the offenses of voluntary and involuntary manslaughter. Definitional and issues instructions were tendered to the jury on murder, voluntary manslaughter (unreasonable belief that the killing was justified), and involuntary manslaughter. The jurors, however, were not informed that they could return a guilty verdict on only one of the offenses.

On appeal, the appellate court vacated all three convictions and remanded the cause for a new trial.

The supreme court affirmed the reversal, rejecting the State's argument that the verdicts could be reconciled because the mental state required for murder "subsumed the lesser mental states required for voluntary manslaughter and involuntary manslaughter." After noting the three offenses differed only in the particular mental culpability required to sustain each, the court concluded the mental states involved are mutually inconsistent. Thus, "[w]here a determination is made that one [of the mental states] exists, the others, to be legally consistent, must be found not to exist."

Subsequently, in *People v. Spears* (1986), 112 Ill.2d 396, 493 N.E.2d 1030, the supreme court applied the *Hoffer* rule despite the State's contention that *Spears* involved separable acts and conduct toward multiple victims and, therefore, the rationale in *Hoffer* did not apply.

Defendant Henry Spears was charged with attempted murder and armed violence (based on the great-bodily-harm form of aggravated battery) in the shooting of his estranged wife, Barbara. Spears was also charged with armed violence in the shooting of Annette Keys. In his jury trial, the State presented evidence that Spears was at his estranged wife's apartment where she, Keys, and two other women had been playing cards. At some point, Spears and Barbara scuffled. Spears drew a gun from a shoulder holster and aimed it at Barbara as she tried to scramble to a side wall. The defendant fired a shot which struck Barbara before she reached the wall. Although Spears was grabbed from behind, he fired a second shot, striking both Barbara and Keys. Spears fired a third shot at Barbara's head, but missed her.

In his defense, Spears testified that Barbara had pushed him and he had stumbled. When someone then grabbed him from behind, he panicked and pulled the gun from the holster. In the ensuing struggle, the gun accidentally fired.

Pattern jury definitional and issues instructions were tendered for attempted murder, armed violence, and two uncharged counts of reckless conduct (Ill. Rev. Stat. 1983, ch. 38, par. 12-5(a)), which, at defendant's request, the jury was instructed to consider as a lesser included offense of the two armed-violence counts. Five verdict forms were provided: one for the attempted murder of Barbara, two for armed violence, and two for reckless conduct as to Barbara and Annette Keys.

The jury found defendant guilty on all five counts. However, the court entered judgment only on the attempted-murder count and one armed-violence count. The appellate court, with one justice dissenting, determined the verdicts were inconsistent and remanded the cause for a new trial.

The supreme court affirmed the reversal. The court agreed, generally, that where a claim of inconsistent guilty verdicts involves multiple shots or victims, the question is whether the trier of fact could rationally find separable acts accompanied by mental states to support all of the verdicts as legally consistent. (*Spears,* 112 Ill.2d at 405, 493 N.E.2d at 1034.) However, the court noted that that principle found no application where the State was attempting to justify guilty verdicts in direct conflict with both its theory of the case at trial and evidence it presented in support of that theory. (*Spears,* 112 Ill.2d at 405, 493 N.E.2d at 1034.) The court stated:

It would be manifestly unfair to allow the State, with the benefit of hindsight, to be able to create separable acts on appeal, neither alleged nor proved at trial. Such an inquiry does not operate in a vacuum. The manner by which a defendant is charged, and the jury is instructed, provides the essential framework for analyzing the consistency of jury verdicts in the troublesome context of multiple shots or victims. We believe that the substance of the allegations charging the defendant, as an unequivocal expression of prosecutorial intent [citation], and what the evidence showed in relation to those charges, are of particular importance in determining whether guilty verdicts could rationally and consistently be based upon separable acts accompanied by the requisite mental states. (Emphasis added.) Spears, 112 Ill.2d at 405–06, 493 N.E.2d at 1034.

The court examined the information and observed that the State had not charged a separate offense for each action or shot fired by defendant. As to conduct toward Barbara, the State had based each of its three charges on the two shots which actually struck her. (*Spears,* 112 Ill.2d at 406, 493 N.E.2d at 1034.) Because the same conduct was used as the basis for those charges, the court found the contention of separate acts untenable. (*Spears,* 112 Ill.2d at 406, 493 N.E.2d at 1034.) More importantly the court noted, even assuming defendant's acts were separable, evidence in the record did not support the State's argument that the defendant's mental state changed during the shootings to support the State's hypothesis. (*Spears,* 112 Ill.2d at 406, 493 N.E.2d at 1034.) Neither the State nor the defense had presented any evidence to suggest defendant's state of mind had varied during his acts. (*Spears,* 112 Ill.2d at 406, 493 N.E.2d at 1034.) Because the jury's verdicts as to defendant's conduct toward Barbara for offenses requiring otherwise mutually inconsistent mental states could not be reconciled based on separable acts or a change in defendant's mental state, the supreme court determined the verdicts were legally inconsistent under *Hoffer. Spears,* 112 Ill.2d at 406–07, 493 N.E.2d at 1034–35.

The supreme court further noted that the *Hoffer* rule also controlled the guilty verdicts for defendant's conduct toward Keys. By its guilty verdict, the jury found, in effect, that defendant had acted both recklessly (reckless conduct) and knowingly (armed violence predicated on aggravated battery) in firing the single shot which struck Keys. Based on that single act, the verdicts were legally inconsistent. *Spears,* 112 Ill.2d at 407, 493 N.E.2d at 1035.

Under the rule in *Hoffer,* the judgments rendered by the circuit court in the instant case appear inconsistent as based on mutually exclusive mental states. However, we must consider whether, under similar analysis used by the supreme court in *Spears,* the judgments are supported by separable acts occurring at different times against different victims by legally different defendants. We therefore begin with a review of the indictments, as they represent the State's prosecutorial intentions in charging defendants, and proceed to evaluate the record of evidence in light of those charges.

The murder indictment states that on February 10, 1983, defendants O'Neil, Kirschbaum, Rodriguez, Pett, and Mackay, acting as individuals and as officers and high managerial agents of Film Recovery, committed murder in that they knowingly created a strong probability of Stefan Golab's death. Specifically, the grand jury charged those individuals had "failed to disclose and make known to [Golab] that he was working with cyanide and substances containing cyanide and failed to instruct him as to matters involving safety procedures and proper handling of said chemicals[.]" Further, those individuals "failed to provide Golab with appropriate and necessary safety and first-aid equipment and sundry health-monitoring systems for his protection while working with and handling cyanide and substances containing cyanide[.]" The murder indictment also states O'Neil, Kirschbaum, Rodriguez, Pett, and Mackay failed to "properly provide for the storage, detoxification and disposition of cyanide and substances containing cyanide [and] failed to advise Golab of the dangerous nature of his work, and the conditions under which he engaged in it[.]"

The involuntary manslaughter indictment against Film Recovery and Metallic Marketing states that, on February 10, 1983, they "unintentionally killed Stefan Golab by authorizing, requesting, commanding and performing certain acts of commission and acts of omission[] by its [*sic*] officers, board of directors and high managerial agents, to wit: Steven J. O'Neil, Michael T. Mackay, Gerald Pett, Charles Kirschbaum, Daniel Rodriguez, and others, who acting within the scope of their employment performed the said acts recklessly in such manner as was likely to cause death and great bodily harm to some individual and caused the death of Stefan Golab[.]" The indictment did not otherwise specify the nature of the acts.

The indictments against all defendants for reckless conduct contain identical charges made in the murder indictment against the individual defendants as summarized above, save for stating that the conduct occurred "on or about March 1982 through March 1983."

With regard to the consistency of the judgments for murder and reckless conduct against defendants O'Neil, Kirschbaum, and Rodriguez, acting solely in their individual capacities, we note the corresponding indictments differ only in one respect. The murder indictment is limited to the individual defendants' conduct on February 10, 1983, while the reckless conduct indictments concern conduct over a period of time from March 1982 through March 1983, which would include the date of Golab's death. In all other respects, the same conduct is used as the foundation for the indictments for both offenses against the individual defendants. Although the indictments for both offenses are therefore based on identical acts of the individual defendants, it is conceivable the apparent inconsistency in the convictions for those offenses, due to the mutual exclusiveness of the mental states required to sustain each, might be reconciled by evidence in the record. After carefully reviewing the record, however, we do not conclude that, as to the individual defendants, evidence existed to establish, separately, defendants' mental states to support separate offenses of murder and reckless conduct.

A total of four witnesses testified exclusively as to events which might establish defendants' mental states on February 10, 1983. Michael W. Lackman, an Elk Grove fireman and paramedic who responded to the emergency call on February 10, 1983, did not testify as to any condition of the plant at Film Recovery and stated only that someone told him cyanide was used at Film Recovery's plant. Kenneth Kvidera, an Elk Grove Village police officer who assisted in the ambulance call, stated that when he went into the plant on February 10, 1983, he smelled a strong, foul odor which made him gag and experienced a burning sensation in his throat. Kvidera also noted that a "yellowish-orange" haze was visible in the plant. Kenneth Kryzywicki, another Elk Grove Village police officer who responded to the emergency call from Film Recovery on February 10, 1983, also testified to experiencing a burning sensation in his throat when inside the plant. He stated he had difficulty breathing, that his chest hurt, and his eyes teared. Kryzywicki also noted the mist in the plant air and observed that workers present wore paper masks over their faces but did not wear any other protective clothing or equipment. Gordon Hollywood, an Elk Grove Village police investigator, testified to substantially the same facts as Kryzywicki.

The only other witness to testify exclusively with respect to events of February 10 1983, was Mohammed Hassan, the emergency room physician at Alexian Brothers Hospital who treated Golab. Hassan did not testify as to any facts which might establish defendants' states of mind on February 10, 1983.

Several other plant workers testified to being in the plant on February 10, 1983, but their testimony does not establish what the conditions were in the plant on that particular day. Roman Guzowski testified that he was working with Golab when Golab became faint. Antonio Roman and Juan Fuentes testified they were working nearby and saw Golab trembling and begin to foam at the mouth. The parties stipulated that Elevterio Salinas would testify to similar facts. Through other stipulations, the parties agreed Mario Rodriquez and Juan Hernandez would testify they were present when Golab died. In addition, Debra Sadzeck, a bookkeeper, stated she was in the plant on February 10, 1983, retrieving payroll cards, when she saw Golab "slumped over" in the lunchroom.

None of the above testimony in any way substantially differs from that otherwise contained in the record regarding conditions in the plant, generally. Thus, we cannot conclude the record supports a determination that the individual defendants possessed different mental states on February 10, 1983, as distinguished from the period of March 1982 to March 1983, such as might support separate offenses of murder and reckless conduct. While we do not believe it helpful to summarize the considerable amount of that testimony in detail here, those who testified as to working conditions in the plant established the following: workers were not told that they were working with cyanide or that the compound put into the vats could be harmful when inhaled; although ceiling fans existed above the vats, ventilation in the plant was poor; workers were not informed they were working with cyanide and were given no safety instruction; workers were given no goggles to protect their eyes; workers were given no protective clothing and, as a result, workers' clothing would become wet with the solution used in the vats; there were small puddles of that solution as well as film chips on the plant floor around the vats; the solution burned exposed skin; a strong and foul odor permeated the plant; the condition of air in the plant made breathing difficult and painful; and, finally, workers experienced dizziness, nausea, headaches, and bouts of vomiting.

Because the offenses of murder and reckless conduct require mutually exclusive mental states, and because we conclude the same evidence of the individual defendants' conduct is used to support both offenses and does not establish, separately, each of the requisite mental states, we conclude that the convictions are legally inconsistent.

With regard to consistency of the judgment for murder against individual defendants O'Neil, Kirschbaum, and Rodriguez and that against the corporate entities for involuntary manslaughter, we observe that the corresponding indictments are both based on Golab's death on February 10, 1983. However, unlike the murder indictment, the indictment for involuntary manslaughter does not specify the "acts of commission and omission" upon which that charge was based. The material difference between the indictments, however, concerns reference to unnamed "others" in the involuntary manslaughter indictment as acting on behalf of the corporations in causing Golab's death in addition to naming the same individuals named in the murder indictment. To the extent the involuntary manslaughter indictment contemplates the conduct of others, as well as the individual defendants convicted of murder, as providing a basis for corporate criminal responsibility, it is possible the judgments against the corporate defendants for involuntary manslaughter could be consistent with the judgments for murder against the individual defendants.

To state it differently, in Illinois, a corporation is criminally responsible for offenses "authorized, requested, commanded, or performed, by the board of directors or by a high managerial agent acting within the scope of his employment." (Emphasis added.) (Ill. Rev. Stat. 1981, ch. 38, par. 5-4(a)(2).) A high managerial agent is defined as "an officer of the corporation, or any other agent who has a position of comparable authority for the formulation of corporate policy or the supervision of subordinate employees in a managerial capacity." (Ill. Rev. Stat. 1981, ch. 38, par. 5-4(c)(2).) Thus, a corporation is criminally responsible whenever any of its high managerial agents possesses the requisite mental state and is responsible for a criminal offense while acting within the scope of his employment. To the extent the record discloses that a high managerial agent of Film Recovery or Metallic Marketing, other than individual defendants O'Neil, Kirschbaum, and Rodriguez, might provide foundation for the charge of involuntary manslaughter, that judgment would not be inconsistent with judgment for murder against the individual defendants.

We first note that, because Pett was acquitted of all charges, we do not believe his conduct can be considered in establishing corporate criminal responsibility. As Pett's acts did not support either the charge against him for murder, requiring intentional conduct, or for reckless conduct, requiring recklessness, we find no basis upon which we could conclude he could have performed the offense of involuntary manslaughter. Further, recognizing Pett's acquittal might not necessarily preclude a determination that, while he may not have performed the offense, he otherwise authorized, requested, or commanded its performance, we observe that the record contains no evidence to support criminal responsibility on that basis.

In addition to O'Neil, Rodriguez, Kirschbaum, and Pett, other directors or high managerial agents of the corporations are identified in the record. Testimony established that Al Tolin was on the board of directors at Film Recovery and that Milton Marks was considered a vice-president of Metallic Marketing. The record also establishes that, for approximately seven months from November 1982 until the summer of 1983, Glenn N. Love was employed as the comptroller at Film Recovery. Further, Thomas VandenLangenberg was employed at Film Recovery for approximately one year, beginning November 1980, as manager of the shipping and receiving department and, thereafter, until January 1983, in the accounts payable department, keeping track of customer accounts. However, beyond testimony identifying those individuals and their positions in the corporations' structures, the record does not contain evidence of any conduct of those individuals such as would provide foundation to establish criminal liability against either of the corporate defendants for involuntary manslaughter.

The record discloses evidence as to only five other individuals whose conduct might conceivably support the charge of involuntary manslaughter such as might provide a basis to reconcile the judgment for that offense against the corporate defendants with the judgment for murder against O'Neil, Rodriguez, and Kirschbaum. Those individuals were Michael T. Mackay, who was indicted but not tried, Richard Stucker, Bob Major, Antonio Roman, and Fred Kopp, who were not named in the indictments. We summarize below, in detail, the nature and extent of evidence in the record with respect to the conduct of those individuals.

Regarding Michael T. Mackay, Susan Bellomo, a secretary at Film Recovery, testified that Mackay was associated with Metallic Marketing. Debra Sadzeck testified that Mackay was on the board of directors at Film Recovery. Sadzeck also stated that Mackay was involved in operations of Silver Recovery Systems, Inc., a company operating out of Salt Lake City, Utah. She acknowledged that she might have taken orders from Mackay during December 1982, or January or February 1983, if he "called in."

Regarding Richard Stucker, Officer Kenneth Kvidera testified that on February 10, 1983, he spoke to Stucker, who identified himself as the vice-president of Film Recovery. Kvidera stated he was told Stucker was present when Golab was carried out of the plant on February 10, 1983, after Golab collapsed. Investigator Gordon Hollywood testified that he spoke to Stucker along with Officer Kvidera on February 10, 1983. After that conversation, he accompanied Stucker through the plant to the warehouse area, where, Stucker explained, Golab had been working. Hollywood stated Stucker did not expressly tell Hollywood that Stucker was vice-president of Film Recovery. Hollywood stated, however, that he saw Stucker "directing people," indicating to him that Stucker was someone "in charge." Debra Sadzeck testified Stucker was sales coordinator for Film Recovery. Kathy Erpito, who had been employed as a receptionist and as an accountant at Film Recovery, testified Stucker was one of her "bosses." She stated Stucker was also a corporate officer of Associate Silver Recyclers, Inc., which operated out of the same premises as Film Recovery. Erpito testified Stucker signed checks for Associate Silver Recyclers, Inc., to Film Recovery and Metallic Marketing.

Regarding Bob Major, Susan Bellomo testified Major was one of the individuals she took orders from. Bellomo stated she had asked Major, along with O'Neil, Kirschbaum, Pett, and Fred Kopp, about fumes that she smelled in the office. She was told by everyone she asked that the smell came from the chemical used in the plant. The smell was attributed to ventilation in the plant or the opening and closing of the plant's doors. Bellomo stated Major was one of the individuals she would advise concerning visits by firemen or fire inspectors. Debra Sadzeck described Major as O'Neil's "right-hand man." Sadzeck stated that Major's title was "director of education" at Film Recovery's plant. Michael Selway, an industrial hygienist for the U.S. Department of Labor Occupational Safety and Health Administration, testified that on February 22, 1983, he spoke to Major when he visited Film Recovery after being assigned to investigate Golab's death. Selway also identified Major as the director of education. Selway testified he understood Major's responsibility to be to "go out into the field and educate people" as to the process used at the plant.

Regarding Antonio Roman, Secundino Boyas, a plant worker at Film Recovery, testified Roman was "like a supervisor." Juan Fuentes stated that Roman was "in charge" of and gave orders to workers grinding film for processing. The parties stipulated that, if called to testify, Jose Campos, also a plant worker, would establish that Roman was his boss when Campos worked in the film grinding room.

In his own testimony, Roman denied that he was a boss. He indicated that, because he could speak English and Spanish, Kirschbaum occasionally would have him tell only Spanish-speaking plant workers what Kirschbaum wanted them to do.

Regarding Fred Kopp, in addition to the reference to Kopp in her testimony noted above, Susan Bellomo testified Kopp was general manager of Film Recovery. Bellomo described Kopp's title as "vice-president." She stated Kopp had "decision-making powers" at Film Recovery and was involved in the day-to-day operations of the plant during 1982. Bellomo testified Kopp left Film Recovery in January 1983 and was not employed with the company when Golab died. Glenn N. Love testified Kopp left Film Recovery in December 1982 and had no further involvement with the corporation. Debra Sadzeck stated Kopp was a vice-president of Metallic Marketing and was on the board of directors of Film Recovery. Kathy Erpito named Kopp as one of her bosses at Film Recovery and stated she complained to him about headaches she experienced while at work.

In his own testimony, Kopp acknowledged that he was general manager at Film Recovery and stated that while he was employed at Film Recovery he was in charge of plant operations. Kopp testified he joined Film Recovery in January of 1980 and worked there until he was terminated in October 1982. Kopp stated his direct involvement in the plant ended in August 1981, although he did return occasionally. Kopp's direct testimony otherwise concerned, generally, efforts taken to insure the safety of workers in the plant, including testing air in the plant, furnishing safety equipment and protective gear for workers, and adding ventilation fans.

On cross-examination by the State, Kopp admitted that when the cyanide compound was first put into the tanks in which the granulated film was soaked, there was a possibility of producing cyanide gas. Kopp stated workers would work over those tanks on the day after the solution was mixed. Kopp admitted that, other than the ceiling fans, there was no local exhaust mechanism on those tanks and that, if cyanide gas was released, the workers working over the tanks had no protection from inhaling cyanide gas.

After carefully considering the above testimony, we cannot conclude the record supports a basis upon which we might reconcile the individual defendants' convictions for murder with the convictions for involuntary manslaughter against Film Recovery and Metallic Marketing.

First, we must dismiss any consideration of the conduct of Antonio Roman because there is no evidence in the record that Roman was in any way responsible for formulating corporate policy or supervising subordinate employees in a managerial capacity for either Film Recovery or Metallic Marketing. Roman's supervisory authority at

Film Recovery was limited to those workers granulating film and amounted to nothing more than translating, into Spanish, directions of Kirschbaum to those workers who could not understand English. Further, there is no evidence linking Roman to the operations of Metallic Marketing.

While the record indicates the other individuals might be considered high managerial agents of one or both of the corporations, we do not find evidence of their conduct in the record to show they committed the offense of involuntary manslaughter to establish criminal responsibility as to the corporate defendants.

The record contains no evidence of any conduct of Michael T. Mackay, either in his association with Metallic Marketing or as a director of Film Recovery, other than to possibly have given orders to Debra Sadzeck. No testimony establishes what such orders might have been.

In similar fashion, although evidence establishes Richard Stucker as a vice-president of Film Recovery with authority to direct subordinate employees, the record fails to contain evidence of any conduct which might form a basis for criminal responsibility against Film Recovery for involuntary manslaughter. Testimony establishes only that Stucker was on the premises on the day Golab died. No evidence links Stucker to the operations of Metallic Marketing.

Although Bob Major was identified as the director of education at Film Recovery and as O'Neil's "right-hand man," the record again fails to contain evidence of any conduct by Major whatsoever which might support a charge of involuntary manslaughter. No evidence links Major to the operations of Metallic Marketing.

The testimony of and about Fred Kopp comes nearest to providing support for the charge of involuntary manslaughter against Film Recovery. That testimony establishes that Kopp was the general manager of Film Recovery and was, while employed there, involved in day-to-day operations in the plant. By his own admission, Kopp stated it was possible that workers working over the tanks in which film was being soaked could inhale any resulting gas fumes produced and were not protected from doing so through a local exhaust system or other protective means. However, the record establishes that Kopp's employment at Film Recovery ended, at the earliest, in August 1982, or, at the latest, in January 1983. In either case, testimony establishes that Kopp was not employed at Film Recovery at the time of Golab's death on February 10, 1983. Even assuming that Kopp's admissions indicate the type of conduct as might otherwise provide foundation for criminal responsibility against Film Recovery for involuntary manslaughter, the record contains no evidence that Kopp's conduct, while employed with Film Recovery, caused Golab's death after Kopp had left the company. No evidence links Kopp with the operations of Metallic Marketing.

Therefore, we find no basis in the record upon which to conclude that the conduct of a high managerial agent, apart from that of the individual defendants found guilty of murder, could provide the basis for establishing criminal responsibility against the corporate defendants for Golab's death. And, because the same conduct is used to support offenses which have mutually exclusive mental states, we conclude the judgments rendered for both offenses are legally inconsistent.

In *Hoffer,* the supreme court affirmed its earlier pronouncement in *People v. Frias* (1983), 99 Ill.2d 193, 457 N.E.2d 1233, and *People v. Hairston* (1970), 46 Ill.2d 348, 263 N.E.2d 840, that, where judgments are legally inconsistent, as they are when rendered for offenses requiring mutually exclusive mental states, reversal and retrial must follow. (*People v. Hoffer* (1985), 106 Ill.2d 186, 195–99, 478 N.E.2d 335, 340–42.) We are mindful, however, the supreme court has also directed that, where, as in the instant case, defendants challenge the sufficiency of evidence at the first trial, it is necessary to address that issue to avoid the risk of subjecting defendants to double jeopardy. (*People v. Taylor* (1979), 76 Ill.2d 289, 391 N.E.2d 366.) Our review of the record does not lead us to conclude that the evidence, as first adduced, was so insufficient as to bar retrial.

Evidence at trial indicated Golab died after inhaling poisonous cyanide fumes while working in a plant operated by Film Recovery and its sister corporation Metallic Marketing where such fumes resulted from a process employed to remove silver from used X-ray and photographic film. The record contains substantial evidence regarding the nature of working conditions inside the plant. Testimony established that air inside the plant was foul smelling and made breathing difficult and painful. Plant workers experienced dizziness, nausea, headaches, and bouts of vomiting. There is evidence that plant workers were not informed they were working with cyanide. Nor were they informed of the presence of, or danger of breathing, cyanide gas. Ventilation in the plant was poor. Plant workers were given neither safety instruction nor adequate protective clothing. Finally, testimony established that defendants O'Neil, Kirschbaum, and Rodriguez were responsible for operating the plant under those conditions. For purposes of our disposition, we find further elaboration on the evidence unnecessary. Moreover, although we have determined evidence in the record is not so insufficient as to bar retrial, our determination of the sufficiency of the evidence should not be in any way interpreted as a finding as to defendants' guilt that would be binding on the court on retrial.

Reversed and remanded.

COCCIA, P.J., and MURRAY, J., concur.

6 Civil Liability

It makes no difference whether a good man has defrauded a bad man or a bad man has defrauded a good man, or whether a good or bad man has committed adultery: The law can look only to the amount of damage done.

Aristotle

God works wonders now and then: Behold! A lawyer and an honest man!

Benjamin Franklin

STUDENT LEARNING OBJECTIVES

1. Analyze and identify the differences between civil and criminal actions.
2. Analyze and assess a tort action.
3. Assess and analyze the elements of a negligence action.
4. Analyze and identify special relationships.
5. Analyze and assess the elements of a contract action.

As criminal laws are designed to protect society and can remove freedom from the offender, civil laws are designed to correct unfairness between parties and correct injustices resulting in money or related non-criminal damages. Civil cases often result from one party damaging the other party, or violating an agreement, or other injustice which the court can remedy through awarding of money or related damages. For safety professionals, civil cases often fall within the category called "tort law" resulting from circumstances such as injuries outside the protections provided under state workers' compensation laws and contract disputes. Safety professionals, as an agent for the company or organizations, are often the defendant or the entity upon which the action is brought against. The individual or entity bring the action which is known as the plaintiff. Civil actions can be brought in state or federal court depending upon the jurisdiction and damage amount.

Tort comes from the Latin word meaning twisted. Tort law is focused on a wrongful act by one party and an award of money damages against the other party. Generally, tort law in the United States has evolved as a body of law and rules such as reasonable care must be used so not to injure another person. The institutional structure through which these laws and rules are applied in the court system is called litigation, and this system is as important as the laws and rules in achieving equity.

In most tort actions, an individual brings an action against another individual or other entity in the appropriate court through the initiation of a formal complaint. The complaint is served on the other party, and an answer is usually required. Discovery, consisting of depositions, motions, expert evaluations, and other actions are taken by the parties under the supervision of the court. Discovery is done in preparation for trial; however, a substantial percentage of tort actions settle prior to a trial. All settlements must be approved by the court, and the agreed upon money is transferred to the appropriate party.

If this action is not settled and moves to the trial, generally, the structure includes jury selection, opening statement by each party, calling of witnesses by each party for direct and cross examination, closing arguments by each party, and the matter is provided to the jury for a decision. This is a very simplistic structure, while the art, science, and strategy of litigation can be very complex. Safety professionals can play many roles in tort litigation ranging from plaintiff to defendant to expert witness depending upon the case. It is important that safety professionals have a firm grasp on the structure and the requirements depending upon their role within the litigation of the specific case.

An area of tort law which safety professionals should recognize is that of mass torts. Mass tort cases involve many injuries or fatalities caused by one incident, such as an explosion, or by a singular source, such as a chemical release from an operation. Mass tort cases, although relatively new, have presented challenges to the court system due to the sheer number of cases. In these very complex cases involving a large number of plaintiffs, the court has developed rules to consolidate and manage these actions. However, as we have seen in many cases, if the company loses the action, the company often files for bankruptcy, and the court must then work to distribute any company assets to the large number of plaintiffs in an equitable manner. The cost of litigation for both the plaintiff and defendant in these types of mass tort cases can be millions of dollars.

Safety professionals should be aware that tort law for physical harm is generally divided into three categories—namely, intentional torts, strict liability, and negligence. An intentional tort is when a person intends to commit the harm. Negligence, in general terms, is carelessness. Strict liability (often product liability) generally creates liability by law for a person or entity who did not mean to harm another and has exercised reasonable care in attempting to avoid the harm however the harm happened. Torts against non-physical interests can include defamation, invasion of privacy, misrepresentation, and intention infliction of emotional harm.

An intentional tort is when a person intends to commit the harm. For example, Person A engage in an altercation with Person B, and Person A intentionally punches Person B on the nose. This would be the intentional tort of assault and battery. Safety professionals can encounter this type of action when employees engage in intentional physical altercations resulting in harm in areas such as the parking lot after work, cafeteria, or even workplace. Wherein workers compensation required that the injury "arise out of or in the course of employment," the pivotal question is whether the altercation is work related. If intentional but not work related, Person B would bring an action involving the intentional of assault and battery and request such damages as medical costs, loss of wages, and related damages.

Negligence is a primary area of importance for safety professionals. Negligence is defined as "the omission to do something which a reasonable man, guided by those ordinary considerations which ordinarily regulate human affairs, would do, or the doing of something which a reasonable and prudent man would not do."* As

---

* Black's Law Dictionary.

PRIMARY ELEMENTS OF NEGLIGENCE:

- DUTY   Has a DUTY been created?
- BREACH   Has the DUTY been BREACHED?
- CAUSATION   Is the BREACH the CAUSE of the injury?
- DAMAGES   How much?

identified in Chapter 5, there is criminal negligence; however, we will be focusing on civil law negligence. The primary elements which must be proven in a *prima facie* case based in negligence include the elements of duty, breach of the duty, causation, and damages.

Safety professionals should provide substantial attention to the first element of a negligence action, namely, has a legal duty been created through the relationship with the plaintiff. Does the Occupational Safety and Health Act create a legal duty to protect the plaintiff? Has the circumstances created a legal duty for the safety professional? In situations such as doctor–patient relationships, the courts have often found a legal duty. Does the safety professional owe the plaintiff a legal duty to act with reasonable care in certain circumstances such as an expectation to operate a motor vehicle safely?

Is a safety professional a "professional" who may owe a duty of care paralleling the attorney–client and doctor–patient relationship?

As a citizen, the courts have found a general duty of reasonable care. For adults, the courts have generally utilized a reasonable person standard of which a person should not place another at foreseeable risk of harm through their actions or conduct. For children, the courts often use a child standard of care; for individuals with disabilities, the standard is a reasonable person with the same abilities. For companies, the manufacturer of goods general duty of care is to act reasonably to protect persons who may come in contact with the product produced if there is a knowledge of probable danger arising from the product, knowledge that danger will be shared by others, and the proximate or remoteness of the relation is a factor to consider. The scope of liability for manufacturer of products scope of potential liability is expanded.

Under the limited duty rule, an individual owes no duty to assist, act or rescue another person. However, there are a number of exceptions to this rule including misfeasance (you caused the harm), special relationship (work relationships and special dependency), and voluntary assumption of duty (including rescue and special skills). This is important for safety professionals to carefully review. Additionally, a duty can be created by statute, prevention of aid by others, and reliance on a promise. In many circumstances, safety professionals may have a duty to respond created by statute, holding self out as possessing special skills, or through their working relationship. Careful analysis of individual situations and state laws by safety professionals should be conducted.

Safety professionals, as the agent of the company, should pay careful attention to any duty created as the owner or occupier of land. In general, the land owner owes no duty of reasonable care to trespassers. However, a duty may be owed if injury occurs to a trespasser due to willful, wanton, or through gross negligence. The land owner is responsible for knowing the conditions of the land as well as any artificial conditions created on the land. Land owners owe a duty to licensees or individual granted access to the land, such as contractors. Land owners owe a duty to warn or make safe of any dangerous conditions as long as the land owner knows of such conditions. Individuals invited on the land, or invitees, must be warned of dangerous conditions by the land owner. Owners can be held liable if he/she should have known about the dangerous conditions. Where the land is open to the public (or public invitees), there is an implied assurance by the land owner that the premises are reasonably safe for entry. Safety professionals, again as the agent of the land owner, should be aware that this duty can be discharged through warning or making the property safe.

Of particular importance to safety professionals is the "Attractive Nuisance Doctrine" involving children. Owners or occupiers of property owe a duty to trespassing children (Example: Construction site). If there is something manmade that attracts children to the land where there is a risk of harm, a duty of care is created requiring the risk or unsafe condition be removed or safeguarded to protect the children.

The Good Samaritan Rule is generally a doctrine that provides protection to a person who comes to the aid of another individual, who is injured or ill, from being sued for contributory negligence, as long as the person offering aid acts with reasonable care. This doctrine is used by rescuers to avoid civil liability for injuries arising from their negligence. Overall, this doctrine is utilized to remove any fear or reluctance of being sued (generally, negligence or wrongful death) when bystanders assist an injured or ill person. In general, the Good Samaritan Doctrine required that the care provided was the result of an emergency, the initial injury was not caused by the rescuer, and the care provided was not provided in a reckless or grossly negligent manner.

If the court find that a duty is created, the second element which must be proved in a negligence action is that of breach. In essence, did the defendant breach his/her duty to the plaintiff? If a duty has not been created, there can be no breach. If a duty has been created, the defendant did breach this duty resulting in the harm to the plaintiff. The court will focus on whether the defendant breached the duty of a "reasonably prudent person" under the circumstances. A "reasonably prudent person" is a legal standard that represents how the average individual would responsibly act in the same or similar circumstances.

Res Ipsa Loquitur or "the thing speaks for itself" is a rebuttable presumption that the defendant was negligent "which arises upon proof that instrumentality causing injury was in defendant's exclusive control, and that the accident was one which ordinarily does not happen in absence of negligence."* Under the Rules of Evidence, the negligence of the defendant can be inferred from the facts of the accident, character of the accident, or circumstances leading to the accident. In essence, the accident could not have occurred, and the thing which caused the injury was under the management and control of the defendant. Safety professionals should also be aware that the Doctrine of *Respondeat Superior* (Let the Master Answer) can be utilized where if the accident occurred and no one knows who was in control, the supervisor or superior over the area can be the target of the action. Additionally, exclusive control

---

* Black's Law Dictionary.

is not usually required; however, the power to control and the opportunity to exercise this control is often sufficient under *Res Ipsa Loquitor* to shift the burden of proof from the plaintiff to the defendant.

If the court find there was a duty and the duty was breached, the third element of a negligence claim is examined, namely causation, or was the negligence the cause of the injury. The court will look for the "causal link" between the acts or omissions of the defendant and the actual injury or harm to the plaintiff. If there is a causal link between the act and the injury, the hurdle of the third element is met. If there is no linkage between the act and the injury, the case is dismissed. However, the court may also look at the foreseeability of the risk and the injury. In essence, whether the defendant could have reasonably foreseen that his/her actions might cause an injury. If the defendant's actions or omissions can be linked to the plaintiff's injuries, although through possible random acts, a linkage could be found. If the acts involved an act of nature or the acts or omissions could not be foreseeable, the defendant would most likely prevail and the action dismissed.

Safety professionals should be aware that ALL elements of the negligence action must be proved prior to moving to the final element of damages. The final element in a negligence action is the damages. The court will compensate the plaintiff for his/her injuries and the resulting costs, such as medical costs, property repair, and other losses through the award of monetary compensation or money. These damages are often called compensatory damages, and proof of damages are usually required. In certain circumstances such as where the defendant's actions were outrageous, showed reckless indifference, or showed willful and wanton disregard, punitive damages may be permitted. Punitive damages serve two general purposes – namely, to punish the defendant for his/her actions and to deter others from similar actions. Punitive damages usually have no limits and is left to the judge or jury.

Safety professionals should be aware of the immunities and defenses in negligence actions, depending on the state. Starting with the immunities, there is Sovereign Immunity which precludes actions against the federal government, state government, and related governmental functions. Most states have abandoned this immunity in favor of permitting tort actions with restrictions and limitations.

An immunity was also available to charities in the past; however, most states have abolished this protection.

Depending on the state, the defenses of contributory negligence and comparable negligence may be available. Contributory negligence, although replaced by comparative negligence in most states, addresses when the plaintiff's actions contributed to the harm and could eliminate or reduce any recovery by the plaintiff. Comparative negligence, in its pure form, is a reduction of the defendant's faulty conduct by the percentage of the plaintiff's fault. Modified Comparative Fault can bar recovery by the plaintiff, if the plaintiff's percentage of fault is greater than the defendant's fault (Example: If plaintiff is 40 percent at fault, the plaintiff could only recover 60 percent from the defendant).

Assumption of the Risk defenses can be expressed or implied. Under the expressed Assumption of the Risk defense, the plaintiff expressly provides oral permission to release the defendant from any obligations of the duty of care. For safety professionals, this is often by contract or waiver. If by contract, safety professionals must ensure that the release is clear and unambiguous within the agreement. If by expressed waiver, safety professionals should be aware that this waiver does not release from liability for reckless or intentional wrongful acts or omissions.

Actions sounding in negligence happen every day in the courtrooms around the country, from the slip and fall accidents in the grocery stores to vehicular accidents. Safety professionals should be cognizant of this area of risk and prepare to minimize or eliminate these risks where possible. Although workers compensation is often the exclusive remedy for work-related injuries and illnesses, contractors, visitors, vendors, and even trespassers present a risk which safety professionals should recognize and address.

Shifting gears, another area of potential civil liability that often enters the domain of the safety professional is that of contracts. A contract, in its basic form, is an OFFER between two or more parties, and ACCEPTANCE by the parties and a trade of some type of CONSIDERATION (money, goods, services, etc.). By definition, a contract is "an agreement between two or more persons which creates an obligation to do or not to do a particular thing. Its essentials are competent parties, subject matter, a legal consideration, mutuality of agreement, and mutuality of obligation."*

Contract

Offer + Acceptance + Consideration = Contract

Contract law addresses all aspects of this codified promise between parties including the making of the contract, the keeping of the promises or terms of the contract, and the breaking of the promises or terms of the agreement. In theory, a contract between two parties is relatively simple and millions of contracts are signed every day. However, the devil is definitely in the details. Contract law addresses the different types of agreements and the specialty type of agreements. For example, a contract to purchase property is also governed by property law as well as contract law, and a collective bargaining agreement would be governed by labor law as well as contract law.

As a safety professional, negotiated contracts are often the way to get things done in the workplace. From a credit card to a consultant and your student loan to purchasing your home, a contract is the mechanism through which work is accomplished. In our society today, contracts abound and contract law is the method through which contracts between parties is structured, secured, and enforced. Most contracts flow freely without difficulties being negotiated by the parties; however, when issues arise between the times, the parties signed the agreement, and performance of the activities or products agreed to in the contract, contract law provides a method of dispute resolution as well as an enforcement mechanism to ensure performance or provide restitution.

Contract law provides the structure and enforcement; however, individuals are provided the freedom and autonomy to negotiate and agree upon the terms and

---

* Black's Law Dictionary.

conditions of a contract. Freedom of contract is an underlying freedom; however, conversely, it also protects against an individual being mandated or compelled to enter into any contract. The basic principles of contract law simply provide what elements are required to make a legally enforceable contract. Usually, a contract can be oral as well as written. For safety professionals, virtually all contracts agreed upon within the scope of the job are required to be in writing and oral contracts are often specifically forbidden.

The Statute of Frauds, originally developed in 1677 in England, has been adopted by every state. In essence, the Statute of Frauds provides a list of contracts that are required to be in writing such as a contract for marriage, a contract for goods over $500.00, and a contract for the sale of land. For this specific class of contracts covered under the Statute of Frauds, certain formalities, such as producing the signed contract, are required before an action is permitted.

Correlating with the Statute of Frauds is the Uniform Commercial Code or U.C.C. The Uniform Commercial Code is "one of the uniform laws drafted by the National Conference of Commissioners on Uniform State Laws governing commercial transactions."[*] Safety professionals should be aware that the U.C.C. governs transitions such as the sale of goods, commercial paper, bank deposits and collections, letters of credit, bulk transfers, warehouse receipts, bills of laden and other investment, business and related secure transactions.[†] For example, U.C.C. Section 2-201 provides that "a contract for the sale of goods for the price of $500 or more is not enforceable by way of action or defense unless there is some writing sufficient to indicate that the contract for sale has been made between the parties and signed by the party against whom enforcement is sought or by his authorized agent or broker."[‡]

Safety professionals should be aware that you often serve as the company or organization's "agent" in forming contractual relationships with other entities. An "agent" is defined as "one who represents and acts for another under the contract or relation of agency. A business representative whose function is to bring about, modify, affect, accept performance of, or terminate contractual obligations between the principle and a third party."[§] Most safety professionals enter into a wide variety of contracts while serving as the agent of their company including such contracts as the purchase of safety equipment, acquisition of consulting services, and acquiring software or computer services. The purchase is for the benefit of the company with the safety professional serving as the agent for the company in the formation and agreement to the contract.

With the safety professional serving as agent, one emerging are a of contract law which recognition should be provided is that of the "adhesion contact." As often seen in insurance contracts, credit card agreements, software contracts, and related contracts, an adhesion contact (or often called a form or standardized contract) is a non-negotiable contract prepared by one party, and the other party must adhere

---

[*] Black's Law Dictionary.
[†] Note: Every state except Louisiana has adopted the U.C.C.)
[‡] Black's Law Dictionary.
[§] Id.

to the terms and language of the contract on a take-it-or-leave-it basis. These types of contracts are common in today's business world; however, enforcement of such contracts can be challenged and courts have created exceptions. Additionally, safety professionals should be aware of "clickwrap" contracts or contracts present the terms of the contract after the purchase is made on a website where "I agree" button before proceeding on the website (often used with computer or software purchases).

Safety professionals should be aware of the issues involving arbitration clauses in contracts. In essence, the arbitration clause forgoes the individual's right to sue for breach and requires arbitration to resolve any disputes. The arbitration clause often dictates the arbitrator or arbitration panel to decide the claim. Although arbitrators often follow the rule of law, most arbitrators are not bound to follow the rules of law and there is often no review in court or appeal process. Safety professionals should be aware that arbitration clauses are often utilized in business-related transactions because of the reduced litigation costs and speed of the process.

A collective bargaining agreement is a contract between the employee's representative (a labor organization or union) and the employer. In addition to the rules of contract, this type of negotiation and agreement is also bound by the rules of the National Labor Relation Act and correlating labor laws. The National Labor Relation Board is the governing agency and disputes/claims are often heard within the National Labor Relations Board system.

When one party to the contract agreement fails to do what he/she promised in the contract or breaches the contract, safety professionals should be aware that litigation or arbitration often frequently happens. The courts seldom mandate performance of the contract, preferring to order payment of monies. When a court requires performance of the contract or "specific performance," the contract usually involves unique skills or products. The courts usually provide money damages due to the fact that money is usually involved, it is practical and expedient and money can be utilized to acquire a substitute for performance.

In summation, safety professionals should identify the potential risks involved in tort actions as well as contract actions. Although not all of the potential risks of civil actions are encompassed in this chapter, safety professionals should be aware that civil liability risks and the resulting injury or breach can provide a far greater monetary risk than workers compensation. Prudent safety professionals should identify the potential risk and take the appropriate actions to minimize or eliminate the risks within this area.

Questions

1. What are the elements that must be proved in a contract action?
2. What are the elements that must be proved in a negligence action?
3. What is *Res Ipsa Loquitor*?
4. How does the Good Samaritan Rule apply to safety professionals?
5. What is immunity, and how does it work?

Case Modified for the Purpose of this Text

315 F.Supp.2d 1197
United States District Court,
N.D. Florida,
Pensacola Division.
Dominic FERACI, individually and on behalf of his minor children, Nicolas
Anthony Feraci and Kristen Nicole Feraci, Plaintiffs,
v.
GRUNDY MARINE CONSTRUCTION COMPANY; P & S Construction
Services, Inc.; Total Leasing Company, Inc.; Ronnie Resmondo; Paul Waynick;
and Ledr Group, Inc., d/b/a TMG Staffing Services, Inc., Defendants.
No. 3:02–CV–525/MCR.
March 11, 2004.

SYNOPSIS

Background: Subcontractor's employee brought action against general contractor, subcontractor, his supervisors, employee leasing company, and marketer that arranged for leasing company to provide workers for subcontractor to recover for personal injuries sustained while working on construction site.

Holdings: On defendants' motions for summary judgment, the District Court, Rodgers, J., held that:

1. Employee leasing company was entitled to workers' compensation immunity;
2. General contractor was entitled to workers' compensation immunity; and
3. Supervisor's negligence did not abrogate his workers' compensation immunity.

Motions granted.

ORDER GRANTING DEFENDANTS' MOTIONS FOR SUMMARY JUDGMENT

District Judge.

Pending before the court are five motions for summary judgment (*see* docs. 199, 205, 207, 213, and 215) and documents in support thereof (*see* docs. 200–01, 206, 208–09, 213–16, 243, 257–58, and 261), which were filed by the following five Defendants: (1) GRUNDY MARINE CONSTRUCTION COMPANY; (2) P & S CONSTRUCTION SERVICES, INC.; (3) TOTAL LEASING COMPANY, INC.; (4) RONNIE RESMONDO; and (5) LEDR GROUP, INC., d/b/a TMG STAFFING SERVICES, INC. Plaintiff DOMINIC FERACI timely filed memoranda and evidentiary materials in opposition to each motion (Docs. 223–27, 232–35). The court has taken the motions under advisement (Doc. 256) and is now prepared to rule on

Defendants' motions. Because of an entitlement to workers' compensation immunity, the following Defendants' motions for summary judgment are GRANTED: (1) GRUNDY MARINE CONSTRUCTION COMPANY; (2) P & S CONSTRUCTION SERVICES, INC.; (3) RONNIE RESMONDO; and (4) LEDR GROUP, INC., d/b/a TMG STAFFING SERVICES, INC. Even though TOTAL LEASING COMPANY, INC., is not entitled to workers' compensation immunity, the company's motion for summary judgment is GRANTED, because Plaintiffs failed to demonstrate a cause of action against the company.

I. STATEMENT OF THE CASE

A. PROCEDURAL HISTORY

On December 23, 2002, Plaintiffs filed the current action in this Court based on diversity jurisdiction.[1] (Doc. 1). Plaintiffs later filed an amended complaint (see doc. 55), to which all Defendants filed timely answers (see docs. 76–77, 82, 84, 96, 99). On April 30, 2003, Plaintiffs filed a motion to dismiss Defendant PAUL WAYNICK without prejudice from the case (see doc. 118), and on May 14, 2003, the Court granted Plaintiffs' motion (see doc. 123). The following three causes of action are *1200 common to all remaining Defendants: (1) unspecified intentional torts; (2) negligence; and (3) gross negligence (Doc. 55).[2] Beginning in mid-August 2002, the five remaining Defendants each filed a motion for summary judgment along with supporting documentation (Docs.199–201, 205–209, 213, 215–216, 243, 257–258). Plaintiffs timely filed materials in opposition to each motion (Docs. 223–27, 232–35). On January 26, 2004, the Court entered an Order and Notice notifying the parties that summary judgment would be taken under advisement beginning on February 2, 2004 (Doc. 256).

B. RELEVANT FACTS

For purposes of ruling on Defendants' motions for summary judgment, the following facts are either undisputed or viewed in the light most favorable to Plaintiffs.[3] This is a personal injury case for damages arising out of an injury to Plaintiff DOMINIC FERACI ("Feraci"), which occurred on October 19, 2001, while he was working at a construction site. At the time of the accident, Defendant GRUNDY MARINE CONSTRUCTION COMPANY ("Grundy") was a prime contractor with the United States Army Corps of Engineers who had entered into a contract to perform construction operations at Hurlburt Field Air Force Base in Okaloosa County, Florida ("the project") (Docs. 209, ¶ 1; 214, ¶ 1). Grundy subcontracted with Defendant P & S CONSTRUCTION SERVICES, INC. ("P & S"), to perform underground utility work on the project, including the installation of concrete and PVC pipe (Docs. 209, ¶ 2; 214, ¶ 2). Pursuant to the terms of the subcontract between Grundy and P & S, P & S was obligated to secure and maintain worker's compensation coverage for the project personnel who were under P & S's direction and control (Doc. 209, ¶ 3).

1On September 30, 2001, Plaintiff DOMINIC FERACI ("Feraci") was hired as a laborer to work for P & S at the Hurlburt Field project (Doc. 55, ¶ 6B). Feraci was employed by Defendants P & S and LEDR GROUP, INC. d/b/a TMG STAFFING SERVICES, INC. ("TMG") (Doc. 214, ¶ 4).[4] TMG is an employee *1201 leasing company who leased Feraci to P & S to work on the project (Doc. 214, ¶ 3). Pursuant to the February 1, 2001, contract between P & S and TMG, TMG was responsible for the "back office" and administrative tasks relevant to its leased personnel, including payment of worker's compensation premiums and payroll (Doc. 209, ¶ 6). Thus, TMG acquired and maintained worker's compensation coverage for Feraci (Docs. 201, ¶ 8; 209, ¶ 7). Throughout the course of the project, TMG did not interfere with P & S's day-to-day operations (Doc. 209, ¶ 9). Pursuant to the terms of the P & S/TMG contract, TMG retained various rights related to safety and risk management; however, P & S was responsible for the direct supervision of the leased employees and for compliance with any relevant safety regulations (Doc. 209, ¶ 10).

On the morning of the accident, Hugh Noa ("Noa"), one of Grundy's superintendents, ordered P & S to move four 48–inch elliptical concrete pipes from one location at the project site to another (Docs. 209, ¶ 17; 214, ¶ 13). Noa did not give P & S any specific instructions as to the methods or procedures to be employed in moving the pipes (Doc. 209, ¶ 18). P & S's foreman, Defendant RONNIE RESMONDO ("Resmondo") ordered Feraci and two co-workers, Paul Waynick ("Waynick") and Kenneth Melvin ("Melvin"), to move the four pipes using a Caterpillar excavator, commonly referred to as a "trac-hoe."[5] (Docs. 209, ¶¶ 12, 19; 216, ¶¶ 2–4).[6] The *1202 pipes were to be hoisted using a steel cable attached to the trachoe's bucket (Doc. 209, ¶ 13).[7] Throughout his time on the project, Feraci had assisted crews using the same hoisting method with smaller pipes (Docs. 209, ¶ 15; 216, ¶¶ 6–7).[8] Waynick operated the trac-hoe while Feraci and Melvin worked as the ground personnel (Doc. 209, ¶ 20). The men moved one of the concrete pipes without incident; however, while moving the second pipe, Feraci suffered injury (Docs.209, ¶¶ 21–22, 214, ¶ 13). Feraci and Melvin had been standing away from the trac-hoe but somehow Feraci became crushed between the second concrete pipe and either the trac-hoe or the hoist cable (Docs. 209, ¶ 22; 214, ¶¶ 13–14).[9] As a result of the accident, CNA Insurance, TMG's worker's compensation carrier, voluntarily paid workers' compensation benefits to Feraci (Docs. 209, ¶ 25; 214, ¶¶ 6–7; 216, ¶ 20).

In Plaintiffs' amended complaint, Plaintiffs aver that the causes of Feraci's injuries were due to the Defendants' "willful and wanton disregard" for Feraci's safety, as well as the following "grossly negligent acts and omissions:"

1. Inadequate supervision over the operations, work environment, and personnel[;]
2. Too many employees unaware of each other's movement and activity[;]
3. Very congested area requiring additional oversight, traffic management, and safety monitoring[;]
4. Inadequately trained operator concerning the safety aspect of ground personnel[;]
5. Inexperienced and/or inadequately trained laborers[;]
6. No established procedures or policies for visual contact at all times with ground personnel assigned to the operator[;]

7. *1203* Improperly adjusted mirrors on the trackhoe equipment to allow visual contact with ground personnel[;]

8. Limited visibility of equipment operator with ground personnel and structures[;]

9. No safety meeting was held before this operation addressing the relevant safety precautions of the job[;]

10. Toolbox safety meetings were not conducted regularly or documented at the worksite[;]

11. Inadequate hazard identification of operations, work tasks, personnel assignments, and the worksite[;]

12. Failure to perform equipment safety inspections of equipment and worksites[;]

13. Failure to provide ground spotters to eliminate blind equipment operations[;]

14. Failure to maintain the working environment, equipment, machinery, supplies, and training for their employees to meet all state and federal Occupational Safety and Health Administration (OSHA) standards[;]

15. Failure to inspect, review, test, and approve safety procedures prior to commencing the subject operation[;]

16. Failure to provide proper supervision and safety monitoring of the task[;]

17. Failure to provide safe work practices and use of protective equipment imposed by controlling federal, state and local government, and for all applicable laws, ordinances, and regulations related to environmental, equipment, machinery, and all other matters which affected the assigned employee's safety[;]

18. Failure to provide a safe work environment involving heavy equipment, human beings, and construction materials and facilities[;]

19. Failure to implement safety policies and procedures[;]

20. Inadequate risk protection and prevention[;]

21. Inadequate training, generally[;]

22. Failure to provide a competent worksite superintendent.

(Doc. 55, ¶ 7A). In addition, Plaintiffs also generally refer to Defendants' knowing and reckless conduct, but they are not specific as to what and whose conduct demonstrates knowledge and recklessness.[10]

II. MOTIONS FOR SUMMARY JUDGMENT

A. STANDARD

Summary judgment is appropriate where the pleadings, depositions, answers to interrogatories, admissions on file, and affidavits, if any, show that no genuine issue of material fact exists and that the party moving is entitled to judgment as a matter of law. *See Celotex Corp. v. Catrett, *1204* 477 U.S. 317, 322, 106 S.Ct. 2548, 2552, 91 L.Ed.2d 265 (1986). The substantive law will identify which facts are material and which are irrelevant. See Anderson v. Liberty Lobby, Inc., 477 U.S. 242, 248, 106 S.Ct. 2505, 2510, 91 L.Ed.2d 202 (1986). An issue of fact is material if it is a*

legal element of the claim under the applicable substantive law which might affect
the outcome of the case. See id.

At the summary judgment stage, a court's function is not to weigh the evidence to determine the truth of the matter, but to determine whether a genuine issue of fact exists for trial. *See Anderson, 477 U.S. at 249, 106 S.Ct. at 2510.* A genuine issue exists only if sufficient evidence is presented favoring the nonmoving party for a jury to return a verdict for that party. *See id.* "If reasonable minds could differ on the inferences arising from undisputed facts, then a court should deny summary judgment." *Miranda v. B & B Cash Grocery Store, Inc.,*975 F.2d 1518, 1534 (11th Cir.1992) (citing *Mercantile Bank & Trust Co. v. Fidelity & Deposit Co.,* 750 F.2d 838, 841 (11th Cir.1985)).

When assessing the sufficiency of the evidence in favor of the nonmoving party, the court must view all the evidence, and all factual inferences reasonably drawn from the evidence, in the light most favorable to the nonmoving party. *See Hairston v. Gainesville Sun Publ'g Co., 9 F.3d 913, 918 (11th Cir.1993).* The court is not obliged, however, to deny summary judgment for the moving party when the evidence favoring the nonmoving party is merely colorable or is not significantly probative. *See Anderson, 477 U.S. at 249, 106 S.Ct. at 2510.* A mere scintilla of evidence in support of the nonmoving party's position will not suffice to demonstrate a material issue of genuine fact that precludes summary judgment. *See Walker v. Darby, 911 F.2d 1573, 1577 (11th Cir.1990).*

B. WORKERS' COMPENSATION IMMUNITY UNDER FLORIDA LAW

In the current motions for summary judgment, all Defendants request the Court to grant summary judgment in their favor under the immunity provision of Florida's workers' compensation statute. *See* FLA. STAT. § 440.11(1) (2002). In response, Plaintiffs claim that the intentional tort exception to workers' compensation immunity applies to preclude summary judgment.

"Florida's Workers' Compensation Law, codified in chapter 440, Florida Statutes, protects workers and compensates them for injuries in the workplace, without examination of fault in the causation of the injury." *Gerth v. Wilson,* 774 So.2d 5, 6 (Fla. 2nd DCA 2000). The Florida legislature intended the statute to provide "quick and efficient delivery of disability and medical benefits to an injured worker and to facilitate the worker's return to gainful reemployment at a reasonable cost to the employer." FLA. STAT. § 440.015 (2002). "Essentially, under this no-fault system, the employee gives up a right to a common-law action for negligence in exchange for strict liability and the rapid recovery of benefits." *Turner v. PCR, Inc.,* 754 So.2d 683, 686 (Fla.2000) (*citing United Parcel Service v. Welsh, 659 So.2d 1234, 1235 (Fla. 5th DCA 1995)*; 2 Arthur Larson & Lex K. Larson, *Larson's Workers' Compensation* § 65.10 (Desk ed.1999)). "The goal of this policy is to avoid lawsuits at the outset, not simply to prevent adverse verdicts against employers and coworkers at the end of lengthy litigation." *Fleetwood Homes of Florida, Inc. v. Reeves,* 833 So.2d 857, 864 (Fla. 2nd DCA 2002).

For those who fall within the statute's purview, "workers' compensation is the exclusive remedy for 'accident[al] injury or *1205* death arising out of work performed in the course and the scope of the employment.' "*Turner,* 754 So.2d at 686 (*quoting* FLA. STAT. § 440.09(1) (1997)). Thus, absent an excepted circumstance, Florida's Workers' Compensation Law generally protects employers from liability for an employee's injuries beyond the workers' compensation benefits. "At the same time …, the statutory scheme itself explicitly recognizes the liability of co-employees [and supervisors] to injured employees under certain limited conditions, including intentional or reckless actions." *Id.* (citing FLA. STAT. § 440.11(1) (1997)).

1. Intentional Tort Exception to Workers' Compensation Immunity

"Notwithstanding the general recognition of tort immunity for employers, the [Supreme Court of Florida] has recognized an intentional tort exception to the worker's compensation statutory scheme." *Turner,* 754 So.2d at 686 (citations omitted). Florida Workers' Compensation Law does not shield an employer from liability for intentional torts against an employee. *See id.* (citations omitted). Under the intentional torts exception, the employee must show that the employer "either [1.] 'exhibite[d] a deliberate intent to injure *or* [2.] engage[d] in conduct which [was] substantially certain to result in injury or death.'" *Id.* at 687 (citation omitted) (emphasis in original); *see also McClanahan,* 854 So.2d at 795; *Gerth,* 774 So.2d at 6.

234When determining whether the substantial certainty standard has been met, the employer's conduct is evaluated under an objective standard. *See Turner,* 754 So.2d at 688–89; *see also McClanahan,* 854 So.2d at 795. "[A]n analysis of the circumstances in a case [is] required to determine whether a reasonable person would understand that the employer's conduct was 'substantially certain' to result in injury or death to the employee." *Turner,* 754 So.2d at 688. When determining substantial certainty, the employer's actual intent is not controlling. *See id.* In order to prove substantial certainty, a plaintiff employee must demonstrate "that the employer engaged in conduct that is at least worse than 'gross negligence.'" "*McClanahan,* 854 So.2d at 795–96; *see also Turner,* 754 So.2d at 687 n. 4; *Tinoco v. Resol, Inc.,* 783 So.2d 309, 310–11 (Fla. 3rd DCA 2001).[11]

There have been several cases in Florida post-*Turner* applying the "substantial certainty" *1206* standard. In the *Tinoco* case, a Florida court determined that, under factual circumstances similar to the instant case, the plaintiff failed to prove the establishment of the intentional tort exception. In *Tinoco,* the plaintiff-employee brought an intentional tort action against his employer for injuries he sustained in a work-related accident. *See Tinoco, 783 So.2d at 310.* In defense, the defendant-employer asserted that it was immune from suit on the basis of workers' compensation immunity. *See id.* On the day of the accident, the plaintiff was working as a pipe fitter, and his work crew was digging a trench and installing pipe in the trench. *See id.* The crew was using a new excavator which had a defect that caused it to lurch forward two or three feet every time the operator tried to move it, and after that initial lurch, the excavator would operate properly. *See id.* The foreman knew of the defect, but concluded that it would be safe to use the machine so long as employees stayed at least three feet away from its forward path. *See id.* The entire crew knew of the defect, and prior to the plaintiff's injury, the excavator had been operated twenty-six or twenty-seven times without incident. *See id.* The plaintiff was in the operator's blind spot, so when the plaintiff stepped in front of the excavator to assist the lowering of a pipe, the operator did not see him. *See id.* As a result, the excavator lurched forward crushing the plaintiff's foot. *See id.*

The trial court in *Tinoco* granted summary judgement in favor of the employer on the basis of workers' compensation immunity. On appeal, the Third District Court of Appeal of Florida affirmed the trial court's ruling on the basis of *Turner. See id. at 310–11.* The court determined that "the facts of this case do not show that the employer exhibite[d] a deliberate intent to injure or engaged in conduct which [was] substantially certain to result in injury or death." *Id.* at 310 (*quoting Turner*, 754 So.2d at 687 n. 4). In addition, the district court noted that "the circumstances here demonstrate negligence, [b]ut under the case law, a showing of negligence, or even gross negligence, is not enough." *Id.* at 310–11 (citing *Turner*, 754 So.2d at 687 & n. 4).[12]

*1207 The case of *Sierra v. Associated Marine Institutes, Inc.*, 850 So.2d 582 (Fla. 2nd DCA 2003), found to the contrary, albeit on a very different set of facts. In *Sierra*, a Florida court determined that the plaintiff pled sufficient facts to preclude the employers' motion to dismiss on workers' compensation immunity grounds. *See id.* Defendant Big Cypress Wilderness Institute, Inc. ("Big Cypress"), contracted with the State of Florida to operate a juvenile detention facility, known as a "boot camp." *See id.* at 585. The juveniles, aged fourteen to eighteen, who were housed there had a history of serious felony offenses. *See id.* They had been placed in the facility due to the risk that they posed to public safety. *See id.*[13] The youths had also been assessed as flight risks; however, before assigning the deceased to guard the youths, the boot camp failed to inform him of the flight risk. *See id.* The boot camp assigned the deceased alone to oversee the youth's performance of heavy manual labor in a secluded area off of the camp's grounds. *See id.* During a break at 8:25 p.m., the youths struck the deceased in the head with their manual labor tools, machetes and a pickaxe. *See id.*

The plaintiff, the wife of the deceased, brought a wrongful death action against her husband's employers, Big Cypress and its parent company, Associated Marine Institutes, Inc. *See id. at 585.* The defendants filed a motion to dismiss arguing that they were shielded from liability under the workers' compensation immunity doctrine. *See id.* The trial court agreed with the defendants and dismissed the complaint with prejudice. *See id.* On appeal, the Second District Court of Appeal for Florida reversed the dismissal of the plaintiff's complaint. *See id.* According to the court, the plaintiff's complaint alleged facts sufficient to except the suit from immunity under the intentional tort exception. *See id.* Based on the facts as plead, the court determined that the defendants should have known that there was a substantial certainty that sending a new counselor alone to guard two serious, escape-risk felons who would be using potentially dangerous tools would result in the counselor's injury or death. *See id.* at 589.

2. Culpable Negligence of a Supervisor/Manager

As the Court indicated above, employers are not the only defendants who are clothed with workers' compensation immunity. Supervisors are also entitled to the same immunity from suit to which the employer is entitled. *See* FLA. STAT. § 440.11(1) (2002). Section 440.11(1), Florida Statutes, provides, in pertinent part:

The same immunity provisions enjoyed by an employer shall also apply to any ... supervisor ... who in the course and scope of his or her duties acts in a managerial or policymaking capacity and *1208 the conduct which caused the alleged injury arose within the course and scope of said managerial or policymaking duties and was not a violation of law, whether or not a violation was charged, for which the maximum penalty which may be imposed does not exceed 60 days' imprisonment as set forth in s. 775.082.

Id. Under § 775.082, Florida Statutes, the only crimes with penalties exceeding 60 days are first-degree misdemeanors. *See Kennedy,* 650 So.2d at 1106. Thus, "when evaluating whether the negligent conduct of [a] managerial [employee] rises to a level sufficient to abrogate their statutory immunity, such negligence must be equivalent to a violation of law constituting a first-degree misdemeanor or higher crime." *Id.* "Thus, pursuant to subsection 440.11(1), there would be no workers' compensation immunity for a managerial employee who, through culpable negligence, actively inflicted injury, but there would be immunity for a managerial employee who passively exposed an employee to injury even if the employee [were culpably negligent]." *Id.; see also Emergency One,* 652 So.2d at 1235. "Culpable negligence is negligence of a gross and flagrant character which evinces a reckless disregard for the safety of others. It is that entire want of care which raises a presumption of indifference to consequences." *Killingsworth v. State,* 584 So.2d 647, 648 (Fla. 1st DCA 1991) *(citing State v. Greene, 348 So.2d 3 (Fla.1977)).*[14]

C. Defendants' Individual Motions for Summary Judgment

1. TMG Staffing Services, Inc.'s Motion for Summary Judgment

In its motion for summary judgment, TMG argues that it is entitled to summary judgment for three reasons: (1) as Feraci's co-employer, it is clothed with workers' compensation immunity for Plaintiffs' various negligence claims; (2) Plaintiffs' evidence is not sufficient to prove an intentional tort; and (3) as an employee leasing company, TMG is not vicariously liable for its leased employees. In response, Plaintiffs claim to have provided evidence sufficient to meet the requirements of the intentional tort exception. Plaintiffs maintain that TMG exhibited "an intentional or wanton disregard" for Feraci's safety by failing to properly manage safety, risk, and hazard control at the project site prior to Feraci's accident.

1209 a. Workers' Compensation Immunity

5In response to TMG's motion, Plaintiffs do not dispute TMG's assertion that it is entitled to workers' compensation immunity for Plaintiffs' negligence claims. As previously noted by the Court, workers' compensation is the exclusive remedy for an injured employee whose injury arose out of work performed in the course and scope of his employment. TMG admits to being a co-employer of Feraci, and TMG leased him to P & S to work at Hurlburt Field. P & S had subcontracted to perform the underground installation of concrete pipe at the project site, and when Feraci was injured, he was assisting other P & S employees in the movement of concrete pipes from one area of the project site to another. Thus, Feraci's injury arose out of work performed in the scope of his employment. In addition, TMG provided workers' compensation insurance for Feraci. As a result, TMG is entitled to workers' compensation immunity and is entitled to summary judgment as a matter of law as to Plaintiffs' negligence claims.

b. Intentional Tort Exception

In response to TMG's motion, Plaintiffs argue that they have brought forth sufficient evidence to meet the intentional tort exception to TMG's workers' compensation immunity defense. Further, Plaintiffs claim that TMG reserved the right of direction and control over the management of safety, risk, and hazard control over its leased employees working at the project site. Because of the retention of that right, Plaintiffs assert that TMG may be held vicariously liable for punitive damages for the intentional torts of its employees Waynick and Resmondo.

6As previously noted by the Court, an employer is not entitled to workers' compensation immunity for intentional torts against an employee. To meet this intentional tort exception, Plaintiffs must show that TMG either exhibited a deliberate intent to injure Feraci or engaged in conduct that was substantially certain to result in injury to Feraci. First, there is no evidence in the record to demonstrate that TMG exhibited a deliberate intent to injure Feraci. Second, there is also no evidence in the record to demonstrate that TMG engaged in conduct which was "substantially certain" to result in injury to Feraci despite Plaintiffs' assertion that TMG did not manage safety, risk, and hazard controls regarding its employees at the project site.

TMG is an employee leasing company that is statutorily required to retain "a right of direction and control over management of safety, risk, and hazard control at the worksite or sites affecting its leased employees." FLA. STAT. § 468.525(4)(e) (2002). In keeping with the statutory requirement, TMG included in its employee leasing contract with P & S a clause which explicitly reserves such a right (Doc. 140, Ex. F, Service Agreement between P & S and TMG, p. 2, § 4, ¶ 1). However, TMG's reservation of that right did not automatically create an obligation on behalf of TMG to exercise that right. At most, it may have created a duty to inspect the project site to ensure that P & S was complying with federal, state, and local safety regulations. Assuming *arguendo* that TMG had such a duty to inspect the safety of the project site, any failure to inspect would amount to either negligence or gross negligence, not reckless or wanton conduct.

Furthermore, Plaintiffs concede that there is no evidence in the record to demonstrate that TMG actually exercised the retained right to direct and control the safety, risk, and hazard control at the project site. Assuming *arguendo* that there were facts to demonstrate TMG's exercise of that right, failure to comply with any ***1210*** duties imposed smacks of negligence, or maybe even gross negligence, tort claims which the Court has already determined cannot be brought against TMG. After analyzing the factual circumstances in this case, Plaintiffs have failed to demonstrate that a reasonable person would understand that TMG's conduct was "substantially certain" to result in injury to Feraci, and based on the evidence in the record, no reasonable jury could conclude otherwise.

In addition, Plaintiffs' argument that TMG is vicariously liable for potential punitive damages based on the conduct of its employees Waynick and Resmondo is equally unavailing. In their response to summary judgment, Plaintiffs cite *Carroll*

Air Systems, Inc. v. Greenbaum, 629 So.2d 914 (Fla. 4th DCA 1993), to support the proposition that TMG is vicariously liable. The court in *Carroll* stated that "an employer may be held liable for vicarious punitive damages under respondeat superior when, in addition to the willful and wanton misconduct by the employee, there is independent fault or negligence on the part of the employer." *Id.* at 917 (citing *Mercury Motors Express, Inc. v. Smith,* 393 So.2d 545 (Fla.1981)). *Carroll,* however, is not analogous to the case at hand. The employer in *Carroll* was held liable for punitive damages to a third-party (*i.e.* non-employees) for injuries which had been caused by an employee. *See Carroll, 629 So.2d at 917.* In that case, workers' compensation did not factor into the liability equation.

7In the case at hand, Feraci, the injured party, was not a third-party outside of the employment relationship. Rather, he was an employee of TMG, and the accident that injured him was covered by Florida's Workers' Compensation Law. Furthermore, it appears that *Carroll* 's vicarious liability rule could not be properly applied to a workers' compensation case. Workers' compensation immunity, when applicable, precludes an employer's liability for negligence in relation to an employee's injury or death. If *Carroll* 's vicarious liability rule could be successfully applied to an employer who is otherwise entitled to worker's compensation immunity, then the employer's own negligence would cause it to be vicariously liable for punitive damages. That would be an illogical result and a backdoor approach for holding an employer liable for negligence in direct contravention of the spirit of Florida's Workers' Compensation Laws.[15]

2. P & S Construction Services, Inc.'s Motion for Summary Judgment

In its motion for summary judgment, P & S argues that it is entitled to summary judgment as to all of Plaintiffs' claims based upon the doctrines of workers' compensation immunity and election of remedies. In response, Plaintiffs argue that their evidence establishes the requirements of the intentional tort exception and that the election of remedies doctrine is inapplicable to the instant case.

a. Workers' Compensation Immunity

In response to P & S's motion, Plaintiffs do not dispute P & S's assertion that it is entitled to workers' compensation immunity for Plaintiffs' negligence claims. As previously noted by the Court, workers' compensation is the exclusive remedy for an injured employee whose injury arose out of work performed in the course and scope of the employment. P & S admits to being a co-employer of Feraci, and Feraci *1211* was leased to P & S to work at Hurlburt Field. As the Court previously explained, Feraci's injury arose out of work performed in the scope of his employment. Therefore, P & S is entitled to workers' compensation immunity and is entitled to summary judgment as a matter of law regarding Plaintiffs' negligence claims.

b. Intentional Tort Exception

In response to P & S's motion, Plaintiffs argue that they have brought forth sufficient evidence to meet the intentional tort exception to workers' compensation immunity. According to Plaintiffs, the facts of this case "indicate a deliberate, intentional, and gross disregard for safety," and the "composite of circumstances was substantially certain to result in death or injury to Feraci." In addition, Plaintiff's argue that P & S is vicariously liable for punitive damages based upon certain actions of its employees.

As previously noted by the Court, an employer is not entitled to workers' compensation immunity for intentional torts against an employee. To meet this intentional tort exception, Plaintiffs must show that P & S either exhibited a deliberate intent to injure Feraci or engaged in conduct that was substantially certain to result in injury to Feraci. First, there is no evidence in the record to demonstrate that P & S exhibited a deliberate intent to injure Feraci. Second, there is also no evidence in the record to demonstrate that P & S engaged in conduct which was "substantially certain" to result in injury to Feraci.

8Plaintiffs attempt to join together twenty-two alleged "grossly negligent actions or omissions," which are listed on pages 6 and 7 of this Order, to maintain that the "composite of the circumstances" was substantially certain to cause injury or death to Feraci. In other words, Plaintiffs are trying to stack numerous instances of alleged negligent (or even grossly negligent) conduct by P & S to arrive at the conclusion that Feraci's injury was substantially certain to result. The Second District Court of Appeal of Florida has expressly rejected such a position. *See Fleetwood Homes, 833 So.2d at 868–69.* In *Fleetwood Homes,* the court stated that "we do not believe that the supreme court in *Turner* intended to allow a plaintiff to add together small risks of injury in order to reach a combined total where the likelihood of injury to some employee sometime was substantially certain." *Id.* Therefore, assuming *arguendo* that the alleged twenty-two "grossly negligent acts or omissions" occurred, Plaintiffs cannot lump them together to demonstrate substantial certainty. At most, those acts or omissions would demonstrate gross negligence. As a result, after analyzing the factual circumstances in this case, the Court finds that Plaintiffs have failed to demonstrate that a reasonable person would understand that P & S's conduct was "substantially certain" to injure Feraci. Based on the evidence in the record, no reasonable jury could conclude otherwise.[16]

In addition, Plaintiffs' argument that P & S is vicariously liable for potential punitive damages for Resmondo's deliberately allowing an intoxicated Waynick to operate the trac-hoe is equally unavailing. In their response to summary judgment, Plaintiffs cite *Carroll Air Systems, Inc. v. Greenbaum,* 629 So.2d 914 (Fla. 4th DCA 1993), to support the proposition that TMG is vicariously liable. For reasons already stated by the Court, *Carroll* is not applicable to this case. Furthermore, the evidence **1212* in the record does not create any question about whether Waynick was under the influence of drugs on the morning of the accident. Thus, there is no evidence demonstrating that Resmondo deliberately allowed Waynick to operate the trac-hoe while Waynick was under the influence of drugs.

3. Grundy Marine Construction Company's Motion for Summary Judgement

In its motion for summary judgment, Grundy argues that it is entitled to summary judgment for two reasons: workers' compensation immunity, and Plaintiffs' failure to establish the intentional tort exception to Grundy's immunity. In response, Plaintiffs argue that the evidence in this case indicates Grundy's "intentional and gross disregard for safety." According to Plaintiffs, that evidence is sufficient to establish the intentional tort exception to Grundys' workers' compensation immunity. Additionally, Plaintiffs assert that Grundy is vicariously liable for the tortious intentional acts of its subcontractor, P & S.

a. Workers' Compensation Immunity

In its motion, Grundy argues that Plaintiffs' negligence claims against it are barred by Florida's workers' compensation immunity doctrine. Even though Grundy is not a direct employer of Feraci, Grundy asserts that, as a general contractor, it is a "statutory employer" under Section 440.10(1)(b), Florida Statutes. Section 440.10(1)(b) provides that:

In case a contractor sublets any part or parts of his contract work to a subcontractor or subcontractors, all of the employees of such contractor and subcontractor or subcontractors engaged on such contract work shall be deemed to be employed in one and the same business or establishment; and the contractor shall be liable for, and shall secure, the payment of compensation to all such employees except to employees of a subcontractor who has secured such payment.

FLA. STAT. § 440.10(1)(b) (2002). Thus, "[a] contractor may be immune from suit where workers' compensation has been paid on behalf of the subcontractor." *Carnegie Gardens Nursing Center v. Banyai,* 852 So.2d 374, 375–76 (Fla. 5th DCA 2003) (citing *Yero v. Miami–Dade County,* 838 So.2d 686, 687 (Fla. 3rd DCA 2003); FLA. STAT. § 440.1(1)(b)). In the case at hand, Grundy was the general contractor of the project, and Grundy hired P & S as a subcontractor to work at Hurlburt Field. P & S secured the workers' compensation benefits for Feraci in the employee leasing agreement between P & S and TMG, and TMG provided those benefits for Feraci. Therefore, the subcontract between Grundy and P & S made Grundy a statutory employer under § 440.10(1)(b), Florida Statutes, thereby entitling Grundy to workers' compensation immunity.[17] As a result, Grundy is entitled to summary judgment as to Plaintiffs' negligence claims.

b. Intentional Tort Exception

In response to Grundy's motion, Plaintiffs argue that they have brought forth sufficient evidence to meet the intentional tort exception to workers' compensation immunity. According to Plaintiffs, the evidence in this case indicates "an intentional or gross disregard" by Grundy for Feraci's safety. In addition, Plaintiffs maintain that Grundy is vicariously liable for the intentional torts of its subcontractors.

*1213 As previously noted by the Court, an employer is not entitled to workers' compensation immunity for intentional torts against an employee. To meet this intentional tort exception, Plaintiffs must show that Grundy either exhibited a deliberate intent to injure Feraci or engaged in conduct that was substantially certain to result in injury to Feraci. First, there is no evidence in the record to demonstrate that Grundy exhibited a deliberate intent to injure Feraci. Second, there is also no evidence in the record to demonstrate that Grundy engaged in conduct which was "substantially certain" to result in injury to Feraci.

Plaintiffs attempt to join twenty-two alleged "grossly negligent actions or omissions," which are listed on pages 6 and 7 of this Order, by Grundy to maintain that the "composite of the circumstances" was substantially certain to cause injury or death to Feraci. As previously explained in this Order, Florida law does not allow Plaintiffs to accumulate several negligent (or grossly negligent) acts or omissions to demonstrate substantial certainty.[18] As a result, after analyzing the factual circumstances in this case, Plaintiffs have failed to demonstrate that a reasonable person would understand that Grundy's conduct was "substantially certain" to result in injury to Feraci. Based on the evidence in the record, no reasonable jury could conclude otherwise.

In addition, Plaintiffs argue (without legal citations in support) that Grundy is vicariously liable for the intentional torts of its subcontractor, P & S. Assuming Grundy could be vicariously liable in such a situation, no vicarious liability would exist in the instant case. The Court has already determined that the evidence in the record does not support a claim for an intentional tort against P & S; therefore, there is no intentional tort claim for which Grundy could be held vicariously liable.

4. Total Leasing Company, Inc.

In its motion for summary judgment, Total asserts that, despite Plaintiffs' contentions to the contrary, Total is not a co-employer of Feraci. Total argues that, in the event if it is considered an employer, it is nonetheless entitled to workers' compensation immunity. In response, Plaintiffs maintain that Total is a co-employer and that Total's immunity is abrogated by the intentional tort exception.

a. Workers' Compensation Immunity

As the Court determined in footnote 4 of this Order, Total is not an employer of Feraci and is not entitled to workers' compensation immunity. Because Total is not immune from suit, there must be sufficient evidence in the record to support Plaintiffs' intentional tort and negligence claims against Total.

At the outset, the Court notes that Plaintiffs do not specify which of their intentional tort allegations apply to Total. However, it is of no consequence because the very nature of an intentional tort requires Plaintiffs to prove Total had: (1) an intent to offer injury to Feraci by force; (2) an intent to injure Feraci; or (3) acted in a manner that amounted to "exaggerated recklessness" as to Feraci's safety. *See e.g. Sullivan v. Atlantic Federal Savings & Loan Association, 454 So.2d 52* (defining the elements of assault and battery); *Caprio v. American Airlines, Inc.,* 848 F.Supp. 1528, 1534 (M.D.Fla.1994) ("In order to submit a claim for punitive damages based upon intentional torts to the jury, Plaintiff must make a threshold showing that Defendant's conduct approaches a level *1214* that 'transcends the level of simple negligence, and even gross negligence, … and enters the realm of wanton intentionality, exaggerated recklessness, or such an extreme degree of negligence as to parallel an intentional and reprehensible act.") (*quoting American Cyanamid Co. v. Roy, 498 So.2d 859, 861 (Fla.1986)*); *see also* 55 Fla. Jur.2d *Torts* § 5 (West 2004). There is no evidence in the record to demonstrate that Total had an intent to either offer to cause harm or to cause harm to Feraci, or had acted with exaggerated recklessness.[19] As a result, Plaintiffs cannot maintain a cause of action against Total for an intentional tort, and based on the evidence in the record, no reasonable jury could conclude otherwise.

In addition to the undefined intentional tort claims, Plaintiffs' amended complaint asserts claims for both negligence and gross negligence. "To sustain a cause of action for negligence, the burden of proof is on the plaintiff to establish that: (1) the defendant had a duty to protect the plaintiff; (2) the defendant breached that duty; and (3) the defendant's breach was the proximate cause of the plaintiff's injuries and resulting damages." *Cooper Hotel Services, Inc. v. MacFarland,* 662 So.2d 710, 712 (Fla. 2nd DCA 1995) (citing *Lake Parker Mall, Inc. v. Carson,* 327 So.2d 121, 123 (Fla. 2nd DCA 1976)). In its motion for summary judgment, Total argues that Plaintiffs cannot maintain a cause of action against Total for negligence, because there is no evidentiary support in the record that Total owed a duty of care to Feraci.

"The duty element of negligence focuses on whether the defendant's conduct forseeably created a broader 'zone of risk' that poses a general threat of harm to others." *Whitt v. Silverman,* 788 So.2d 210, 216 (Fla.2001) (*quoting McCain v. Florida Power Corp., 593 So.2d 500, 502–03 (Fla.1992)*). "Foreseeability clearly is crucial in defining the scope of the general duty placed on every person to avoid negligent acts or omissions." *McCain,* 593 So.2d at 503. "Florida, like other jurisdictions, recognizes that a legal duty will arise whenever a human endeavor creates a generalized and foreseeable risk of harming others." *Id.* "Where a defendant's conduct creates a *foreseeable zone of risk,* the law generally will recognize a duty placed upon defendant either to lessen the risk or see that sufficient precautions are taken to protect others from the harm that the risk poses. *Id.* (*quoting Kaisner v. Kolb, 543 So.2d 732, 735 (Fla.1989)* (emphasis in original)). The Supreme Court of Florida has also noted that every risk need not be set out in a statute or by case law in order to give rise to a duty of care:

[E]ach defendant who creates a risk is required to exercise prudent foresight whenever others may be injured as a result. This requirement of reasonable, general foresight is the core of the duty element. For these same reasons, duty exists as a matter of law and is not a factual question for the jury to decide: Duty is the standard of conduct given to the jury for gauging the defendant's factual conduct. As a corollary, the trial and appellate courts cannot find a lack of duty if a foreseeable zone of risk more likely than not was created by the defendant.

*1215 Whitt, 788 So.2d at 217 (*quoting McCain,* 593 So.2d at 503).

10As previously noted, Total is not a co-employer of Feraci. Total is an independent contractor that is engaged in the business of marketing employee management services. In its contract with TMG, Total merely agreed to solicit client companies desiring risk management, human resources, employee benefits, and payroll management on behalf of TMG. Total in fact solicited P & S, a client company, on behalf of TMG, and TMG leased its employees to P & S to work on the project at Hurlburt Field. There is no evidence in the record to indicate that Total owed any duty to Feraci. Plaintiffs have not demonstrated that Total actually controlled anyone or anything at the project site at any point in time (especially on the day of the accident). Further, Plaintiffs have not demonstrated that Total was legally obligated in any manner to control safety at the job site. Total located P & S, a client company who was in need of employees to work on the project, and put P & S into contact with TMG. Putting the two companies in contact with each other did not create a duty for Total to protect Feraci's (or any other TMG employees') safety, and Total's actions did not create a foreseeable zone of risk. As a result, based on the evidence in the record, Total owed no duty to Feraci, and Total is entitled to summary judgment as a matter of law on all of Plaintiffs' negligence claims.[20]

Assuming *arguendo* that Total is a co-employer of Feraci, Total would be entitled to workers' compensation immunity for Plaintiffs' negligence claims for the same reasons as P & S and TMG. As to the intentional tort exception, Plaintiffs have failed to establish the requirements necessary to avoid workers' compensation immunity. As the Court has already explained in this Order, even assuming that all twenty-two alleged actions or omissions were committed by Total, they would amount to nothing more than gross negligence. Since the intentional tort exception requires Plaintiffs to demonstrate more than gross negligence, Plaintiffs would be unable to maintain an intentional tort action against Total.

5.   Ronnie Resmondo's Motion for Summary Judgment

In his motion for summary judgment, Resmondo argues that, as an employee of P & S, he is immune from suit for Feraci's injuries. Resmondo was an employee of P & S who worked in a supervisory capacity at the project site. At the time of Feraci's accident, Resmondo was Feraci's supervisor. On the day of the accident, Resmondo had received orders from Grundy to move four 48–eight inch elliptical concrete pipes from one location to another. Acting in the course and scope of his employment, Resmondo delegated the job to Feraci, Melvin, and Waynick. Because Resmondo's boss, Steve Smith, had ordered the removal of the Fiat Ellis loader, which had been previously used to move the concrete pipe, Feraci, Melvin, and Waynick had to use the trac-hoe. Waynick had experience operating the trac-hoe, albeit not for the movement of the 48–inch elliptical concrete pipes, and Feraci had experience in moving similar concrete pipes as a ground ***1216*** person with the Fiat Ellis loader. In addition, Feraci had experience moving pipe of smaller size with a trachoe using the exact same procedure as was employed on the day of the accident.

11Plaintiffs argue that Resmondo's culpable negligence under the facts of this case abrogates his immunity. First, Plaintiffs claim that engaging in and allowing others to engage in drug use at the project site amounts to culpable negligence. Plaintiffs assert that Resmondo failed to have Waynick, the operator, screened for drugs immediately following the accident. They also maintain that Resmondo "committed the criminal act of falsely completing a document required by OSHA regarding site drug use." As already noted by the Court in footnote 6 of this Order, there is no evidence that either Resmondo or Waynick were under the influence of illegal drugs on the day of Feraci's accident. Thus, Resmondo is not culpably negligent for the use of drugs himself or for allowing others to use drugs on the job site.[21]

Second, Plaintiffs claim that Resmondo's failure to ensure ground communication between Waynick and the ground personnel, Feraci and Melvin, through the use of a spotter, amounts to culpable negligence. There is conflicting evidence in the record regarding whether or not a spotter was used at the time of Feraci's accident; however, construing the evidence in a light most favorable to Plaintiffs, the Court will assume Resmondo failed to check whether or not a spotter was being used before the pipe moving operation began. At most, that failure amounts to nothing more than simple negligence. It is not negligence of a gross and flagrant character which evinces a reckless disregard for the safety of others.

Third, Plaintiffs argue that Resmondo had a duty to implement a hazard analysis to determine the location of possible pinch points, *i.e.* areas where workers could be pinched between construction equipment. Plaintiffs also maintain that Feraci was never trained how to recognize such pinch points. Plaintiffs assert that such hazard analysis was required by OSHA and that TMG was responsible for ensuring that P & S adhered to OSHA regulations. There is no evidence in the record demonstrating that Resmondo was in fact responsible for implementing a pinch point analysis and for training Feraci on how to recognize such pinch points. TMG's safety professional, Frank Ruckles, testified that, to his knowledge, the hazard analysis was performed by Grundy Marine. Plaintiffs cannot demonstrate that Resmondo had a responsibility regarding the implementation of hazard analysis and the training of Feraci on how to recognize pinch points. Thus, Plaintiffs cannot show that any negligence by Resmondo was of a gross and flagrant character so as to evince a reckless disregard for the safety of others.[22] *1217* As a result, Resmondo was not culpably negligent, and based on the evidence in the record, no reasonable jury could conclude otherwise.[23] Accordingly, Resmondo's workers' compensation immunity is not abrogated, and he is entitled to judgment as a matter of law.[24]

Accordingly, it is hereby ordered:

1. Defendant TOTAL LEASING COMPANY, INC.'s motion for summary judgment (*see* doc. 199) is GRANTED.
2. Defendant LEDR GROUP, INC., d/b/a TMG STAFFING SERVICES, INC.'s motion for summary judgment (*see* doc. 205) is GRANTED.
3. Defendant GRUNDY MARINE CONSTRUCTION COMPANY's motion for summary judgment (*see* doc. 207) is GRANTED.
4. Defendant P & S CONSTRUCTION SERVICES, INC.'s motion for summary judgment (*see* doc. 213) is GRANTED.
5. Defendant RONNIE RESMONDO's motion for summary judgment (*see* doc. 215) is GRANTED.
6. Consistent with this order, the Clerk of Court is directed to enter final judgment as to all claims in favor of Defendants GRUNDY MARINE CONSTRUCTION COMPANY; P & S CONSTRUCTION SERVICES, INC.; TOTAL LEASING COMPANY, INC.; LEDR GROUP, INC., d/b/a TMG STAFFING SERVICES, INC.; and RONNIE RESMONDO. Plaintiffs shall take nothing by this action and go hence without day.
7. The Clerk of Court is directed to close the file in this case.

7 Case Law

Laws should be like clothes. They should be made to fit the people they are meant to serve.

Clarence Darrow

It usually takes a hundred years to make a law, and then, after it is done its work, it usually takes another hundred years to get rid of it.

Henry Ward Beecher

STUDENT LEARNING OBJECTIVES

1. Analyze and assess the process of developing case law.
2. Analyze and assess the court hierarchy and impact on case law.
3. Analyze and assess a Complaint and Answer.

Case law is "the aggregate of reported cases as forming a body of jurisprudence, or the law of a particular subject as evidenced or formed by the adjudged cases, in distinction to statutes, regulations, and other sources of law."[*] Although the executive and legislative branches "make" the laws and regulations, it is the judicial branch that interprets and applies the laws and regulations, Through the numerous and varied cases hear before the courts, case law has developed doctrines that provides guidance as to the application of a particular law or regulation.

Safety professionals should make the distinction between state and federal laws and courts. Federal courts interpret federal statutes and regulations and decide matters of federal common law. State courts decide state laws and statutes and establish rules for their specific state. Similarly, appellate courts hear appeal cases from the federal level, and state appellate courts hear state appeal cases. Trial court, or district court, both on the federal or state levels, is the initial entry level and handle the largest inflow of judicial business. On the state level in most states, the district courts not only handle the litigation but also maintain wills, deeds, and related documents. Some district courts have added family courts, drug courts, and related specialty courts to handle the volume of cases presented to the district court. (Note: Safety professionals should be aware that the trial court goes by different names in different states, including circuit court, district court, superior court, and courts of common pleas.)

Correlating to the federal court structure, all states possess a highest court or a court that has the last word in interpreting state laws. In most states, this court is called the state Supreme Court. However, safety professionals should be aware that the name of the court may vary depending on the state, such as the Supreme

---

[*] Black's Law dictionary.

Judicial Court in the state of Maine. It should also be noted that 10 states have only a two-tiered judicial system with only a trial court and Supreme Court. Other states have implemented an intermediate appellate court structure; however, safety professionals should be aware of the scope and jurisdiction of this level of courts. Most courts parallel the federal system with an automatic right of appeal and discretionary review at the Supreme Court level. In other states, the appellate courts are assigned appeal cases from the state Supreme Court. Additionally, safety professionals should be aware that in some states, such as Texas, have two supreme courts which are separated based on the subject matter of the appeal (civil or criminal) and in two states, namely Alabama and Tennessee, have courts of criminal appeal.

Case law is created on a daily basis by all levels of the court system. Generally, larger states produce more case law because there are more cases. Historically, courts would publish their decisions, and these decisions were bound into series of books according to the state, region, or particular court. These cases could be referenced by finding and citing the particular case with decisions by courts in the same state or region carrying more weight than cases outside of the state or region. Trial courts rarely publish their decisions; thus, most published decision are appellate decisions. State court decisions are published in a different book series that contains federal appellate and Supreme Court decisions. In general, trial courts decide how to apply the law and how appellate courts create and refine the law for future application by lower courts.

Historically, appellate cases were published according to court and region, such as the *Supreme Court Reporter, Federal Reporter, and South Western Reporter.* These reporter series are usually found in your local court house or law library. To find a case where the safety professional possessed the case cite (such as 3 Sup Court 85), the first step would be to find the reporter series (Sup. Court). The number 3 reflects the book number, and the number 85 would be the page number of the case. However, today there are several databases such as *Westlaw and Lexis-Nexis* as well as internet sources and individual state networks that can provide immediate access to federal and state cases.

Safety professionals should be cognizant of the hierarchy of courts (identified in Chapters 1 and 2), as well as the fact that case law encompasses both criminal as well as civil cases. In our civil system, litigation is the method through which disputes are settled between private parties. The courts have established laws and rules, known as criminal and civil procedure that serve as the mechanism through which to maintain order, present cases, and resolve matters. Upon resolution of the case, the case information is summarized and codified and then published, and this becomes the basis for what is known as "case law."

However, safety professionals should be aware that it may have been several years in a civil action from the time of the incident or injury to the time the case is finalized, summarized, and published. The initial step in most civil actions is when the injured person (or plaintiff) files a complaint against the other individual or organization (known as the defendant). A complaint is "†the original or initial pleading

---

* The major publisher of state court decisions is the West Group.
† Black's Law Dictionary.

by which an action is commenced under codes or Rules of Civil Procedure.... Such complaint (whether it be the original claim, counterclaim, cross-claim, or third-party claim) shall contain: (1) a short and plain statement of the grounds upon which the court's jurisdiction depends, unless the court already has jurisdiction and the claim needs no new grounds of jurisdiction to support it, (2) a short and plain statement of the claim showing that the pleader is entitled to relief, and (3) a demand for judgment for the relief to which he deems himself entitled. Relief in the alternative or of such different types may be demanded." This complaint document is required to be filed with the court and served upon the defendant. The defendant, as proscribed by the Rules of Civil Procedure, is required to provide a written Answer document within a specified time to the plaintiff and court and often denies the allegations. This starts the Discovery phase of most civil actions. Discovery "in a general sense, ascertainment of that which was previously unknown."[*] Discovery is usually by agreement of the parties or their legal counsel and can consist of a number of legal activities including, but not limited to depositions and interrogatories. In civil actions, as the facts of the situation emerge through the discovery process, settlement often results.

Deposition: "The testimony of a witness taken upon interrogatories, not in open court, but in pursuance of a commission to take testimony issued by a court, or under a general law or court rule on the subject, and reduced to writing and duly authenticated, and intended to be used upon the trial of a civil action or criminal prosecution. A discovery device by which one party asks oral questions of the other party or of a witness for the other party. The person who is deposed is called the deponent. The deposition is conducted under oath outside of the courtroom, usually in one of the lawyer's offices. A transcription (word-for-word account) is made of the deposition."[†]

Safety professional should be aware of the process utilized by most trial courts in civil actions. After a Complaint, Answer and the Discovery process (which can take several months or even years), the judge will rule on the motions by the parties and schedule a trial date. The parties will submit their witness lists and if a jury trial, the jury candidates will be notified. Prior to the trial, the jury pool will be assembled, and each side will be provided a number of strikes through which potential jury members can be removed by either side. The judge can also remove jury candidates for cause. Upon acquisition of the appropriate number of jurors and alternates, the judge will call the trial to order.

The process in a civil trial in most courts following the pattern of opening statements by both parties, witnesses for direct and cross examination, closing arguments by the parties, judges instructions, and the matter goes to the jury for deliberation and decision. Although the process sounds straightforward, the lawyers have dissected every component, witness, jury member, and question in an effort to win the case. The lawyers, a combination of artist, scholar, and persuader, conduct this process under the careful guidance and direction of the judge. At the end of the process with a decision provided by the jury, this case can be reported and could become part of our case law for future review and utilization when addressing similar issues in future cases.

---

[*] Id.

[†] Id.

Questions

1. What is case law and how is it made?
2. What is the hierarchy of federal courts and who creates case law?
3. What is the difference between state and federal case law?
4. What is a deposition?
5. What is a motion?

Selected Case Study

Case modified for the purposes of this text

U.S. Supreme Court
Chaplinsky v. New Hampshire, 315 U.S. 568 (1942)
Chaplinsky v. New Hampshire
No. 255
Argued February 5, 1942
Decided March 9, 1942
315 U.S. 568
APPEAL FROM THE SUPREME COURT OF NEW HAMPSHIRE

SYNOPSIS

1. That part of c. 378, § 2, of the Public Law of New Hampshire which forbids under penalty that any person shall address "any offensive, derisive or annoying word to any other person who is lawfully in any street or other public place," or "call him by any offensive or derisive name," was construed by the Supreme Court of the State, in this case and before this case arose, as limited to the use in a public place of words directly tending to cause a breach of the peace by provoking the person addressed to acts of violence.

Held

1. That, so construed, it is sufficiently definite and specific to comply with requirements of due process of law. P. 315 U. S. 573.
2. That, as applied to a person who, on a public street, addressed another as a "damned Fascist" and a "damned racketeer," it does not substantially or unreasonably impinge upon freedom of speech. P. 315 U. S. 574.
3. The refusal of the state court to admit evidence offered by the defendant tending to prove provocation and evidence bearing on the truth or falsity of the utterances charged is open to no constitutional objection. P. 315 U. S. 574.

2. The Court notices judicially that the appellations "damned racketeer" and "damned Fascist" are epithets likely to provoke the average person to retaliation, and thereby cause a breach of the peace. P. 315 U. S. 574

91 N.H. 310, 18 A.2d 754, affirmed.

APPEAL from a judgment affirming a conviction under a state law denouncing the use of offensive words when addressed by one person to another in a public place.

MR. JUSTICE MURPHY delivered the opinion of the Court.

Appellant, a member of the sect known as Jehovah's Witnesses, was convicted in the municipal court of Rochester, New Hampshire, for violation of Chapter 378, § 2, of the Public Laws of New Hampshire:

> No person shall address any offensive, derisive or annoying word to any other person who is lawfully in any street or other public place, nor call him by any offensive or derisive name, nor make any noise or exclamation in his presence and hearing with intent to deride, offend or annoy him, or to prevent him from pursuing his lawful business or occupation.

The complaint charged that appellant,

> with force and arms, in a certain public place in said city of Rochester, to-wit, on the public sidewalk on the easterly side of Wakefield Street, near unto the entrance of the City Hall, did unlawfully repeat the words following, addressed to the complainant, that is to say, 'You are a God damned racketeer' and 'a damned Fascist and the whole government of Rochester are Fascists or agents of Fascists, ' the same being offensive, derisive and annoying words and names.

Upon appeal, there was a trial *de novo* of appellant before a jury in the Superior Court. He was found guilty, and the judgment of conviction was affirmed by the Supreme Court of the State. 91 N.H. 310, 18 A.2d 754.

By motions and exceptions, appellant raised the questions that the statute was invalid under the Fourteenth Amendment of the Constitution of the United States in that it placed an unreasonable restraint on freedom of speech, freedom of the press, and freedom of worship, and because it was vague and indefinite. These contentions were overruled, and the case comes here on appeal.

There is no substantial dispute over the facts. Chaplinsky was distributing the literature of his sect on the streets of Rochester on a busy Saturday afternoon. Members of the local citizenry complained to the City Marshal, Bowering, that Chaplinsky was denouncing all religion as a "racket." Bowering told them that Chaplinsky was lawfully engaged, and then warned Chaplinsky that the crowd was getting restless. Some time later, a disturbance occurred and the traffic officer on duty at the busy intersection started with Chaplinsky for the police station, but did not inform him that he was under arrest or that he was going to be arrested. On the way, they encountered Marshal Bowering, who had been advised that a riot was under way and was therefore hurrying to the scene. Bowering repeated his earlier warning to Chaplinsky, who then addressed to Bowering the words set forth in the complaint.

Chaplinsky's version of the affair was slightly different. He testified that, when he met Bowering, he asked him to arrest the ones responsible for the disturbance. In reply, Bowering cursed him and told him to come along. Appellant admitted that he said the words charged in the complaint, with the exception of the name of the Deity.

Over appellant's objection, the trial court excluded, as immaterial, testimony relating to appellant's mission "to preach the true facts of the Bible," his treatment at the hands of the crowd, and the alleged neglect of duty on the part of the police. This action was approved by the court below, which held that neither provocation nor the truth of the utterance would constitute a defense to the charge.

It is now clear that

> Freedom of speech and freedom of the press, which are protected by the First Amendment from infringement by Congress, are among the fundamental personal rights and liberties which are protected by the Fourteenth Amendment from invasion by state action.

Appellant assails the statute as a violation of all three freedoms, speech, press, and worship, but only an attack on the basis of free speech is warranted. The spoken, not the written, word is involved. And we cannot conceive that cursing a public officer is the exercise of religion in any sense of the term. But even if the activities of the appellant which preceded the incident could be viewed as religious in character, and therefore entitled to the protection of the Fourteenth Amendment, they would not cloak him with immunity from the legal consequences for concomitant acts committed in violation of a valid criminal statute. We turn, therefore, to an examination of the statute itself.

Allowing the broadest scope to the language and purpose of the Fourteenth Amendment, it is well understood that the right of free speech is not absolute at all times and under all circumstances. There are certain well-defined and narrowly limited classes of speech, the prevention and punishment of which have never been thought to raise any Constitutional problem. These include the lewd and obscene, the profane, the libelous, and the insulting or "fighting" words – those which, by their very utterance, inflict injury or tend to incite an immediate breach of the peace. [Footnote 4] It has been well observed that such utterances are no essential part of any exposition of ideas, and are of such slight social value as a step to truth that any benefit that may be derived from them is clearly outweighed by the social interest in order and morality. [Footnote 5]

> Resort to epithets or personal abuse is not in any proper sense communication of information or opinion safeguarded by the Constitution, and its punishment as a criminal act would raise no question under that instrument.

The state statute here challenged comes to us authoritatively construed by the highest court of New Hampshire. It has two provisions – the first relates to words or names addressed to another in a public place; the second refers to noises and exclamations. The court said:

> "The two provisions are distinct. One may stand separately from the other. Assuming, without holding, that the second were unconstitutional, the first could stand if constitutional."

We accept that construction of severability and limit our consideration to the first provision of the statute.

On the authority of its earlier decisions, the state court declared that the statute's purpose was to preserve the public peace, no words being "forbidden except such as have a direct tendency to cause acts of violence by the persons to whom, individually, the remark is addressed." [Footnote 7] It was further said:

> The word 'offensive' is not to be defined in terms of what a particular addressee thinks.... The test is what men of common intelligence would understand would be words likely to cause an average addressee to fight.... The English language has a number of words and expressions which, by general consent, are 'fighting words' when said without a disarming smile.... [S]uch words, as ordinary men know, are likely to cause a fight. So are threatening, profane or obscene revilings. Derisive and annoying words can be taken as coming within the purview of the statute as heretofore interpreted only when they have this characteristic of plainly tending to excite the addressee to a breach of the peace.... The statute, as construed, does no more than prohibit the face-to-face words plainly likely to cause a breach of the peace by the addressee, words whose speaking constitutes a breach of the peace by the speaker -- including 'classical fighting words,' words in current use less 'classical' but equally likely to cause violence, and other disorderly words, including profanity, obscenity and threats.

We are unable to say that the limited scope of the statute as thus construed contravenes the Constitutional right of free expression. It is a statute narrowly drawn and limited to define and punish specific conduct lying within the domain of state power, the use in a public place of words likely to cause a breach of the peace.

This conclusion necessarily disposes of appellant's contention that the statute is so vague and indefinite as to render a conviction thereunder a violation of due process. A statute punishing verbal acts, carefully drawn so as not unduly to impair liberty of expression, is not too vague for a criminal law. Nor can we say that the application of the statute to the facts disclosed by the record substantially or unreasonably impinges upon the privilege of free speech. Argument is unnecessary to demonstrate that the appellations "damned racketeer" and "damned Fascist" are epithets likely to provoke the average person to retaliation, and thereby cause a breach of the peace.

The refusal of the state court to admit evidence of provocation and evidence bearing on the truth or falsity of the utterances is open to no Constitutional objection. Whether the facts sought to be proved by such evidence constitute a defense to the charge, or may be shown in mitigation, are questions for the state court to determine. Our function is fulfilled by a determination that the challenged statute, on its face and as applied, does not contravene the Fourteenth Amendment.

Affirmed.

8 Administrative Law

The best thing about the future is that it comes one day at a time.

Abraham Lincoln

The pendulum of the mind oscillates between sense and nonsense, not between right and wrong.

Carl Jung

STUDENT LEARNING OBJECTIVES

1. Analyze and assess administrative law.
2. Analyze and assess the OSH Act and applicable administrative processes.
3. Analyze and assess promulgation of an OSHA standard.
4. Analyze and understand the penalties under the OSH Act.
5. Analyze and understand state plans under the OSH Act.

Administrative law is defined as a "body of law created by administrative agencies to implement their powers and duties in the form of rules, regulations, orders, and decisions." For safety professionals, the primary federal governmental agency is the Occupational Safety and Health Administration (OSHA) which was one of three agencies (including National Institute for Occupational Safety and Health [NIOSH] and Occupational Safety and Health Review Commission [OSHRC]) created under the Occupational Safety and Health Act of 1970.[*] OSHA's mission is to ensure safe and healthful workplaces within the scope of their jurisdiction. The Occupational Safety and Health Act (hereinafter "OSH Act") requires "every employer engaged in interstate commerce to furnish employees 'a place of employment … free from recognized hazards that are causing, or are likely to cause, death or serious harm to employees.'"[†]

OSHA generally applies to all employers with one or more employees. OSHA employs three basic strategies which have been authorized under the OSH Act to achieve its mission, namely the following: (1) Strong, fair, and effective enforcement of standards; (2) Education, training, and compliance assistance; and (3) Partnerships, alliances, and other cooperative and voluntary programs. The OSH Act grants the Secretary of Labor (through the Assistance Secretary for OSHA) the authority to promulgate, modify, and revoke safety and health standards to conduct inspections and investigations and to issue citations, including proposed penalties; to require employers to keep records of safety and health data; to petition the courts to restrain imminent danger situations; and to approve or reject plans from states

---

[*] 29 C.F.R. Section 1975.
[†] 29 U.S.C.A. Section 654(a)(1).

proposing to assume jurisdiction from federal OSHA over private sector and state and local governments (known as "state plan" states). Under Executive Order 12196, all federal agencies must comply with the OSHA standards and OSHA possesses authority to inspect federal agency worksites and issue notices of violation. Annual reports are filed with each agency identifying the deficiencies as well as the positive safety and health elements within the agency's safety and health program. In general, the OSH Act exempts residential domestic household workers, businesses operating on Indian reservations, state and local government workers, and workers in specific industries, such as mining, which are covered by another agency (such as MSHA).

Safety professionals should be aware that Section 4 of the OSH Act provides jurisdiction over workplace safety and health in the United States and all of its territories. Section 18 of the OSH Act encourages states to develop and operate their own safety and health programs, and the state plan program must be as effective as the federal program. OSHA approves and monitors state plans and provides up to 50 percent of the state plan's operating costs. State plan programs must promulgate standards that are as effective as or more effective than the federal standards. Most state plan programs have adopted the federal standards with some modifications and enhancements to make the standards more applicable to the industries functioning in the state. State plans may promulgate standards unique to their state or industries if OSHA has not addressed in the federal standards.

OSHA is granted authority under the OSH Act to promulgate standards. For a two-year period following the effective date of the OSH Act in 1971, the Secretary of Labor was empowered to promulgate national consensus standards. In essence, the Secretary was empowered to adopt other standards from nationally recognized organizations (such as The American National Standards Institute [ANSI]). The Secretary is also empowered to enact an emergency temporary standard for a period of six months and then must go through the rulemaking process. The usual method to promulgate a standard is very extensive and lengthy requiring publication, substantial public meetings, notice, and comment. The burden is on OSHA to show that a significant risk to workers exists and that there are feasible measures employers can take to protect their employees.

The OSHA standard are codified in the Code of Federal Regulations, along with amendments, corrections, and deletions. General industry standards are codified in 29 CFR Part 1910. Construction standards are in 29 CFR Part 1926. Shipbuilding, repairing, and breaking are in 29 CFR Parts 1915, 1916, and 1917. Federal Service and supply contract standards are in 29 CFR Parts 1925 and 41 CFR Part 50-204. Agricultural operations standards are in 29 CFR Part 1928. OSHA standards can be design-specific standards (minimum construction criteria or performance-based standards reduce worker exposure to hazard with flexibility to achieve goal) as well as being vertical (particular industry) or horizontal standards (applies to all workplaces).

Safety professionals should be aware that the OSH Act imposes upon employers the general duty to furnish to each of their employees both employment and places of employment which are free from recognized hazards that are causing or are likely to cause death or serious harm to their employees.[*] This is generally referred to as the

---

[*] 29 U.S. C.A. Section 654(a)(1).

"General Duty Clause." In essence, the general duty clause was designed by congress to apply to only "recognized" hazards and should not be applied where there is a promulgated standard.

Safety professionals should be aware that they, as the agent for the employer, may challenge the validity of an OSHA standard by filing a petition with a U.S. Court of Appeals' court within sixty days following the promulgation of the standard by the Secretary of Labor. Generally, the standard will be upheld by the U.S. Court of Appeals if the standard is supported by substantial evidence in the record and considered as a whole.[*] However, safety professionals should be aware that a petition can be made to the Secretary of Labor for a permanent or temporary variance from a particular OSHA standard. In short, safety professionals must notify employees of the variance application so they have a chance to participate in the hearing, and they must show that the alternative method will provide employees with employment as safe and healthful as would prevail if he or she was to comply immediately with the standard.[†]

In promulgating a standard, OSHA has established a specific "roadmap" to provide guidance through this extensive and elongated process. This "roadmap" includes the following:

Step 1: Pre-Rulemaking Activities

There are many ways an OSHA standard can be initiated including recommendations from a national committee (such as National Advisory Committee on Occupational Safety and Health), review of enforcement data, recommendations from NIOSH or other agencies, court decisions, petitions from labor organizations or industry groups, and catastrophic events. At this stage, OSHA determines whether a standard is needed and preliminary rulemaking projects are announced. OSHA may also develop a Request for Information or an Advanced Notice of Proposed Rulemaking.

Step 2: Development of the Proposed Rule

After determination that a standard or rule is needed, a Notice of Proposed Rulemaking (NPRM) is developed. OSHA will continue to collect data and may consult with internal and external stakeholders. OSHA is required to conduct a risk analysis to determine the significance of the risk or a health effects analysis for health-related rulemaking. Additionally, OSH is required to conduct an economic analysis to determine the economic costs as well as a technological feasibility analysis and an informational collection analysis. Lastly, OSHA is required to submit all significant regulatory actions to the White House Office of Management and Budget (OMB) within 90 days for review and comment under Executive Order 12866.

Step 3: Publication of the Proposed Rule

A NPRM is required for any new standard being created, any changes to current standards, or removal of a standard or regulation and the notice must contain a request for public comment. Once approved, the Notice of Proposed Rulemaking

---

[*] 29 U.S.C.A. Section 655 (f).
[†] 29 CFR Section 1905.10(b).

must be published in the *Federal Register* and the public is usually provided 60–90 days to comment. In cases where OSHA does not expect significant comment, OSHA can choose to publish a direct final rule (DFR) at the same time as the Notice of Proposed Rulemaking. If adverse comments are received, OSHA can withdraw the DFR. If no adverse comments, the DFR become effective.

Step 4: Development of the Final Rule

The final rule creates, changes, or removes the standard or regulation. OMB again reviews the final rule to determine whether or not the rule is considered "significant regulatory action" and solicits comment from other government agencies affected by the final rule.

Step 5: Publication of the Final Rule

Upon approval by OMB, the final rule is published in the *Federal Register* and filed with Congress and the Government Accountability Office (GAO) in accordance with the Congressional Review Act (CRA). If OMB determines the standard or rule to be major, OSHA must delay the effective date by 60 days after the publication date in the *Federal Register.* During this 60 day period, GAO provides Congress with a brief report and members of Congress can introduce a resolution of disapproval that, if adopted by both houses and signed by the president, can nullify the OSHA standard or rule.

Once the final rule has been published and the 60 day period has elapsed, OSHA is permitted to enforce the standard or rule. Safety professionals should be aware that there are criminal sanctions as well as civil or monetary penalties for violation of the OSH Act. Safety professionals should be aware of the receipt increase in the OSHA penalties as well as the annual increase in the monetary penalty schedule amounts.

OSHA PENALTIES

Below are the penalty amounts adjusted for inflation as of January 13, 2017 (Table 8.1).

State Plan States

States that operate their own Occupational Safety and Health Plans are required to adopt maximum penalty levels that are at least as effective as Federal OSHA.*

TABLE 8.1
OSHA Penalty Schedule

Type of Violation	Penalty
Serious other-than-serious posting requirements	$12,675 per violation
Failure to abate	$12,675 per day beyond the abatement date
Willful or repeated	$126,749 per violation

* OSHA website located at www.osha.gov.

In summation, safety professionals should become knowledgeable in the administrative processes and procedures involving the Occupational Safety and Health Administration as well as other governmental agencies which have enforcement responsibilities that impact your workplace. Safety professionals should become the site expert in all aspects of the administrative processes of the agencies in order to be "ahead of the game" in preparing and addressing new standards or standard modifications that can impact your safety program (Table 8.2).

TABLE 8.2
State Plan Contact Information

Alaska Occupational Safety and Health (AKOSH)

- 3301 Eagle Street, Room 305
- Anchorage, AK 99503
- (907) 465-2700 | (800) 656-4972
- (907) 269-4950

Alaska State Plan

Arizona Division of Occupational Safety and Health (ADOSH)

- 800 W Washington Street
- Phoenix, AZ 85007
- **Toll-Free** (855) 268-5251
- (602) 542-5795
- (602) 542-1614

Arizona State Plan

Division of Occupational Safety and Health (DOSH)

- 1515 Clay Street, 19th Floor
- Oakland, California 94612
- (510) 622-8965
- (510) 286-7037

California State Plan

Connecticut Occupational Safety and Health Division (CONN-OSHA)

- 38 Wolcott Hill Rd
- Wethersfield, CT 06109
- (860) 263-6900
- (860) 263-6940

Connecticut State Plan

Hawaii Occupational Safety and Health Division (HIOSH)

- 830 Punchbowl Street, Suite 321
- Honolulu, HI 96813
- (808) 586-8841
- (808) 586-9116

Hawaii State Plan

(Continued)

TABLE 8.2 (*Continued*)
State Plan Contact Information

Illinois Department of Labor Safety Inspection and Education Division

- 900 South Spring Street
- Springfield, IL 62704
- (217) 782-9386
- (217) 785-8776

Illinois State Plan

Indiana Occupational Safety and Health Administration (IOSHA)

- 402 West Washington Street, Room W195
- Indianapolis, IN 46204
- (317) 232-2693
- (317) 233-3790

Indiana State Plan

Iowa Occupational Safety and Health Administration

- 1000 E Grand Avenue
- Des Moines, IA 50319-0209
- (515) 242-5870
- (515) 281-7995

Iowa State Plan

Kentucky Occupational Safety and Health

- 1047 US HWY 127 South, Suite 4
- Frankfort, KY 40601
- (502) 564-3070
- (502) 696-1902

Kentucky State Plan

Maryland Occupational Safety and Health (MOSH)

- 10946 Golden West Drive, Suite 160
- Hunt Valley, MD 21031
- (410) 527-4499
- (410) 527-4481

Maryland State Plan

Michigan Occupational Safety & Health Administration (MIOSHA)

- 530 W. Allegan Street
- P.O. Box 30643
- Lansing, Michigan 48909-8143
- **Toll-Free** (800) 866-4674
- (517) 284-7778
- (517) 284-7725

Michigan State Plan

(*Continued*)

TABLE 8.2 (*Continued*)
State Plan Contact Information

Minnesota Occupational Safety and Health Administration

- 443 Lafayette Road North
- St. Paul, MN 55155-4307
- **Toll Free** (877) 470-6742
- (651) 284-5050
- (651) 284-5741

Minnesota State Plan

Nevada Occupational Safety and Health Administration

- 1301 N Green Valley Pkwy, Suite 200
- Henderson, NV 89074
- (702) 486-9020
- (702) 990-0358

Nevada State Plan

New Jersey Public Employees Occupational Safety and Health (PEOSH)

- PO Box 369
- Trenton, NJ 08625-0369
- (609) 633-3896
- (609) 292-3749

New Jersey State Plan

New Mexico Occupational Health & Safety Bureau (OHSB)

- 525 Camino de los Marquez, Suite 3
- Santa Fe, NM 87502
- (505) 476-8700
- (505) 476-8734

New Mexico State Plan

Public Employees Safety and Health (PESH) Bureau

- Governor W. Averell Harriman State Building Campus,
- Building 12, Room 158
- Albany, NY 12240
- (518) 457-1263
- (518) 457-5545

New York State Plan

North Carolina Department of Labor Occupational Safety and Health Division

- 1101 Mail Service Center
- Raleigh, NC 27699-1101
- (919) 807-2900

North Carolina State Plan

(*Continued*)

TABLE 8.2 (*Continued*)
State Plan Contact Information

Oregon Occupational Safety and Health Division (Oregon OSHA)

- Salem Central Office
- PO Box 14480
- 350 Winter Street, NE, Rm. 430
- Salem, OR 97309-0405
- (503) 378-3272
- (503) 947-7461

Oregon State Plan

Puerto Rico Occupational Safety and Health Administration (PR OSHA)

- Prudencio Rivera Martinez Building, 20th Floor
- 505 Muñoz Rivera Avenue, 20th floor
- Hato Rey, Puerto Rico 00918
- (787) 754-2172
- (787) 767-6051

Puerto Rico State Plan

South Carolina Department of Labor, Licensing & Regulation
Division of Occupational Safety and Health (SC OSHA)

- P.O. Box 11329
- Columbia, SC 29211-1329
- (803) 896-7665
- (803) 896-7670

South Carolina State Plan

Tennessee Occupational and Safety and Health Administration (TOSHA)

- 220 French Landing Drive
- Nashville, TN 37243-1002
- (615) 741-2793
- (615) 741-3325

Tennessee State Plan

Utah Occupational Safety and Health Administration (Utah OSHA)

- PO Box 146600
- 160 East 300 South
- Salt Lake City, Utah 84114-6650
- (801) 530-6800
- (801) 530-6044

Utah State Plan

Vermont Occupational Safety and Health Administration (VOSHA)

- PO Box 488
- 5 Green Mountain Drive

(*Continued*)

TABLE 8.2 (*Continued*)
State Plan Contact Information

- Montpelier, VT 05601-0488
- (800) 287-2765

Vermont State Plan

Virgin Islands Division of Occupational Safety and Health (VIDOSH)

- 4401 Sion Farm
- Christiansted, St. Croix, VI 00820
- (340) 773-1994 | (340) 773-1440
- (340) 773-0094

Virgin Islands State Plan

Virginia Occupational Safety and Health (VOSH) Headquarters Main Street Centre

- 600 East Main Street, Suite 207
- Richmond, VA 23219
- (804) 371-2327
- (804) 371-6524

Virginia State Plan

Division of Occupational Safety and Health (DOSH)

- 7273 Linderson Way SW
- Tumwater, WA 98501-5414
- (360) 902-5580
- (360) 902-5619

Washington State Plan

Wyoming Department of Workforce Services - Wyoming Safety (OSHA)

- Herschler Building
- 1510 East Pershing Boulevard,
- West Wing
- Cheyenne, WY 82002
- (307) 777-7786
- (307) 777-3646

Wyoming State Plan[a]

[a] OSHA website located at www.osha.gov.

Questions

1. What is the process to promulgate an OSHA standard?
2. What is a Notice of Proposed Rulemaking?
3. What is the *Federal Register*?
4. What is a willful violation, and what is the penalty?
5. What is a Failure to Abate violation, and what is the maximum penalty?

Cases Modified for the Purpose of this Text

COMMONWEALTH OF KENTUCKY
OCCUPATIONAL SAFETY AND HEALTH REVIEW COMMISSION

KOSHRC 5045-13
SECRETARY OF LABOR COMMONWEALTH OF KENTUCKY –
COMPLAINANT v AMAZING CONTRACTORS LLC – RESPONDENT

Frankfort, for the Secretary. Lexington, for Amazing Contractors. DECISION AND ORDER OF THIS REVIEW COMMISSION. This case comes to us on Amazing Contractor's petition for discretionary review.

Our hearing officer in her recommended order affirmed two citations: a repeat serious citation[*] alleging Amazing failed to protect its employees against falls from a roof and a serious citation[†] which alleged a failure to provide fall protection training. When he arrived to conduct his inspection, the Secretary's compliance officer found six Amazing employees working on the roof which was fifteen feet, ten inches above the ground below. Recommended order, pages 3 and 5 (RO 3 and 5) and transcript of the evidence, page 19 (TE 19). According to information gleaned from photographs taken by an Amazing employee, the employer provided an insufficient number of roof anchors which employees used to secure their lanyards which in turn were attached to their fall protection harnesses. As the compliance officer, explained, the cited standard requires a roof anchor to support five thousand pounds per employee. TE 26. In her recommended order, our hearing officer found "There were three anchors that were nailed down on the roof" for six employees; she concluded that was a violation of the standard.

RO 4, 5, and 10. Before our hearing officer, Amazing argued it had no employees and thus was not subject to citation. Our hearing officer "concluded that Lackaby (Amazing's representative on site and at the trial) was 'an employee.'"

RO 9. In neither its petition for discretionary review nor its briefs to the Commission did Amazing Contractors argue it was not an employer and so it has abandoned that argument. The Kentucky General Assembly created the Review Commission and authorized it to "hear and rule on appeals from citations." KRS 338.071 (4). The first step in this process is a hearing on the merits. A party aggrieved by a hearing officer's recommended order may file a Petition for Discretionary Review (PDR) with the Review Commission; the Review Commission may grant the PDR, deny the PDR, or elect to call the case for review on its own motion. Section 47 (3), 803 KAR 50:010. When the Commission takes a case on review, it may make its own findings of fact and conclusions of law. In Brennan, Secretary of Labor v OSHRC and Interstate Glass,[‡] 487 F2d 438,441 (CA8 1973), CCH OSHD 16,799 page 21,538, BNA 1 OSHC 1372, 1374, the eighth circuit said when the Commission hears a

---

[*] Our hearing officer sustained a $7,000 penalty for the repeat serious citation.

[†] Our hearing officer sustained a $3,500 penalty for the serious citation.

[‡] In Kentucky Labor Cabinet v Graham, Ky, 43 SW3d 247, 253 (2001), the Kentucky Supreme Court said because Kentucky's occupational safety and health law is patterned after the federal, it should be interpreted consistently with the federal act.

case it does so "de novo." See also Accu-Namics, Inc v OSHRG, 515 F2d 828, 834 (CA5 1975), CCH OSHD 19,802, page 23,611, BNA 3 OSHC 1299, 1302, where the Court said "the Commission is the fact-finder, and the judge is an arm of the Commission...."[*]

Our supreme court in Secretary, Labor Cabinet v Boston Gear, Inc, Ky, 25 SW3d 130, 133 (2000), CCH OSHD 32,182, page 48,639, said "The review commission is the ultimate decision-maker in occupational safety and health cases ... the Commission is not bound by the decision of the hearing officer." In Terminix International, Inc v Secretary of Labor, Ky App, 92 SW3d 743,750 (2002), the Kentucky Court of Appeals said, "The Commission, as the ultimate fact-finder involving disputes such as this, may believe certain evidence and disbelieve other evidence and accord more weight to one piece of evidence than another." The repeat serious fall protection citation. The Cabinet's repeat serious fall protection citation carried a proposed penalty of $7,000;[†] it is based on an allegation the six workers on the roof did not have enough roof anchors to go around. According to the Cabinet and the cited standard, the 5,000 rated anchor points were only to be used by one worker. The disputed photographs, Amazing argues they were admitted into evidence in error, show the three anchors on the roof were rated at 5,000 pounds each. One photograph, exhibit 8, shows two lanyards attached to one D ring. Photographic exhibit 6 depicts an anchor with two D rings; Amazing Contractors has argued the two D rings on the 5,000 rated anchor were confusing; while we agree with Amazing on this point, the standard specifically limits each 5,000 pound anchor to one employee. As the photographs show, exhibits 5, 6, 7, and 8, the anchors are clearly rated at 5,000 pounds. For the repeat serious citation, the Cabinet cited to standard 29 CFR 1926.502 (d) (15);[‡] it says: Anchorages used for attachment of personal fall arrest equipment shall be independent of any anchorage being used to support or suspend platforms and capable of supporting at least 5,000 pounds ... per employee attached.... Then, the citation[§] alleges: Anchorage used for attachment for personal fall arrest equipment was not capable of supporting at least 5,000 pounds ... per employee.... a) ... six ... employees of Amazing Contractors, LLC were exposed to a fifteen (15) foot ten (10) inch fall hazard ... without adequate fall protection.... For the cases which come before us, the Kentucky Labor Cabinet has the burden of proof. 803 KAR 50:010, section 43

---

[*] See federal commission rule 92 (a), 29 CFR 2200.

[†] Compliance officer Dickerson rated this violation as high serious because a potential fall from height could result in death and greater probability of an injury because the roofers had been working on the roof for five to six hours that day. Dickerson assigned an unadjusted penalty of $14,000. TE 42. He told the hearing officer the $7,000 unadjusted penalty was increased to $14,000 because it was a repeat. TE 78 and KRS 338.991 (1). Compliance officer Dickerson said he awarded a credit of 50% for size, the number of employees, because Amazing employed eight workers. TE 47. Good faith was not awarded because of the high serious/greater probability characterization. No history credit was awarded; the CO was not asked why. TE 47. The $14,000 unadjusted penalty was reduced to $7,000 by the 50% credit for size.

To prove the elements of a repeat, the Cabinet must show a prior citation for a substantially similar violation was now a final order. Potlatch Corporation, CCH OSHD 23,294, BNA 7 OSHC 1061 (1979). The repeat serious citation stated the prior citation used to prove the repeat was a final order; Amazing did not challenge this allegation. Labor proved this citation was a repeat violation.

[‡] Kentucky has adopted the federal standard at 803 KAR 2:412, section 2 (1).

[§] Exhibit 4.

(1) (ROP 43 (1)). For our Commission to sustain a citation, the Cabinet must prove the four elements set out in Ormet Corporation, CCH OSHD 29,254, page 39,199, BNA 14 OSHC 2134, 2135 (1991), where the federal review commission said: In order to prove that an employer violated a standard, the Secretary must show that: (1) the standard applies to the cited condition; (2) the terms of the standard were violated; (3) one or more of the employer's employees had access to the cited conditions; and (4) the employer knew,* or with the exercise of reasonable diligence, could have known of the violative conditions. Whether the standard applies? Amazing Contractors, on the day of the inspection, was engaged in roofing which is construction work and we so find. TE 17. Amazing worked as a subcontractor for Craftsman Restoration, LLC. Exhibit 2, the contract between Amazing and Craftsman, TE 21 and TE 103. We find Amazing was properly cited according to 1926.502 and 1926.503 which are found in the construction standards. Ormet, supra. Whether Amazing violated the terms of the standard? Our hearing officer found the standard was awkwardly cited; we agree. The citation's instance description speaks about a lack of "adequate fall protection," without defining the term, while the standard says an anchor must be capable of supporting 5,000 pounds per employee exposed. As our hearing officer stated in her recommended order,† the violation rested on six roofers relying on three anchors which were individually rated at 5,000 pounds each. RO 5. For 5,000 pound anchors, each employee must be tied off to a separate anchor, a detail left out of the instance description.

Compliance officer David Dickerson said he used a Leica Disto meter to measure the height of the roof where he saw employees working; he took photographs of the men on the roof. Photographic exhibits 9, 10, and 11. He testified the "left-hand corner of the house" measured fifteen feet, ten inches from the ground. TE 19. Individual fall protection, a harness and lanyard tied off to an anchor, is required when an employee engaged in construction is working at an unprotected height of six feet for a steep roof according to the compliance officer. TE 83. An employer has the option of providing guard rails or safety nets. CO Dickerson said "I didn't see anything along the edge" which we infer to mean he observed no safety nets or guardrails. TE 19. Labor's repeat serious citation did not set out why fall protection was required. To prove a violation of the cited standard, the Cabinet must establish the six employees on the roof were not individually tied off to an anchor capable of supporting 5,000 pounds. 1926.502 (d) (15). During his walk around inspection, CO Dickerson said he observed one employee working "right at the edge." He then walked around the house and took photographs. He said there "were four people in the photographs I took on the back of the house." TE 19. Mr. Dickerson said during his inspection he found six employees on the roof; our hearing officer found six employees on the roof as well. TE 51 and RO 3. CO Dickerson, relying on photographic exhibits 5, 6, 7, and 8, determined there were only three 5,000 pound anchors. Three anchors are, according to the cited standard, insufficient for five or six employees. TE 26 and 40. For us, the crux of this case is whether the Cabinet 6 proved Amazing had installed only

---

* The comma should come after the word "or," not before it. Nevertheless this is how it is punctuated by OSHRC on line as well as CCH and BNA.
† We adopt our hearing officer's findings of fact to the extent they support our decision.

three anchors on the roof for the six employees; without those critical facts, we must dismiss the repeat serious citation as we shall. Compliance officer Dickerson said he did not go up on the roof because he had no fall protection; he said compliance officers generally do not have fall protection harnesses with them when they conduct inspections. TE 27 and 53. This means he was, confined to the ground, unable to count or to inspect the roof anchors himself. CO Dickerson had no hard hat with him either and so he maintained a ten foot distance between himself and the edge of the roof; he said the employees continued their work on the roof while he photographed them. Mr. Dickerson was concerned about objects falling from the roof and, we suppose, hitting him on his head. TE 19. In its brief to our Review Commission, the Secretary relied exclusively on photographs 5, 6, 7, and 8 to prove the number of roof anchors - three. Amazing has preserved its objection to these photographs. We find the photographs were admitted as evidence, over the objection of Amazing in error. Because CO Dickerson could not go up on the roof to inspect and count the roof anchors, he asked an employee of Amazing Contractors to take his camera to the roof to take the photographs. CO Dickerson said he could not remember the employee's name; the employee did not testify. TE 28. Dickerson, when asked if he observed the taking of the photographs, said "I did not visible see him take the photographs because I was on the ground and I was conducting employee interviews at that point." TE 29. When asked on direct examination when the exhibits, 5, 6, 7, and 8, appeared on his 7 camera, Dickerson said they were "present when he returned with the camera." TE 30. As Amazing Contractors has argued, a piece of evidence, a photograph, must be authenticated by the person offering the evidence at a trial. KRE 901 (a). That rule states: General provision. The requirement of authentication or identification as a condition precedent to admissibility is satisfied by evidence sufficient to support a finding that the matter in question is what its proponent claims. In her recommended order, our hearing officer admitted the photos; she said, "Dickerson watched the photographs being taken." RO 4. Mr. Dickerson, however, said he was busy interviewing employees when the photos were taken. TE 29. Our hearing officer then "found that the resulting photographs were true and accurate representations of the anchors as attached to the roof." RO 4. Certainly, the employee photographer, or others who observed the roof anchors, could have testified his photos were "true and accurate presentations of the anchors" which he had observed; but he did not testify. CO Dickerson could not make that representation because he did not go onto the roof and never personally observed the anchors. Equally troubling to us is the compliance officer's inability to tell whether two employees were actually tied off to the anchor depicted in photographic exhibit 8; he could not see if anyone was attached to the anchor shown in exhibit 8 because he was not on the roof. CO Dickerson admitted he asked no questions about the number of employees tied off to the exhibit 8 anchor. TE 75–76. Here is what Professor Lawson[*] has to say about authentication of photographs: Authentication is a 'condition precedent' to admissibility of a photograph, meaning that an offering party is required by KRE 901 to produce 'evidence sufficient to support a finding that (what is depicted in the photograph) is what its proponent claims.' In Gorman v Hunt, Ky, 19 SW3d 662, 669 (2000) our Kentucky

---

[*] Fifth edition, 2013, page 830.

Supreme Court set down the requirements for admitting a photograph into evidence: First, the photographs shall be properly authenticated. 'An authentic photograph is one that constitutes a fair and accurate representation of what it purports to depict.' Thus, 'the photograph must be … verified testimonially as a fair and accurate portrayal of (what) it is supposed to represent (emphasis added). While the employee photographer, or others, could have authenticated the photographs because they observed the anchors; they did not testify. CO Dickerson could not authenticate the photos because he never saw the anchors, only the photos. We conclude our hearing officer erred when she admitted photographs 5, 6, 7, and 8. We strike exhibits 5, 6, 7, and 8 from the record; we shall place these exhibits in a separate, sealed envelope. KRE 103 (a) (1). In its brief the Cabinet cited to a case which it said would permit the admission of the roof photographs taken by an Amazing employee even though the admitting compliance officer could not testify the photos, 5 through 8, accurately represented the actual anchor brackets. In Litton v Commonwealth, Ky, 597 SW2d 616,618 (1980), the trial judge in a burglary case admitted photographs taken by a security camera: a "witness is only required to state whether the photograph fairly and accurately depicts the scene about which he is testifying." In that case the "owner (of the building) identified the background in the photographs as being a fair and accurate representation of the area behind his pharmacy counter, an area not open to patrons." Litton. In Litton, the owner identified the scene of the photograph. The same cannot be said of the compliance officer in our case; he was not on the roof, he did not see the anchors and he testified he was interviewing witnesses when the Amazing employee photographer was on the roof taking the pictures. Stevie Lockaby testified he was "a member of the LLC, known as Amazing Contractors." TE 91–92. Mr. Lockaby said he never saw the anchors depicted in photographic exhibits 5, 6, 7, and 8. He said he was not on the roof on the day of the inspection and did not install the anchors. TE 97. When asked, Mr. Lockaby could not authenticate photos 5 through 8 because he was not on the roof. TE 101. Neither on direct examination nor on cross was Lockaby asked about the number of anchors on the roof. Several times CO Dickerson said Mr. Lockaby told him there were three anchors on the roof. TE 26, 27, and 40. Later, however, Mr. Dickerson contradicted himself. When asked on redirect how many anchors were on the roof, he said "Three according to the photographs that were given to me." TE 71. CO Dickerson's reliance on the photographs explains why the Cabinet in its brief to the Commission focused exclusively on the disputed photographs, photographs Dickerson did not take and could not authenticate, to prove the number of anchors. We assign little weight to the CO's statements about what Mr. Lockaby told him about the anchors. Terminix, supra, at 92 SW3d 750. Mr. Lockaby was not on the roof, did not install the anchors and could not authenticate the photographs. Because Mr. Lockaby had not gone on the roof, we have no confidence in his ability to report on the number of anchors independent of the photographs which had been provided to respondent prior to the trial. Transcript of the record, item 19. (TR 19). We hold that the Cabinet, without the photographs, has failed to prove the number of anchors in use on the roof, the essential piece of evidence for the repeat serious citation, and so we dismiss the citation. Whether Amazing's roofing employees had access to the cited condition? We have already ruled that Amazing has abandoned its argument it had no employees on the work site. We find the employees on the roof worked for Amazing and had access to the cited condition. Whether with the exercise of reasonable diligence the employer could have known of the violative condition? Assuming for the fourth element required by Ormet, supra, a violative condition, we find Mr. Lockaby could have, with the exercise of reasonable diligence, easily determined whether his roofing employees were protected from the hazard of falling off the roof. KRS 338.991 (11). The serious, failure to train citation. Our hearing officer in her recommended order affirmed this failure to train citation and the penalty of $3,500.* In the citation, the Cabinet alleged: Six employees of Amazing Contractors, LLC were not properly trained in the use of fall protection equipment, namely anchors, while performing roofing work.... Two employees were observed tied off to one anchor with a load rating of 5,000 pounds per person. This application would have required a 10,000 pound anchor. According to the compliance officer he issued this failure to train citation because the employees on the roof were not observing the rule that only one employee could be tied off to a 5,000 pound anchor; this, to the CO, was proof of improper training. TE 44 and RO 7. Oddly, the compliance officer in his testimony made no mention of employee interviews about training. In its petition for discretionary review Amazing Contractors elected not to ask this Commission to reverse the hearing officer and dismiss this citation. Amazing made no mention of this serious, failure to train citation in its brief to the Commission. We found two federal commission cases which have ruled that instances where employees are not complying with a standard are not evidence of a failure to train. James Construction, a federal ALJ decision, CCH OSHD 31,140, BNA 17 OSHC 12 2173, 2176 (1996). Superior Rigging & Erecting Co, a federal ALJ decision, CCH 31,534, page 44,955 (1998).

Because Amazing Contractors did not petition our Commission to dismiss this failure to train citation, it is now a final and unappealable order. ROP 48 (3) and KRS 338.091 (1). This case was ill-conceived from the start. Asking an employee to take photographs for the compliance officer and then not calling the employee photographer is difficult for us to understand, given the law on the admission of photographs in Kentucky. Similarly, writing a failure to train citation where the only proof consisted of an apparent violation of a standard without more is nonsensical in light of the case law on the subject. Compliance officer Dickerson said he interviewed employees, and in fact was interviewing when the employee photographer took the pictures for him, but he did not inquire about training. But for Amazing's failure to preserve this argument in its appeal to us, we would have reversed this citation. However, Amazing has waived its right to challenge this failure to train citation, and so we affirm. It is so ordered. April 7, 2015.

---

* Dickerson said the violation was serious because, according to the CO, the lack of training exposed employees to a 15 foot fall. Compliance officer Dickerson rated this violation as high serious because of a potential fall from height and greater probability of in injury because the roofers had been working on the roof for five to six hours that day. Dickerson assigned an unadjusted penalty of $7,000. TE 46. He awarded a credit of 50% for size, the number of employees. TE 47. Good faith was not awarded because of the high serious/greater probability characterization. No history credit was awarded. TE 47. The 50% credit resulted in a proposed penalty of $3,500.

9 Occupational Safety and Health Act

The best possible way to prepare for tomorrow is to concentrate with all your intelligence, all your enthusiasm, on doing today's work superbly today. That is the only possible way you can prepare for the future.

Dale Carnegie

Never try to be better than someone else. Learn from others, and try to be the best you can be. Success is the by-product of that preparation.

John Wooden

STUDENT LEARNING OBJECTIVES

1. Analyze and understand the Occupational Safety and Health (OSH) Act.
2. Analyze and understand the functions of National Institute for Occupational Safety and Health (NIOSH), Occupational Safety and Health Administration (OSHA), and Occupational Safety and Health Review Commission (OSHRC).
3. Analyze and assess federal OSHA's jurisdiction.
4. Analyze and assess OSHA's recordkeeping requirements.
5. Analyze and assess employer and employee rights under the OSH Act.

Before the federal OSH Act was enacted and became effective on April 28, 1971,* safety and health issues were not addressed by employers or were limited to safety and health laws for specific industries or laws that governed federal contractors. It was during this period, prior to the enactment of the OSH Act, Congress gradually began to regulate specific areas of safety and health in the workplace through lows such as the Walsh-Healey Public Contracts Act of 1936, the Labor Management Relations Act (Taft-Hartley Act) of 1947, the Coal Mine Safety Act of 1952, and the McNamara-O'Hara Public Service Contract Act of 1965.

The beginnings of the safety profession started with the passage of the then controversial OSH Act in 1907. Through this law, federal and state government agencies were formed and became actively involved in the management of safety and health in the public and private sectors of the American workplace. Employers were placed on notice that unsafe and unhealthful conditions and acts would no longer be permitted in the American workplace. In certain circles, the OSHA became synonymous

---

* 29 U.S.C.A. Section 651, *et. seq.*

149

with the "safety police" and employers were often forced, under penalty of law, to address safety and health issues and conditions in their workplace. Employers often challenged and litigated issues and violations issued by OSHA.

In addition to the OSH Act creating OSHA, the OSH Act also created the NIOSH as well as the OSHRC. NIOSH, now part of the Center for Disease Control, is the research arm with a mission "to develop new knowledge in the field of occupational safety and health and transfer that knowledge into practice."* OSHRC is the judicial administrative arm developed to hear appeals from citations issued by OSHA. In essence, the OSH Act created a three-prong directive wherein OSHA is the enforcement arm, NIOSH is the research arm, and OSHRC is the judicial arm within this administrative structure.

Section 4 of the OSH Act provides OSHA with jurisdiction over workplace safety throughout the United States as well as U.S. territories including all 50 states, the District of Columbia, Puerto Rico, Guam, the Virgin Islands, American Samoa, and the Trust Territory of the Pacific Islands. Section 18 of the OSH Act encourages states to develop and operate their own plans known as "state plan" states (Figure 9.1).

The OSH Act also directs the Secretary of Labor (in cooperation with the Secretary of Health and Human Services) to issue regulations which require

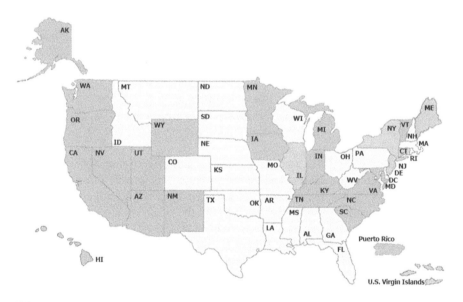

FIGURE 9.1   State plan states.

Note: Twenty-six states, Puerto Rico, and the Virgin Islands have OSHA-approved state plans. Twenty-two state plans (21 states and one U.S. territory) cover both private and state and local government workplaces. The remaining six state plans (five states and one U.S. territory) cover state and local government workers only.†

---

* NIOSH website located at www.CDC.gov-NIOSH.
† OSHA website located at www.osha.gov.

employers to collect and maintain records with regards to work-related deaths, injuries, and illnesses, as well as exposures to potentially toxic materials or harmful physical agents. Additionally, the OSH Act requires the Secretary of Labor to develop and maintain an effective program of collection, compilation, and analysis of statistics related to occupational safety and health.[*] Specifically, for safety professionals, this requires each employer to compile and post an annual summary of occupational injuries and illnesses for each establishment and requires the log to be maintained. Safety professionals should be aware that recordable injuries and illnesses are required to be entered in the log "as early as practicable, but not later than six working days after receiving information on the injury or illness."[†] Safety professionals should be aware that the OSHA Injury and Illness Recordkeeping and Reporting Requirements are currently being revised and updated. Safety professionals should also take note of the Notice-Posting Requirements requiring the posting, in conspicuous placed, the Notices provided by OSHA informing employees of their rights, how to contact OSHA and how to obtain assistance.

OSHA INJURY AND ILLNESS RECORDKEEPING AND REPORTING REQUIREMENTS

RECORDKEEPING REQUIREMENTS

Many employers with more than 10 employees are required to keep a record of serious work-related injuries and illnesses. (Certain low-risk industries are exempted.) Minor injuries requiring first aid only do not need to be recorded.

- How does OSHA define a recordable injury or illness?
- How does OSHA define first aid?

This information helps employers, workers, and OSHA evaluate the safety of a workplace, understand industry hazards, and implement worker protections to reduce and eliminate hazards—preventing future workplace injuries and illnesses.

MAINTAINING AND POSTING RECORDS

The records must be maintained at the worksite for at least five years. Each February through April, employers must post a summary of the injuries and illnesses recorded the previous year. Also, if requested, copies of the records must be provided to current and former employees, or their representatives.

- Get recordkeeping forms 300, 300A, 301, and additional instructions.
- Read the full OSHA Recordkeeping regulation (29 CFR 1904).

---

[*] 29 USCA Sections 657 and 673.
[†] 29 CFR Section 1904.2(a).

UPDATED ELECTRONIC SUBMISSION OF RECORDS

The Injury Tracking Application (ITA) is accessible from the ITA launch page, where you can provide the agency with your 2016 OSHA Form 300A information. OSHA also published a notice of proposed rulemaking to extend the date by which certain employers are required to submit the information from their completed 2016 Form 300A electronically from July 1, 2017 to December 1, 2017.

- Learn about OSHA's rule on submitting injury and illness records electronically.

SEVERE INJURY REPORTING

Employers must report any worker fatality within 8 hours and any amputation, loss of an eye, or hospitalization of a worker within 24 hours.

- Learn details and how to report online or by phone.*

Safety professionals should be aware that the data recorded is accurate to ensure uniformity and consistency for OSHA's analysis. OSHA uses the submitted injury and illness data for the purposes of inspection targeting, performance measurement, standard development resource allocation and related analysis. Safety professionals with a own injury and illness record may want to consider applying for the Voluntary Protection Program and Safety and Health Recognition Program to assist and recognize the safety and health efforts of the organization.

The OSH Act creates employee rights within the area of safety and health. Employees are entitled to working conditions that do not pose a risk of serious harm, as well as the right to:

- Ask OSHA to inspect their workplaces;
- Use their rights under the OSH Act without retaliation or discrimination;
- Receive information and training about hazards, methods of preventing harm, and the OSHA standards that apply to their workplace (Note: Training must be provided in native language or language employee understands);
- Get copies of test results done to find hazards in the workplace;
- Review records of work-related injuries and illnesses; and
- Acquire copies of their personal medical records.

The OSH Act also creates responsibilities for employers. As noted above, employers are required to maintain accurate injury and illness records; post OSHA citations, injury and illness summary data and post the OSHA "Job Safety and Health – It's the Law" poster in a conspicuous location for employees; find and correct safety and health hazards; follow all OSHA standards; inform employees of chemical hazards through training; notify OSHA within

---

* OSHA website located at www.osha.gov.

8 hours of a workplace fatality or when three or more workers are hospitalized; and provide personal protective equipment at no cost to employees (with limited exceptions). Additionally, employers are prohibited from discriminating or retaliating against employees for using their rights provided under the law.

Safety professionals should be aware that OSHA administers the whistleblower or anti-retaliation provisions of 21 different whistleblower protection statutes, including Section 11(c) of the OSH Act which prohibits termination or any manner of retaliation against an employee for exercising his/her rights under the OSH Act. A complaint of retaliation file by an employee with OSHA must allege that the employee engaged in a protected activity (e.g., contacting OSHA); the employer knew of the activity (e.g., contacting OSHA); the employer subjected the employee to an adverse action (e.g., demoting the employee); and the protected activity motivated or contributed to the adverse action (e.g., demotion linked to contacting OSHA). An adverse action is generally defined as any action that would dissuade a reasonable employee from engaging in the protected activity. Adverse actions can include termination or layoff, blacklisting, demotion, denying overtime or promotion, disciplinary action, denial of benefits, failure to hire or rehire, and intimidation.

Questions

1. What is the difference between a state plan and federal OSHA state?
2. What are the requirements under the OSHA Recordkeeping Standard?
3. When must a safety professional contact OSHA or a state plan?
4. What is a whistleblower and what protections are afforded to this individual under the OSH Act?
5. What are the three agencies created under the OSH Act and what do they do?

STATUTES

The statutes enforced by OSHA are listed below. They contain whistleblower or anti-retaliation provisions that generally provide that employers may not discharge or retaliate against an employee because the employee has filed a complaint or otherwise exercised any rights provided to employees. Each law requires that complaints be filed within a certain number of days after the alleged retaliation. Complaints may be filed orally or in writing, and OSHA will accept the complaint in any language. Click on any statute to see the whistleblower provisions (Table 9.1):

The OSH Act provided the Secretary of Labor with powers to make inspections of *employer workplaces* to determine whether OSHA standards are being met (subject to the search and seizure safeguards of the fourth amendment to the U.S. Constitution. See *Marshall v. Barlows, Inc.*, 436 U.S. 307 (1978) in this text). OSHA inspections and investigations are required to be conducted during working hours, or there reasonable times and within a reasonable manner.* If an employer objects to an OSHA inspection

---

* 29 USCA Section 657(a).

TABLE 9.1
Safety Related Laws

Statute	Title
49 U.S.C. § 20109	Accord Regarding BNSF Policies
29 U.S.C. 218C	Affordable Care Act (ACA), Section 1558
15 U.S.C. §2651	Asbestos Hazard Emergency Response Act (AHERA)
42 U.S.C. §7622	Clean Air Act (CAA)
42 U.S.C. §9610	Comprehensive Environmental Response, Compensation and Liability Act (CERCLA)
12 U.S.C.A. §5567	Consumer Financial Protection Act of 2010 (CFPA), Section 1057 of the Dodd-Frank Wall Street Reform and Consumer Protection Act of 2010
15 U.S.C. §2087	Consumer Product Safety Improvement Act (CPSIA)
42 U.S.C. §5851	Energy Reorganization Act (ERA)
21 U.S.C. 399d	FDA Food Safety Modernization Act (FSMA), Section 402
49 U.S.C. §20109	Federal Railroad Safety Act (FRSA)
33 U.S.C. §1367	Federal Water Pollution Control Act (FWPCA)
46 U.S.C. §80507	International Safe Container Act (ISCA)
49 U.S.C. §30171	Moving Ahead for Progress in the 21st Century Act (MAP-21)
6 U.S.C. §1142	National Transit Systems Security Act (NTSSA)
29 U.S.C. §660	Occupational Safety and Health Act (OSH Act), Section 11(c)
49 U.S.C. §60129	Pipeline Safety Improvement Act (PSIA)
42 U.S.C. §300j-9(i)	Safe Drinking Water Act (SDWA)
18 U.S.C.A. §1514A	Sarbanes-Oxley Act (SOX)
46 U.S.C. §2114	Seaman's Protection Act (SPA), as amended by Section 611 of the Coast Guard Authorization Act of 2010, P.L. 111-281
42 U.S.C. §6971	Solid Waste Disposal Act (SWDA)
49 U.S.C. §31105	Surface Transportation Assistance Act (STAA)
15 U.S.C. §2622	Toxic Substances Control Act (TSCA)
49 U.S.C. §42121	Wendell H. Ford Aviation Investment and Reform Act for the 21st Century (AIR21)[a]

[a] OSHA website located at www.osha.gov

at his/her workplace, the Secretary of Labor is required to obtain a search warrant prior to proceeding with the investigation or inspection. An OSHA inspection or search warrant usually must show probable cause to believe OSHA violations are occurring in the workplace or a showing that reasonable legislative or administrative standards for conducting the inspection are satisfied with regard to the specific employer.

As safety professionals are aware, the OSH Act permits the OSHA agency (or compliance officer) to identify hazards which are in violation of the OSHA standards or General Duty Clause and report these hazards to the area or regional director. The director will categorize these hazards, attach the appropriate proposed penalty and codify this information in a citation document which is sent to the employer (See Chapter 10 for further details). The OSH Act permits monetary penalties as well as criminal referrals (to the Department of Justice or correlating state plan prosecutors). The current monetary penalties are below:

TABLE 9.2
OSHA Penalty Schedule

Type of Violation	Penalty
Serious Other-Than-Serious Posting Requirements	$12,934 per violation
Failure to Abate	$12,934 per day beyond the abatement date
Willful or Repeated	$129,336 per violation

OSHA PENALTIES

Above are the penalty amounts adjusted for inflation as of January 13, 2017 (Table 9.2).

The OSH Act has provided the possible use of criminal sanctions since its inception in 1970. An employer who willfully violates the OSH Act, resulting in the death of an employee, faces criminal penalties of up to $10,000 and up to six months in prison. OSHA does not have the authority to directly prosecute an employer or agent of the employer; however, the case can be referred to the U.S. Department of Justice for review and acceptance. Since 1970, there have been relatively few cases under the OSH Act which have been prosecuted. Safety professionals should be aware that there has been activity around the enhancement and expansion of the criminal penalties under the OSH Act. (See Chapter 10 for additional information).

In summation, the OSH Act was the beginning of today's safety profession. Although few changes have been made to the OSH Act itself over the years, it remains the foundational law for OSHA, NIOSH, and OSHRC. Prudent safety professionals should become well acquainted with the OSH Act as well as the standards, regulations and requirements of the OSHA. The goal and reason for the OSH Act parallels that of today's safety profession is to create and maintain a safe and healthful work environment for all employees everyday on the job!

Questions

1. What elements must OSHA prove for a serious violation?
2. What information is required on an OSHA 300 log?
3. What is the OSHA "General Duty" Clause?
4. What is the difference between OSHA and a state plan state?
5. What protections are afforded to an employee under the Whistleblower statute?

Case modified for the Purpose of this Text

361 F.3d 364
United States Court of Appeals,
Seventh Circuit.
UNITED STATES of America, Plaintiff-Appellant,
v.
MYR GROUP, INC., Defendant-Appellee.
No. 03-3250.
Argued February 19, 2004.Decided March 16, 2004.

SYNOPSIS

Background: Federal government indicted parent corporation and its wholly owned subsidiary for willfully violating Occupational Safety and Health (OSH) Act in connection with electrocution deaths of two of subsidiary's employees. The U.S. District Court for the Northern District of Illinois, 274 F.Supp.2d 945, Elaine E. Bucklo, J., dismissed indictment as to parent corporation and government appealed.

Holding: The Court of Appeals, Circuit Judge, held that parent could not be held criminally liable for willful violations of OSHA regulations on theory that duties created by regulations ran to any employees, not just employees of company accused of violating them.

Affirmed.

OPINION

The district judge dismissed an indictment that charged MYR Group, Inc., with violating section 17(e) of the Occupational Safety and Health Act, 29 U.S.C. § 666(e), and the government appeals. The factual record is limited to the facts alleged in the indictment, according to which MYR has a wholly owned subsidiary named L.E. Myers Company (the parties call it "LEM"), which repairs high-voltage lines. MYR oversees the safety programs of its subsidiaries, provides safety manuals and other safety instructions to the employees of the subsidiaries, and jointly with the subsidiaries is responsible for training those employees with regard to safety matters, including how to repair high-voltage lines without being electrocuted. Nevertheless, on two separate occasions, employees of LEM were electrocuted while repairing such lines. The indictment charges both MYR and LEM with two counts of causing the death of an employee by willfully violating rules promulgated under OSHA. 29 U.S.C. § 666(e). MYR is charged with violating regulations requiring, in essence, that employees be properly trained in safe working procedures. 29 C.F.R. §§ 1910.269(a)(2)(i), (ii). LEM is charged with violations of other rules as well, and is awaiting trial in the district court. The government's argument is a simple one. MYR is an employer, albeit not of the two workers who were electrocuted; the two workers were employees; the regulations in question state simply that "employees shall be trained in" safe working procedures. Therefore, the argument concludes, the duties created by the regulations run to anyone's employees, not merely employees of the employer accused of having violated the regulations. In its opening brief, the government tried to make something of the fact that MYR and LEM are corporate affiliates, citing Esmark, Inc. v. NLRB, 887 F.2d 739 (7th Cir.1989). That, however, was a veil-piercing case, where we said that "it is solely where a parent disregards the separate legal personality of its subsidiary (and the subsidiary's own decision making 'paraphernalia'), and exercises direct control over a specific transaction, that derivative liability for the subsidiary's unfair labor practices will be imposed under the theory adopted by the Board in the present case." Id. at 757. At argument, the government made clear that it is not attempting to pierce the corporate veil and by doing so attribute the subsidiary's acts to the parent, consistent with the principles of corporate law. Breathtaking vistas of both criminal and civil liabilities (the latter not dependent on proof that the violation was willful, 29 U.S.C. §§ 666(b), (c); S.A. Healy Co. v. OSHRC, 138 F.3d 686, 688 (7th Cir.1998)) open before our eyes. Were LEM to hire the Illinois Institute of Technology (IIT) to train LEM's employees in the hazards of uninsulated high voltage electrical cables, and IIT fell down on the job and an employee of LEM was electrocuted as a result, IIT would, if the government is right, be either criminally or civilly liable for having violated OSH Act. It would be so merely by virtue of having employees, even though those were not the workers endangered by its violation. It is true that LEM and IIT are not affiliates, but the government's lawyer acknowledged that this would make no difference, for remember that it is not arguing that MYR did anything that would justify treating LEM as if it were really just a division of MYR rather than a separate corporation. The government's argument is not limited to service providers. A firm (provided only that it had employees) that sold a defective espresso machine to a coffee shop would be subject to OSHA liability if the machine exploded and scalded a waiter. OSHA would become a products-liability statute-with criminal sanctions for its willful violation. The government points to our decision in United States v. Pitt-Des Moines, Inc., 168 F.3d 976, 984–85 (7th Cir.1999), which holds that a contractor at a construction site can be prosecuted under section 666(e) if by violating an OSHA regulation he causes the death of an employee of another contractor at the same site. However, the point of this "multi-employer" gloss (cf. Universal Construction Co. v. OSHRC, 182 F.3d 726, 728–30 (10th Cir.1999); R.P. Carbone Construction Co. v. OSHRC, 166 F.3d 815, 818 (6th Cir.1998); Beatty Equipment Leasing, Inc. v. Secretary of Labor, 577 F.2d 534, 536–37 (9th Cir.1978); Marshall v. Knutson Construction Co., 566 F.2d 596, 599–600 (8th Cir.1977) (per curiam); Brennan v. OSHRC, 513 F.2d 1032, 1037–39 (2d Cir.1975); but see Melerine v. Avondale Shipyards, Inc., 659 F.2d 706, 710–11 (5th Cir.1981)) is that since the contractor is subject to OSHA's regulations of safety in construction by virtue of being engaged in the construction business, and has to comply with those regulations in order to protect his own workers at the site, it is sensible to think of him as assuming the same duty to the other workers at the site who might be injured or killed if he violated the regulations. From a safety standpoint, it is a joint-employment case. A crane operator might be killed because the contractor responsible for leveling the ground at the worksite violated a regulation requiring that the surface beneath the crane be planed smooth, and a bulldozer driver might be killed when a crane fell on him because the crane contractor had failed to comply with regulations governing the safe operation of cranes. Each employer at the worksite controls a part of the dangerous activities occurring at the site and is the logical person to be made responsible for protecting everyone at the site from the dangers that are within his power to control. See Universal Construction Co. v. OSHRC, supra, 182 F.3d at 730; Brennan v. OSHRC, supra, 513 F.2d at 1038. This case is not like that. No employee of MYR was engaged in repairing high-voltage lines, any more than a professor of electrical engineering at IIT who trained employees in the hazards of electricity would be present at the worksite. The government's attempt to stretch the statute by filing a criminal indictment is especially questionable. Surely, the proper way to proceed, if the government really thinks the statute can be stretched this far, would be to amend the regulations to bring the third-party case under them. And who by the way is "the government" in this case?

No representative of the Occupational Safety and Health Administration, or for that matter anyone outside the office of the U.S. Attorney for this district, signed the government's brief. The Solicitor General of the United States had to approve the appeal, 28 C.F.R. § 0.20(b); but we have not even been told whether OSHA approves, or for that matter knows of, the extension of liability urged by the U.S. Attorney.

The dismissal of the indictment against the MYR Group is AFFIRMED.

10 OSHA Standards and Enforcement

Big thinkers are specialists in creating positive, forward-looking, optimistic pictures in their minds and in the minds of others.

David J. Schwartz

All great achievements require time.

Maya Angelou

STUDENT LEARNING OBJECTIVES

1. Analyze and assess the requirements of an Occupational Safety and Health Administration (OSHA) standard.
2. Analyze and assess the categories of OSHA standards.
3. Analyze and understand horizontal and vertical standards.
4. Analyze and understand the elements of a compliance inspection.
5. Analyze and assess an OSHA citation for alleged violations and proposed penalties.

As defined in Section 3(8) of the Occupational Safety and Health (OSH) Act, an occupational safety and health standard is "a standard which requires conditions, or the adoption or use of one or more practices, means, methods, operations, or processes reasonably necessary or appropriate to provide safe or healthful employment or places of employment."[*] The OSH Act requires an employer to comply with specific occupational safety and health standards. Section 6(b) of the OSHA Act authorizes the Secretary of Labor to "promulgate, modify, or revoke any safety and health standard, provides procedures for doing so, and established criteria for those standards."[†] Section 6(f) establishes the standard of review of OSHA promulgated standards by the federal courts of appeal.

When combining the sections of the OSH Act, as well as the interpretations of a number of court decisions, these provisions establish the legal framework and the following requirements for an OSHA standard:

1. The standard must substantially reduce a significant risk of material harm;
2. Compliance must be technologically feasible in the sense that the protective measures being required by the standard already exist, can be brought into

---

[*] 29 U.S.C. Section 3(8).
[†] 29 U.S.C. Section 6(b).

existence with available technology, or can be created with technology that can reasonably be developed;

3. Compliance with the OSHA standard must be economically feasible in the sense that the standard will not threaten the industry's long-term profitability or substantially alter its competitive structure;
4. Health standards must eliminate significant risk, or reduce a significant risk to the extent feasible, and safety standards must be highly protective;
5. OSHA Standards must employ the lost cost-effective protective measures capable of reducing or eliminating significant risk; and
6. OSHA Standards must be supported by substantial evidence in the rulemaking record and be consistent with prior agency practice or supported by some justification for departing from that practice.

OSHA standard standards are categorized by General industry, Construction, Maritime, and Agriculture. For most safety professionals, General industry and Construction are the most widely utilized. OSHA standards can be narrowly focused on a specific industry, known as vertical standards, or broadly focused for the vast majority of the industries, known as horizontal standards. The early OSHA standards, or National Consensus Standards, often parallel other voluntary codes (such as NFPA and NEC); however, when adopted by OSHA, these voluntary requirements became mandatory. Many of the early standards were design or specification standards providing minimum criteria to achieve compliance. In recent years, OSHA has moved to more performance-based standards providing more employer flexibility to achieve compliance.

Within the General industry standards (29 CFR 1910), every industry or operation will be unique; however, there are several "horizontal" standards common among and between most industries, including the following:

1. Control of Hazardous Energy (Lockout/Tagout)
2. Emergency and Disaster Preparedness.
3. Hazard Communications Standard (Haz Com)
4. Respiratory Protection
5. Fall Protection
6. Personal Protective Equipment
7. Bloodborne Pathogens Standard

Compliance with these types of horizontal standards, as well as other vertical standards, must be identified by the safety professional, and compliance must be achieved and maintained. OSHA does not provide the safety professional what to do but simply provides standards identifying the minimum requirements to achieve compliance. And, as most safety professionals will identify, simply achieving and maintaining compliance with the OSHA standards does not make a successful safety program. Compliance with the OSHA standards is the "bare bones" minimum necessary to avoid the potential penalties under the OSH Act.

For most safety professionals, the probability of a compliance inspection is fairly small when comparing the number of compliance officers with the number of employers and workplaces in the United States. However, if the safety professional is in a targeted industry, earned a high injury and illness rate or incurring a fatality or multiple injury situation, the probability of inspection increases. And remember, the safety professional must contact OSHA if a workplace fatality occurs or three or more employees are transported to the hospital. These types of incidents usually mandate an investigation or inspection. So what generally happens during a typical compliance inspection?

PRIOR TO A COMPLIANCE INSPECTION

Safety professionals should be aware that OSHA provides no notice prior to the inspection. In fact, it is a crime punishable by a fine of up to $1000 and/or imprisonment for up to six months if advance notice is provided to an employer without the authorization of the Secretary of Labor or designee.[*] However, there are times when an inspection can be scheduled, namely voluntary inspection through state plan education and training divisions, voluntary inspections for Voluntary Protection Program or Safety and Health Recognition Program and other voluntary situations. Additionally, the OSHA compliance officer must come to the operations during working hours; however, if the shift or location operated outside of traditional working hours, the safety professional can contact the area or regional director to possibly schedule other times to inspect the specific location. These are exceptions rather than the rule.

As noted, compliance inspections are virtually always conducted without advance notice. However, in special circumstances, OSHA can provide notice to the employer however notice is normally served less than 24 hours. These circumstances include the following:

- Imminent dangerous circumstances requiring immediate correction;
- Accident investigations where the safety professional notified OSHA of a fatality or catastrophe;
- Inspection after regular business hours or requiring special preparation;
- Situations where notice is required to ensure that the employer and employee representatives or other personnel will be present;
- Situations where the inspection must be delayed more than five days where there is good cause;
- And situations where the OSHA Area Director (AD) determines that advance notice would produce a more thorough or effective investigation.

Additionally, safety professionals should be aware of the programmed inspections, which include the following:

- Site-Specific Targeting Program inspections;
- Construction Inspections;
- Special Emphasis Inspections; and
- Severe Violator Enforcement Program inspections.[†]

---

[*] 29 USCA Section 1903.6.

[†] Note: OSHA's priorities for inspection usually provide imminent danger situations top priority, followed by fatality/catastrophe, complaint/referral, and programmed inspection.

As a result of the Supreme Court decision in *Marshall v. Barlow's, Inc.*,* employers possess the right to require a search warrant prior to entry into the operations and conducting of a compliance inspection. In *Barlow's*, the Supreme Court held that Section 8(a) of the OSH Act, which empowered OSHA compliance officers to search the work area of any employment facility within OSHA's jurisdiction without a search warrant was unconstitutional. The Court concluded that "the concern expressed by the Secretary (of Labor) do not suffice to justify warrantless inspections under OSHA or vitiate the general constitutional requirement that for a search to be reasonable a warrant must be obtained."† Safety professionals should be aware that there are exceptions to the search warrant requirement for OSHA including the consent exception, Plain View exception, and Emergency exception. A fourth and controversial exception is the licensure or *Colonnade-Biswell* exception which has been applied to the OSH Act.‡

> If you think OSHA is a small town in Wisconsin, you're in trouble.
>
> **Unknown**

KNOCK AT THE DOOR

With no prior knowledge, the safety professional will receive the proverbial "knock at the door" and the OSHA compliance officer(s) will present himself/herself to the company at the security entrance or front desk. The reason for the inspection could be varied from a random inspection to a targeted inspection to a complaint inspection. Employee complaints have historically been the top category through which a compliance inspection is generated. The compliance officer will produce their credentials and often inform the safety professional the nature, purpose, and scope of inspection or specific location he/she would like to conduct the inspection.

The OSH Act specifies that a representative of the employer (i.e. safety professional) and a representative of the employees (i.e. labor organization representative or selected employee in non-union operation) must be given an opportunity to accompany the OSHA compliance officer on the inspection. The employer is not required to pay the employee their regular wages for the time spent during the inspection (although most companies do pay the employee's wages for the time spent during the inspection).§ The employer representative must be an employee and not a third party.

INSPECTION

With the consent of the safety professional or other agent of the employer, the inspection usually starts with a review of the OSHA recordkeeping documents and specific

---

* 436 U.S. 307 (1978).
† Id.
‡ *Colonnade Catering Corp. v. United States*, 397 U.S. 72 (1970) (warrantless nonconsensual searches of liquor stores) and *United States v. Biswell*, 406 U.S. 311 (1972).(nonconsensual warrantless searches of pawn shops).
§ *Chamber of Commerce v. OSHA, 636* F.2d 464 (CA-DC, 1980).

requested compliance programs, records, or documents. The compliance officer often inspects equipment, views processes, and talks with employees during the inspection. The compliance officer has the right to consult with employees concerning safety and health matters and also provides that employees shall have the right to bring OSHA violations to the attention of the compliance officer during the inspection.[*]

OSHA compliance officers are required to conduct their inspections in such a manner as to avoid disrupting the employer's business operations. Compliance officers are also required to wear and use appropriate protective equipment and clothing and must comply with the employer's safety and health rules while present in the workplace. Of particular importance, when compliance officers take photographs and sample, compliance officers must take precautions so not to create or cause hazardous conditions in the workplace. Additionally, compliance officers must treat trade secrets as confidential. This is especially important with photographs or other company documents or information which may be available from OSHA under the Freedom of Information Act.

It is important that safety professional and members of the safety team accompany the compliance officer(s) and document the same equipment, items, documents, etc. and photograph the same items as the compliance officer. In short, OSHA is collecting evidence for possible use if violations are identified, and OSHA is not required to provide the employer with this information. Safety professionals should be collecting the same evidence during the inspection to prepare and defend against the violation if issued. As noted later in this chapter, safety professionals will only be provided 15 working days to appeal and may have less time if an informal conference is requested. Every aspect of the compliance officer's inspection should be well documented for possible utilization in the event of a challenge to a violation. It is better to have the documentation and not need it rather than needing the documentation and not having it!

CLOSING CONFERENCE

When the compliance officer(s) determine the compliance inspection is completed, OSHA regulations provide that the compliance officer should confer with the safety professional or employer representatives and inform of any apparent safety and health violations identified during the inspection. Safety professionals should be aware that the compliance officer(s) is/are required to present their findings to the AD for review and approval before the identified violations would be included in the citation. When the closing conference is completed and the compliance officer(s) depart the property, the time starts for OSHA to issue the citation. OSHA is provided six months to issue the written citation.

CITATION

Under Section 9(a) of the OSH Act, if the Secretary of Labor believes that an employer "has violated a requirement under Section 5 of this Act, of any standard,

---

[*] 29 USCA Section 657(a)(2).

rule or order promulgated pursuant to Section 6 of this Act, or of any regulation prescribed pursuant to this Act, he shall within reasonable promptness issue a citation to
the employer."* Safety professionals should be aware that "reasonable promptness"
has been determined as within six months from the occurrence of the violation.†

Safety professionals should be aware that Section 9 of the OSH Act requires the
citation to be in writing and "describe with particularity the nature of the violation,
including a reference to the provision of the Act, standard, rule regulation, or order
alleged to have been violated."‡ Most citation documents are of four columns which
include the standard allegedly violated, a description of the violation, the category of
the citation, and the proposed monetary penalty. There is no specific method of service of the citations required by the OSH Act; however, most citations are sent to the
employer via certified mail with return verification to OSHA. Safety professionals
should be aware that the 15 working days for appeal starts when a representative of
the employer receives and signed for the certified mail.

Under Section 10 of the Act, after the citation is issued, the employer, any employee,
and any authorized union representative has 15 working days to file a notice of contest.§ Safety professionals should be aware that the citation document must be posted
for employee review. If the employer does not contest the violation, abatement date,
or proposed penalties within the 15 working days, the citation becomes final and
therefore not subject to review by any court or agency. If a timely notice of contest is
filed in good faith, the abatement requirement is met and a hearing is scheduled with
the Occupational Safety and Health Review Commission (OSHRC). An employer
may contest any part or all of the citations, proposed penalties, or abatement dates.
Employees have the right to elect party status after an employer has filed a notice of
contest. Safety professionals should be aware that the Notice of Contest also requires
posting for employees.

Of particular importance for safety professionals is the format for a Notice of
Contest. The Notice of Contest does not have to be in any particular form or format and must be sent to the OSHA AD who issued the citation. The OSHA AD is
required to forward the Notice of Contest to the OSHRC, which is required to docket
the case for hearing. It should be noted that several state plan programs offer fill-in-
the-blank forms to assist employers in filing a Notice of Contest.

Safety professionals should carefully review each and every word and aspect of
the citation and ensure the correctness of the alleged violation, categorization, and
penalty. One avenue through which a safety professional can check the appropriateness of the citation information is through a review of the OSHA Field Manual,
which is available on the OSHA website. This manual is utilized by the compliance
officers as a directive when addressing the appropriate categorization and requirements for alleged violations. After review, appropriate defenses can be developed
with supporting evidence acquired and prepared for hearing.

---

* 29 USC Section 651 *et. seq.*
† Id. Note: the statute of limitations contained in Section 9 (c) will not be vacated on reasonable prompt-
  ness grounds unless the employer was prejudiced by the delay.
‡ Id.
§ Id.

Safety professionals should be prepared for a compliance inspection before, during, and after the inspection. Before an inspection by the compliance officer, safety professionals should prepare their teams, methods to acquire and document evidence, and have the equipment to document the same evidence, such as photographs. At the time of inspection, safety professionals should know the type of inspection requirements, ALWAYS be professional, and how the inspection and closing conference is conducted. After the inspection, time is of the essence with the 15 working day time limitation. Safety professionals should be prepared if requesting an informal conference, pursuing a settlement agreement of appealing all of part of the citation. Remember, if the 15 working day limitation for appeal is not addressed, your company will, in essence, lose all appeal rights. Be prepared and ALWAYS be professional!

Questions

1. What is the normal process of an OSHA compliance inspection?
2. How long does a safety professional have to appeal the citation upon receipt?
3. What are the categories of OSHA standards?
4. What is the difference between a horizontal and vertical standard?
5. Explain what information is on an OSHA citation.

Selected Case Study

Case may be modified for the purposes of this text.
SECRETARY OF LABOR, Complainant, v. THE DAVEY TREE SURGERY
COMPANY, Respondent.
OSHRC Docket No. 12-0096 (2016)

DECISION AND ORDER

I. BACKGROUND: On June 27, 2011, an employee of the Davey Tree Surgery Company ("Davey Tree") was killed while cutting trees in a utility easement right-of-way that belonged to the Idaho Power Company. This utility easement was located on federal government property in the Boise National Forest. On December 27, 2011, the Secretary cited Respondent for failing to comply with several sections of the logging operations standard found at 29 C.F.R § 1910.266 and the reporting requirements found at 29 C.F.R. § 1904.39. The Secretary characterized the logging violations as serious, the reporting violations as other-than-serious, and proposed a penalty of $31,175.00.

II. DISCUSSION OF RECENT CASE LAW: On February 26, 2016, the OSHRC issued decisions in two companion cases that are relevant to the instant case, as they provide binding 2 precedent. Both cases are entitled The Davey Tree Expert Company and are listed as Docket Nos. 12-1324 and 11-2556. The Commission's holdings in these two companion cases will be discussed infra. Additionally, for purposes of brevity, the Parties' respective arguments and legal positions shall be summarized.

III. THE SECRETARY'S ARGUMENTS: The Secretary's theory of the case is that Respondent was engaged in logging operations on June 27, 2011. The Secretary believes it has established that Davey Tree Surgery Company's "large-scale tree removal project" for Idaho Power is covered by OSHA's logging operations standard. The Secretary asserts that its interpretation of the logging standard is entitled to deference. OSHA received notification of Mr. Butterfield's fatal workplace accident on June 28, 2011 via a phone message that was left on the Boise Area Office answering machine around 8:00 p.m. on June 27, 2011 (Tr. 52). AD Kearns assigned Cecil Tipton, an experienced Compliance Safety and Health Officer, to lead OSHA's investigation. AD Tipton* contacted Davey Tree's representative on June 28 and arranged to inspect the accident scene where Mr. Butterfield was fatally injured (Tr. 58). AD Tipton met Davey Tree area manager James Hartzell and safety manager Pat McDermott in Boise and drove to Respondent's staging area in Idaho City. From the staging area in Idaho City, they travelled to the worksite in the same manner as Respondent's employees. It took about an hour to get to the worksite from Boise. When AD Tipton got to the worksite, he spoke to the Boise County Sheriff's deputy and took video and measurements of the accident site, the hazard tree† that struck Mr. Butterfield, and the distance from other trees on the worksite. The hazard tree was 103-feet tall, and Mr. Butterfield was only about 70 feet away from this tree when he was struck. This same tree was approximately 100 feet from the power line. OSHA also met with Davey Tree management, returned another time to the worksite to take more detailed photographs and measurements, and conducted employee interviews. A couple weeks after the fatal accident, OSHA observed a different Davey Tree crew felling trees also using a rope come-along system. OSHA alleged that Davey Tree violated several provisions of the logging operations standard. OSHA determined that the logging operations standard applied to Davey Tree's worksite because the employees were conducting manual felling, and the logging operations standard addresses manual felling. Additionally, OSHA consulted a compliance directive related to the application of the logging operations standard for tree care operations. AD Tipton testified that he considered the application of 1910.269, OSHA's Electrical Power Generation, Transmission, and Distribution standard, but determined that it did not apply. AD Tipton determined that 1910.269 did not apply because the work crew was not working within ten feet of the power lines and they were exposed to struck-by hazards, not electrical hazards. AD Tipton did not consider the work that Mr. Butterfield and Mr. Slaven were performing

---

* 1. Mr. Tipton has since been promoted and is now the Area Director in Portland, Oregon.
† Herein, the tree that fatally struck Mr. Butterfield will be designated "the hazard tree."

to be arboriculture because they were not trimming trees, they were not using herbicides, and they were not piecing out trees – they were felling trees whole, from the stump.

Citation 1, Item 1. OSHA's investigation revealed that Davey Tree's first aid kit was missing the following required items listed in 1910.266, Appendix A: roller bandages, triangle bandages, scissors, a blanket, tweezers, tape, elastic wrap, splints, and directions for requesting emergency assistance. OSHA determined that Davey Tree did not have a written plan for what to do in case of an emergency. AD Tipton explained that because there was no communication method at the worksite, Davey Tree was "relying on traveling down a path and getting in the car and traveling down a dirt road and then hoping that somebody is going to be at home in one of these houses so you can make a phone call if there is an emergency" (Tr. 61–62). There was no plan, written or otherwise, about what the crew would do in an emergency. In other circumstances, Mr. Slaven had employed the "nearest phone"policy. Prior to commencing previous jobs, he had contacted a nearby resident and made arrangements to use the homeowner's telephone in the case of an emergency. But Davey Tree did not make prior arrangements with a nearby resident before starting the work on the instant job in Boise National Forest, and there was no cell phone coverage in the area.

Citation 1, Item 2. OSHA also determined that Davey Tree violated 1910.266(d)(6)(i), which requires employees to be spaced properly so that one employee does not present a danger to any other. Mr. Butterfield and Mr. Slaven were both working within the drop zone of the hazard tree. Because a tree being felled can strike another tree, workers other than the sawyer need to be two-tree lengths away from the tree being felled.

Citation 1, Item 3. OSHA determined that Davey Tree violated 1910.266(h)(2)(ii), which requires a hazard evaluation to be conducted before the felling of a tree. (Citation 2, Item 3). OSHA determined that Mr. Slaven failed to do an appropriate hazard evaluation by not evaluating the lean of the hazard tree and the other trees in the area. OSHA found that Davey Tree could have felled the hazard tree more uphill instead of to the side of the hill, could have used ropes properly, could have used the rope come-along system, and could have used wedges (Tr. 81).

Citation 1, Item 4a and 4b. OSHA determined that Davey Tree violated the training requirements at 1910.266(i)(3)(ii) and (iii). OSHA reviewed Davey Tree's safety manual and conducted employee interviews to understand the information and training Davey Tree provided to its employees (Tr. 66–67; Govt. Ex. 11). OSHA determined that Davey Tree did not train its employees on how to use the rope come along system; instead, employees learned how to use it through trial-and-error. Davey Tree has no written instructions related to using the rope come-along system. And, based on review of the manual and employee interviews, OSHA determined that Davey Tree did not provide any training on how to determine the height of a tree that was going to be felled. AD Tipton conducted several interviews with employees, who told him that that they guessed and relied on experience to determine tree height. AD Tipton testified that Davey Tree employees could have measured the height of the hazard tree with a laser range finder, a clinometer, or a rope. Based on his employee interviews, AD Tipton testified that employees were not trained on the "stick trick" before Mr. Butterfield was fatally struck by the tree. AD Tipton testified that the first he heard about the "stick trick" was from James Hartzell showing him what it was with a different crew. The stick trick involves holding up a stick and trying to figure out if you are in the six fall shadow of a tree. Davey Tree does not have any written instructions related to using the stick trick.

Citation 2, Item 1a and 1b. OSHA alleges that Davey Tree failed to comply with the reporting requirements at 1904.39(a) and (b)(1) (Tr. 87–88; Govt. Ex. 1). OSHA was notified about the fatal accident the following workday from a voicemail left by Mr. Pat McDermott. There was no record of calls made by Davey Tree to the 1–800 number as required by the regulations, although other callers were able to access the 1–800 number and were routed to the Boise Area office in a timely manner. Mr. McDermott testified that he attempted to call the 1–800 number and could not get through, but his phone records show only calls to the local area office. In support of its citations, OSHA consulted with a logging expert, Jeff Funke, to provide his analysis of the performance standards at issue. Mr. Funke is the AD for OSHA's Omaha Area Office in Nebraska. AD Funke has been involved in the logging industry since 1990. He got his start as an employee of his family's business, Funke Brothers Logging. Throughout AD Funke's career at OSHA, he developed specialized experience in logging. Funke conducted the majority of the logging inspections when he was a compliance officer in Montana and Idaho and provided training to compliance officers in OSHA about the logging industry. As AD Funke advanced in OSHA, he continued to hone his experience in logging through the supervision of compliance officers and by providing training to the industry. In the course of his career at OSHA, AD Funke has personally inspected at least a hundred cases involving felling operations where trees were removed from the stump (Tr. 521). From his work at Funke Brothers Logging and throughout his career at OSHA, AD Funke has gained expertise in felling techniques in this seven specialized area and he testified that there are widely accepted safe directional felling methods in the industry, including accepted distances for workers. AD Funke has been qualified and has testified as an expert in two matters before the Commission.

Based on the foregoing, the Secretary argues as follows: 1. Davey Tree's argument that the logging standard applies only if trees are felled, moved, and turned into a forest product is in direct conflict with the plain language of the standard, with this Court's order in Pettey Oil Field Servs., Inc., 2006 WL 2050961 at *1, 4–5 (No. 05-1039, 2006), and with OSHA guidance and interpretation. 2. The logging operations standard provides the regulated community adequate notice that tree removal operations are covered by the standard, even if the removal operation was performed outside the commercial tree-harvesting industry. 3. By its plain language, the logging operations standard covers Davey Tree's manual felling operations.

THE SECRETARY'S CONCLUSION: The Secretary urged the Court to reject Davey Tree's affirmative defenses, uphold the OSHA citations, and promote the necessary safeguards to prevent future fatal accidents.

RESPONDENT'S ARGUMENTS Respondent's basic theory of the case is that The Secretary "inappropriately attempted to apply the logging standard to a wholly separate and distinct industry, to wit, the utility line clearance industry." See Davey Tree's Response to the Secretary of Labor's Post-Hearing Brief at 3 (emphasis added). Respondent asserts that the logging standard simply does not apply to line-clearance operations. Id. Respondent asserts the following general, salient points: 1. Davey Tree is in the arboricultural industry. 8 2. A subset of arboricultural operations is line-clearance. 3. Line-clearance arborists are regulated by 29 C.F.R § 1910.269; the Electric Power Generation, Transmission and Distribution standard. 3. The American National Standards Institute (ANSI) standard Z133.1 contains arboricultural safety requirements for removing trees in the vicinity of electrical power lines. 4. Arborists are not loggers. See 59 Fed. Reg. 51672 (Oct. 12, 1994). 5. Respondent was performing line-clearance operations on June 27, 2011.

Respondent articulates the following, specific arguments as to why the logging standard, in particular, is inappropriate: 1. The logging standard's language is clear and unambiguous: "These types of logging include, but are not limited to, pulpwood and timber harvesting and the logging of sawlogs, veneer bolts, poles, pilings, and other forest products." See 29 C.F.R § 1910.266(b)(2). The Secretary's interpretations have been inconsistent. 2. Respondent lacked adequate notice of the Secretary's interpretation. 3. The Secretary's interpretation lacks evidence of pertinent policy considerations. 4. The August 2008 Directive in invalid for lack of notice and comment rulemaking. 5. No reasonable person could conclude that Respondent was engaged in logging operations. 6. The scale and complexity of the project demonstrates that Respondent was engaged in typical line-clearance operations on June 27, 2011. 7. Respondent did not harvest trees for usable wood. 8. Respondent did not use any heavy machinery. 9 9. The location of the tree removal project was not atypical for line-clearance work. 10. Respondent was not performing tree removals on large tracts of land. 11. The Secretary's interpretation is not entitled to deference. VI. ANALYSIS This Court has carefully reviewed the hearing transcript, the case file and the parties' post-hearing submissions. Additionally, this Court has carefully read the Commission's decisions in The Davey Tree Expert Company cases, Docket Nos. 11-2556 and 12-1324. The threshold issue before the Court is whether the logging standard applied to the work that was being performed by Davey Tree at the cited worksite on June 27, 2011. This Court finds that the totality of the evidence establishes that Respondent was not engaged in logging trees for harvest as forest products, and that the logging standard does not apply. Rather, the Court finds that Respondent was engaged in line clearance operations for Idaho Power. Following the precedent articulated by the Commission in The Davey Tree Expert Company line of cases, this Court cannot conclude that Respondent's work on the date cited in this Complaint was covered by the logging standard. The facts of this case are nearly identical to the recently decided Davey Tree line of cases, wherein the Commission determined that the logging operations standard did not apply. Accordingly, the Court finds that the logging standard's requirements do not apply to the conditions found here in Citation 1. Having decided that the logging standard does not apply, the following analyses provide additional bases for vacating certain Citations. In Citation 1, Item 1, Respondent was cited for a serious violation, pursuant to 29 C.F.R. 1910.266(d)(2)(ii): Each first aid kit did not contain the items listed in Appendix A at all times. However, AD Tipton testified that if the logging standard should be found not to apply, then 10 Respondent's first aid kit would have been in compliance with 29 C.F.R. 1910.269 (Tr. 178–79). Accordingly, the Secretary has not met his burden of persuading the Court that this Citation item should be affirmed. In Citation 1, Item 2, Respondent was cited for a serious violation, pursuant to 29 C.F.R. 1910.266(d)(6)(i): Employees were not spaced and the duties of each employee were not organized so that the actions of one employee will not create a hazard for any other employee. However, since the Court has determined that the logging standard does not apply, the Secretary has not met his burden of persuading the Court that this Citation item should be affirmed. In Citation 1, Item 3, Respondent was cited for a serious violation, pursuant to 29 C.F.R. 1910.266(h)(2)(ii): Conditions such as, but not limited to, snow and ice accumulation, the wind, the lean of the tree, dead limbs and the location of other trees, were not evaluated by the feller and precautions were not taken so a hazard in not created for an employee before each tree is felled. Mr. Harry Slaven, a Davey Tree employee, testified as a witness for the Respondent. Mr. Slaven was the feller of the tree that killed Mr. Butterfield. During direct examination, Mr. Slaven related that he had fourteen years of experience with Respondent and was a certified line clearance crew leader. He also stated that he was a member of the International Society of Arborists. He identified his copy of the Davey Tree Company Operations Manual. The witness advised that the Operations Manual has always been kept in his truck. (Id.). Mr. Slaven continued with an extensive account of the hazard evaluation process prior to the felling of this particular tree. He related that the day before the fatality, his crew, consisting of himself, Rob Butterfield and Darrell Sheepskin, conducted a walkthrough of the area. They 11 found steep terrain, burned trees and other standing trees that were dead. He related that for each tree to be felled, his crew took soundings to determine whether the tree was hollow or partially rotted. In addition, the crew noted the lean of the tree and its estimated weight. Mr. Slaven explained that they took the time to do soundings on the trees to be felled because such a tree "has the potential to be a very hazardous tree and it sends up a red flag, and it requires more attention and care to bring this tree down" (Tr. 686). Accordingly, the Secretary has not met his burden of proving that the standard applies or that its terms were violated. In Citation 1, Item 4a, Respondent was cited for a serious violation, pursuant to 29 C.F.R. 1910.266(i)(3)(ii): Training did not consist of safe use operation and maintenance of tools, machines and vehicles the employee uses or operates, including emphasis on understanding and following the manufacturer's operating and maintenance instructions, warnings, and precautions. This item refers to the alleged failure to train employees on the use of a rope come-along system. Mr. Patrick McDermott testified for Respondent. He related that he had been with Davey Tree Company for many years (1970–1975 and 1982–present), and that he was now a senior safety coordinator. His duties included safety policy, safety enforcement and safety training. Mr. McDermott discussed those safety classes he conducted for Davey Tree at four different locations in Idaho. Some of these training presentations included "Notching and Felling," "Communications," "Ropes and Knots," "Policy on Ropes in Trees," and "Hazard Trees." The substance of these five classes appears to dovetail perfectly with the duties of line clearance crews. Mr. Slaven's testimony was rich with discussions of his training in the uses of a rope come-along. Beginning in 2001, Mr. Slaven received come-along training from Brett Dixon. 12 He subsequently became familiar with using a come-along to fell trees while working with other individuals (Tr. 677–78). The testimony from Mr. McDermott and Mr. Slaven made it clear that Respondent provided the disputed training and that such training is provided in multiple locations throughout Idaho. Accordingly, the Secretary has not met his burden of persuading the Court that this citation item should be affirmed. In Citation 1, Item 4b, Respondent was cited for a serious violation, pursuant to 29 C.F.R. 1910.266(i)(3)(iii): Training did not consist of recognition of safety and health hazards associated with the employee's specific work tasks, including the use of measures and work practices to prevent or control those hazards. This Item refers to the alleged failure to train employees on how to determine the height of a tree or the tree length from the stump. During the testimony of Mr. McDermott, he testified about the stick trick. He testified, "It is a method we use to determine the height of a tree." He recalled performing this training in 2009. Mr. Slaven's testimony included his training on the use of the stick trick in March 2009. When asked on direct examination if, on the day of the accident, he knew how to use the stick trick, Mr. Slaven replied, "Yes I did." The testimony from Mr. McDermott and Mr. Slaven makes it is clear that the latter was adequately trained in an accepted method of estimating tree height. Further, on the day of the accident, Mr. Slaven knew how to use the stick trick method. Accordingly, the Secretary has not met his burden of persuading the Court that this Citation item should be affirmed.

In Citation 2, Item 1a, Respondent was cited for an other-than-serious violation, pursuant to 29 C.F.R. 1904.39(a): Within eight (8) hours after the death of any employee from a work-13 related incident or the in-patient hospitalization of three or more employees as a result of a work-related incident, the employer did not orally report the fatality/multiple hospitalization by telephone or in person to the Area Office of the Occupational Safety and Health Administration (OSHA), U.S. Department of Labor, that is nearest to the site of the incident. The employer did not use the OSHA toll-free central telephone number, 1-800-321-OSHA (1-800-321-6742). This item refers to the alleged failure of Respondent to timely report the fatality to OSHA. In fact, however, the Secretary acknowledges that Respondent telephonically notified the OSHA Area Office in Boise; to wit: "A voice message was left on the local office telephone." Citation 2, Item 1a. Also, AD Cecil Tipton testified as follows: "A telephone message was left on our answering machine at our office at approximately 8:00 that night, on the 27th" (Tr. 52, 88–89). Accordingly, the Secretary has not met his burden of persuading the Court that this citation item should be affirmed. In Citation 2, Item 1b, Respondent was cited for an Other-than-Serious violation, pursuant to 29 C.F.R. 1904.39(b)(1): On or about June 27, 2011 and at times prior thereto, the employer did not report a fatal accident to the 800 number after no one was available at the area office. This Item refers to the alleged failure of Respondent to timely report the fatality to the OSHA toll-free central number. Respondent argues that Patrick McDermott, Davey Tree's senior safety coordinator, twice received a busy signal on the central telephone number. Mr. Hartzel was present when Mr. McDermott attempted to call the central number and was not able to get through. But, Mr. McDermott's phone records showed only calls to the local area office. The Secretary has also shown that Davey Tree employees did not 14 make prior arrangements with a nearby resident for emergency telephone services before starting the work on the instant job in Boise National Forest, and there was no cell phone coverage in the area. On balance, however, the Court finds that the Secretary has carried his burden of proof regarding Citation 2, Item 1b, by establishing sufficient evidence of a violation, which Respondent was unable to rebut. Accordingly, Citation 2, Item 1b shall be AFFIRMED.

IV. ORDER This Court concurs with and is bound by the analyses conducted and the decisions reached by the Commission in The Davey Tree Expert Company line of cases; Docket Nos. 12-1324 and 11-2556. This Court finds that the logging standard does not apply to the instant case. Instead, the Court finds that Respondent was engaged in line clearance operations on June 27, 2011 at the cited worksite. The foregoing Decision constitutes the Findings of Fact and Conclusions of Law in accordance with Rule 52(a) of the Federal Rules of Civil Procedure. Based upon the foregoing Findings of Fact and Conclusions of Law, it is ORDERED that:

1. Citation 1, Item 1 is hereby VACATED, with no penalty assessed.
2. Citation 1, Item 2 is hereby VACATED, with no penalty assessed.
3. Citation 1, Item 3 is hereby VACATED, with no penalty assessed.
4. Citation 1, Items 4a and 4b are hereby VACATED, with no penalty assessed.
5. Citation 2, Item 1a is hereby VACATED, with no penalty assessed.
6. Citation 2, Item 1b is AFFIRMED, and a $300.00 penalty is ASSESSED.

11 Occupational Safety and Health Review Commission (OSHRC)

Nearly all men can stand adversity, but if you want to test a man's character, give him power.

Abraham Lincoln

Successful leaders see the opportunities in every difficulty rather than the difficulty in every opportunity.

Reed Markham

STUDENT LEARNING OBJECTIVES

1. Analyze and assess the purposes of the (Occupational Safety and Health Review Commission) OSHRC.
2. Analyze and assess the processes of the OSHRC.
3. Analyze and assess the rules of the OSHRC.

Upon receipt of the safety professional's timely notice of contest or appeal of an Occupational Safety and Health Administration (OSHA) citation (including proposed penalties), the OSHA Area Director (AD) is required to notify the OSHRC of the notice of contest in order that the OSHRC can properly schedule or docket a hearing. Scheduling or docketing a case would include appointment of a judge, scheduling a courtroom, and scheduling the date and time of hearing.

Within 20 days after receipt of the safety professional's Notice of Contest to an OSHA citation, the Secretary of Labor must file a written complaint document (known as a "complaint") with the OSHRC identifying the location, time, and circumstances of the alleged violation and specify the circumstances upon which the proposed penalties are founded.[*] Upon receipt of the complaint, the safety professional, usually through legal counsel, are provided 15 days after receipt to file a written "Answer" to the complaint with the OSHRC. Safety professionals should note that these documents usually are required to be posted and employees or union representatives are provided an opportunity to participate in an OSHA hearing if they properly petition the OSHRC to intervene as parties of interest.

---

[*] 29 CFR Section 2200.33.

Safety professionals should be aware that, in most circumstances, the employer will acquire legal counsel for the OSHRC hearing. However, the safety professional, who possesses the most knowledge regarding the inspection and alleged violations, will be an important and essential component of the legal defense team. It is essential that the safety professional provide all evidence, including inspection notes, documents, photographs, and other evidence collected during the inspection to legal counsel. Safety professionals should also be aware that the OSHRC has authority to issue subpoenas requiring attendance and testimony of witnesses and the production of documents upon application of any party to this OSHA proceeding.

OSHA hearings are conducted by Administrative Law Judges (known as "ALJ") who are assigned by the chairperson of the OSHRC. The ALJ possesses many of the same powers as a federal district court judge and often requires the parties to participate in prehearing conference(s) primarily for the purpose of exploring and facilitating settlement of the issues or simplifying the issues prior to the hearing. The mechanics of het OSHRC hearing parallel the rules of evidence applicable to the federal district court. OSHA, or the Secretary of Labor, has the burden of proof in any hearing involving a citation or proposed penalties. OSHA's attorney(s) as well as the employer's attorney(s) are entitled to a reasonable period of time for oral arguments at the close of the hearing upon proper request. All parties are permitted to, upon proper request prior to the close of the hearing, to file briefs in support of their position as well as finds of fact and conclusions of law.

Safety professionals should be aware that there is a simplified OSHRC proceeding, as well as mediation, which may be offered by the OSHRC. Simplified proceedings are designed to save time and expense with many of the formal pleadings, such as complaint and answer, being eliminated and the Federal Rules of Evidence would not be applicable. Interlocutory appeals and discovery are not permitted. The ALJ will conduct the simplified hearing and issue a written decision. In mediation, OSHA and the company are brought together in an attempt to settle the various issues in question. If the parties agree, a settlement document will be drafted for review and approval by the OSHRC.

In short, safety professionals should be aware that the OSHRC hearing parallel's the processes in federal district court. After the Complaint and Answer, there may be motions as well as discovery and other preliminary matters. The hearing is scheduled before the ALJ usually at the local federal courthouse or other appropriate location. There is NO JURY. At the hearing, there may be opening statements by the parties followed by witnesses testifying under oath and being cross-examined by the other party. A verbatim transcript is usually made of the hearing and the Federal Rules of Evidence apply. The parties often provide a closing statement and then the ALJ will close the hearing. The parties may submit briefs after the hearing which the ALJ will review. After a period of time, the ALJ will issue a written decision that contains a finding of facts, conclusions of law, and either affirms the citation and penalties, vacates the citation, or modifies the citation, proposed penalties and/or abatement requirements. The ALJ's decision is filed with the OSHRC and may be directed for review by any OSHRC member *sua sponte* or in response to a party's petition for discretionary review. Safety professionals should be aware that failure to file a petition for discretionary review precludes subsequent judicial review by the courts. This petition for discretionary review must be filed within 20 days after the ALJ's mailing of a copy of the decision to the parties.[*]

Questions:

1. What is the purpose of the OSHRC?
2. What is an ALJ and what do they do?
3. What is an Answer and what information is contained within this document?
4. What are the powers of an ALJ?
5. Who possesses the burden of proof in a case before the OSHRC and why?

OSHRC - RULES OF PROCEDURE

The OSHRC is empowered to issue an order affirming the ALJ's decision, modifying the ALJ's decision or vacating the citation and/or proposed penalties (Table 11.1). Although the OSHRC has the authority to direct "other appropriate relief" upon review of the ALJ's decision, the OSHRC does not have the authority to award attorney fees or assess costs against a party. Safety professionals should be aware that the OSHRC is not bound by the ALJ's finding of facts; however, the OSHRC is required to substantiate its contentions should it reject the ALJ's decision in a case. Parties who were adversely affected by a decision or order from the OSHRC may obtain review of the decision or order in an appropriate U.S. Court of Appeal. As permitted under Section 11(a) of the OSH Act, any person adversely affected by the OSHRC's final order may file, within 60 days of the decision, a petition for review in the U.S. Court of Appeals for the circuit in which the alleged violations occurred or in the U.S. Court of Appeal for the District of Columbia.[†]

Safety professionals should be aware of the rules and requirements in order to provide their companies or organizations the protections afforded to them under the law. Safety professionals should not fear an inspection by OSHA; however, preparation is necessary to ensure that all legal rights are protected. With most citations and penalties, effective preparation and communications lead to a cost effective and amicable settlement at informal conference. However, it is imperative that safety professionals review each and every detail of the citation and proposed penalties in preparation for any appeal. This preparation starts well before theknock at the door!

---

[*] 29 CFR Section 2200.91.
[†] 29 CFR Section 651 *et. seq.*

TABLE 11.1

Occupational Safety and Health Review Commission (Updated as of 01/15/10)

PART 2200 – RULES OF PROCEDURE

Subpart A – General Provisions

2200.1 Definitions.

2200.2 Scope of rules; applicability of Federal Rules of Civil Procedure; construction.

2200.3 Use of gender and number.

2200.4 Computation of time.

2200.5 Extensions of time.

2200.6 Record address.

2200.7 Service and notice.

2200.8 Filing.

2200.9 Consolidation.

2200.10 Severance.

2200.11 [Reserved]

2200.12 References to cases.

Subpart B – Parties and Representatives

2200.20 Party status.

2200.21 Intervention; Appearance by non-parties.

2200.22 Representation of parties and intervenors.

2200.23 Appearances and withdrawals.

2200.24 Brief of an amicus curiae.

Subpart C – Pleadings and Motions

2200.30 General rules.

2200.31 Caption; Titles of cases.

2200.32 Signing of pleadings and motions.

2200.33 Notices of contest.

2200.34 Employer contests.

2200.35 Disclosure of corporate parents, subsidiaries, and affiliates.

2200.36 [Reserved]

2200.37 Petitions for modification of the abatement period.

2200.38 Employee contests.

2200.39 Statement of position.

2200.40 Motions and requests.

2200.41 [Reserved]

Subpart D – Prehearing Procedures and Discovery

2200.50 [Reserved]

2200.51 Prehearing conferences and orders.

2200.52 General provisions governing discovery.

2200.53 Production of documents and things.

2200.54 Requests for admissions.

2200.55 Interrogatories.

(Continued)

TABLE 11.1 (*Continued*)
Occupational Safety and Health Review Commission (Updated as of 01/15/10)

Subpart D – Prehearing Procedures and Discovery
2200.56 Depositions.
2200.57 Issuance of subpoenas; Petitions to revoke or modify subpoenas; Right to inspect or copy data.

Subpart E – Hearings
2200.60 Notice of hearing; Location.
2200.61 Submission without hearing.
2200.62 Postponement of hearing.
2200.63 Stay of proceedings.
2200.64 Failure to appear.
2200.65 Payment of witness fees and mileage; Fees of persons taking depositions.
2200.66 Transcript of testimony.
2200.67 Duties and powers of Judges.
2200.68 Disqualification of the Judge.
2200.69 Examination of witnesses.
2200.70 Exhibits.
2200.71 Rules of evidence.
2200.72 Objections.
2200.73 Interlocutory review.
2200.74 Filing of briefs and proposed findings with the Judge; Oral argument at the hearing.

Subpart F – Posthearing Procedures
2200.90 Decisions of Judges.
2200.91 Discretionary review; Petitions for discretionary review; Statements in opposition to petitions.
2200.92 Review by the Commission.
2200.93 Briefs before the Commission.
2200.94 Stay of final order.
2200.95 Oral argument before the Commission.
2200.96 Commission receipt pursuant to 28 U.S.C. 2112(a)(1) of copies of petitions for judicial review of Commission orders when petitions for review are filed in two or more courts of appeals with respect to the same order.

Subpart G – Miscellaneous Provisions
2200.100 Settlement.
2200.101 Failure to obey rules.
2200.102 Withdrawal.
2200.103 Expedited proceeding.
2200.104 Standards of conduct.
2200.105 Ex parte communication.
2200.106 Amendment to rules.
2200.107 Special circumstances; waiver of rules.
2200.108 Official Seal of the Occupational Safety and Health Review Commission.

Subpart H – Settlement Part
2200.120 Settlement procedure.

TABLE 11.1 (*Continued*)

Occupational Safety and Health Review Commission (Updated as of 01/15/10)

Subpart I-L – [Reserved]

Subpart M – Simplified Proceedings

2200.200 Purpose.
2200.201 Application.
2200.202 Eligibility for Simplified Proceedings.
2200.203 Commencing Simplified Proceedings.
2200.204 Discontinuance of Simplified Proceedings.
2200.205 Filing of pleadings.
2200.206 Disclosure of Information.
2200.207 Pre-hearing conference.
2200.208 Discovery.
2200.209 Hearing.
2200.210 Review of Judge's decision.
2200.211 Applicability of Subparts A through G.

PART 2204 – RULES IMPLEMENTING THE EQUAL ACCESS TO JUSTICE ACT

Subpart A – General Provisions

2204.101 Purpose of these rules.
2204.102 Definitions.
2204.103 When the EAJA applies.
2204.104 Proceedings covered.
2204.105 Eligibility of applicants.
2204.106 Standards for awards.
2204.107 Allowable fees and expenses.
2204.108 Delegation of authority.

Subpart B – Information Required from Applicants

2204.201 Contents of application.
2204.202 Net worth exhibit.
2204.203 Documentation of fees and expenses.

Subpart C – Procedures for Considering Applications

2204.301 Filing and service of documents.
2204.302 When an application may be filed.
2204.303 Answer to application.
2204.304 Reply.
2204.305 Comments by other parties.
2204.306 Settlement.
2204.307 Further proceedings.
2204.308 Decision.
2204.309 Commission review.
2204.310 Waiver.
2204.311 Payment of award[a].

[a]OSHRC website located at www.oshrc.gov.

GUIDE TO REVIEW COMMISSION PROCEDURES
OCCUPATIONAL SAFETY AND HEALTH REVIEW COMMISSION
NOVEMBER **2007**

TABLE OF CONTENTS

SECTION 1 – INTRODUCTION

THE REVIEW COMMISSION

The Occupational Safety and Health Review Commission ("Review Commission") is an independent agency of the U.S. Government that was established by the Occupational Safety and Health Act of 1970 ("Act") to be like a court that resolves certain disputes under the Act. The Review Commission is composed of three members who are appointed by the President of the United States and confirmed by the Senate for six-year terms. It employs Administrative Law Judges to hear cases.

The Act was passed by Congress to "assure safe and healthful working conditions for working men and women." The Act also established another agency, the Occupational Safety and Health Administration (OSHA), which is part of the U.S. Department of Labor, to enforce the law. OSHA issues regulations setting occupational safety and health standards that an employer must follow. As part of its enforcement responsibilities, OSHA may also conduct an inspection of a workplace. If OSHA's inspectors find what they believe are unsafe or unhealthy conditions, they may issue a citation to an employer. A citation includes allegations of workplace safety or health violations, proposed penalties, and proposed dates by which an employer must correct the alleged hazardous conditions.

If the cited employer or any of its employees or an employee representative disagrees with the citation, they may then file a timely **notice of contest.** The Review Commission (which is **completely independent** of OSHA) then comes into the picture to resolve the dispute over the citation.

PURPOSE OF THIS GUIDE

This Guide is intended to inform employers, employees, and other interested persons about Review Commission proceedings. It provides an overview of the proceedings conducted before the Administrative Law Judges and the Commission Members and it is primarily intended to assist persons in defending their business or their employer's business after having contested an OSHA citation. It will also be useful to other persons who desire a general overview of the Review Commission and its procedures.

The Review Commission also publishes a Guide to Simplified Proceedings and an Employee Guide to Review Commission Procedures that may be obtained at the Review Commission website, located at http://www.oshrc.gov, or by writing or calling:

Executive Secretary
U.S. Occupational Safety and Health Review Commission
1120 20th Street, N.W., 9th Floor
Washington, D.C. 20036-3457
(202) 606-5400

RULES OF PROCEDURE

The Review Commission's Rules of Procedure are published in Part 2200 of Title 29, Code of Federal Regulations ("C.F.R."). These Rules may be available in a local library. They can also be obtained at the Review Commission Website, http://www.oshrc.gov, or by contacting the Review Commission's Office of The Executive Secretary at the address or telephone number above. References to the Rules in this Guide state, "See Rule" and the appropriate number (For example, "See Rule 4" refers to 29 C.F.R. § 2200.4).

This guide is intended to provide an overview of the Review Commission's procedures and it is not intended to be a substitute for the Rules of Procedure, which are followed in the Review Commission's proceedings in deciding cases. Parties to cases should review the Rules and follow them in proceedings before judges and the Commission members.

Using This Guide

This guide describes many of the documents and steps in proceedings before the Commission members and judges. Throughout this Guide, important terms are shown in bold italics and many are included in the **Glossary**.

Parties May Represent Themselves

The Review Commission's Rules do not require that a **party** – an employer, a union, or affected employee(s) – be represented by a lawyer. However, proceedings before the Review Commission are legal in nature. Certain legal formalities must be followed. OSHA will be represented by lawyers from the **Solicitor of Labor's Office,** the employer may be represented by a lawyer, and the decision in the case may have consequences beyond the amount of the penalty. For example, a decision may require corrective actions at a worksite. Parties to cases should consider carefully whether to hire a lawyer to represent them in their case.

Time is of the Essence

Many of the documents parties are required to file, such as those needed to disagree with an OSHA citation or proposed penalty, must be filed within a specific time period. Failure to file documents as required could result in a citation becoming a final order without an opportunity to appeal. Therefore, parties to cases must respond promptly to communications received from the judge, the Commission, or any of the other parties to the dispute.

Sample Legal Documents

The Appendixes contain forms and sample correspondence that may be used or referred to in preparing a case. These are mentioned as appropriate throughout the Guide.

Questions Regarding Proper Procedure

Parties to cases having questions regarding the Commission's procedures in cases pending before a judge should call the judge's office. At other stages of the proceedings, inquiries should be directed to the Executive Secretary's Office at 202-606-5400. Commission employees cannot give legal advice or advise a party how to proceed. However, they can provide information about the Rules of Procedure and the Commission's methods of processing cases.

SECTION 2 – PRESERVING RIGHTS AND CHOOSING A PROCEEDING

OSHA Citation

Cases that come before a Review Commission judge arise from inspections conducted by OSHA, an agency of the United States Department of Labor. When OSHA finds what it believes to be a **violation** at a worksite, it will notify the employer in writing of the alleged violation and the period of time it thinks reasonable for correction by issuing a written **citation** to the employer.

The period of time stated in the citation for an employer to correct the alleged violation is the **abatement period.** OSHA likely will also propose that the employer pay a monetary penalty.

The Act requires that the employer **immediately post a copy of the citation** in a place where **affected employees** will see it, to have legal notice of it. An affected employee is an employee who has been exposed to or could be exposed to any hazard arising from the cited violations.

Employer's Notice of Contest

If an employer disagrees with any part of the OSHA citation – the alleged violation, the abatement period, or proposed penalty – **it must notify OSHA in writing of that disagreement within 15 working days** (Mondays through Fridays, excluding Federal holidays) of receiving the citation. This written notification is referred to as a notice of contest, and if it is filed late with OSHA, the employer is not usually entitled to have the dispute resolved by the Commission.

The notice of contest must be delivered in writing to the AD of the OSHA office that mailed the citation. The AD's name and address will be listed on the citation. A notice of contest must not be sent to the Commission.

Informal Conference with OSHA

If a citation is issued, an employer may schedule an informal conference or engage in settlement discussions with the OSHA AD, **but this does not delay the 15 working day deadlinefor** filing a notice of contest. Thus, if an informal conference is conducted that does not result in a written settlement agreement, if a notice of contest is not filed within the 15 working day deadline all citation items must be abated and all penalties must be paid.

Content and Effect of Notice of Contest

The notice of contest is a statement that an employer intends to contest (1) the alleged violations, (2) the specific abatement periods, and/or (3) the penalties proposed by OSHA. The notice should state in detail those matters being contested (see Appendices 1A, 1B).

For example, if there are two citations and the employer wishes to contest only one of them, the citation being contested should be identified. If there are six different items alleged as violations in a single citation and the employer wishes to contest items 3, 4, and 6, those items should be specified.

If the employer wishes to contest the entire penalty, or only the amount for one citation or specific items of one citation, or only the abatement period for some or all of the violations alleged, this should also be specified.

For any item (violation) not contested, the abatement requirements must be fully satisfied and any related penalty must be paid to the Department of Labor. If the employer contests whether a violation occurred, the abatement period and the proposed penalty for that item is suspended until the Commission issues a final decision.

NOTICE OF DOCKETING

The OSHA AD sends the notice of contest to the Commission. The Executive Secretary's Office then notifies the employer that the case has been received and assigns a docket number. This docket number must be printed on all documents sent to the Commission.

EMPLOYEE NOTIFICATION

At the time the employer receives the Notice of Docketing that the case has been filed and given a docket number, the Commission will furnish a copy of a notice to be used to inform affected employees of the case. A pre-printed post card is sent to the employer with this notice; the employer returns the post card to the Commission to inform it that affected employees have been notified.

EMPLOYEES MAY CONTEST ABATEMENT PERIOD

Unions or **affected employees** wishing to participate in a dispute may file a notice of contest (see Appendix 1C) challenging the reasonableness of the period of time given to the employer for abating (correcting) an alleged violation.

Even if the employer does not contest the citation, unions or affected employees can object to the abatement period. **This must be done within 15 working days of the employer's receipt of the citation**. The notice of contest should state that the signer is an affected employee or a union that represents affected employees and that the signer wishes to contest the reasonableness of the abatement period.

The employee or the union must mail the notice of contest to the AD of the OSHA office that mailed the citation, not the Commission. The AD's name and address will be listed on the citation (see Section 10 of the Act and Rules 20, 22 and 33).

EMPLOYEES MAY ELECT PARTY STATUS

Employees may also elect party status to a case by filing a written notice of election at least ten days before the hearing. A notice of election filed less than 10 days prior to the hearing is ineffective unless good cause is shown for not timely filing the notice. It must be served on all other parties in accordance with Rule 7 (see Rule 20).

PARTY REQUESTS FOR SIMPLIFIED PROCEEDINGS

Cases heard by Administrative Law Judges may proceed in one of two ways: conventional proceedings or simplified proceedings. Each method is described in detail in Sections 3 and 4 of this Guide. The Chief Administrative Law Judge may designate a case for simplified proceedings soon after the notice of contest is received at the Review Commission. Parties may also request simplified proceedings within 20 days of the date on the notice of docketing. If a case is not designated for simplified proceedings, conventional proceedings are in effect.

CHOOSING SIMPLIFIED PROCEEDINGS OR CONVENTIONAL PROCEEDINGS

Simplified proceedings are appropriate for cases that involve less complex issues and for which more formal procedures used in conventional proceedings are deemed unnecessary to assure the parties a fair and complete contest. Simplified proceedings are covered in Section 4 of this Guide and the Commission has developed a Guide to Simplified Proceedings that is published on the Commission's website at http://www. oshrc.gov or may be obtained by writing or calling:

Executive Secretary
U.S. Occupational Safety and Health
Review Commission
1120 20th Street, N.W., 9th Floor
Washington, D.C. 20036-3457
(202) 606-5400

SECTION 3 – AN OVERVIEW OF HEARINGS CONDUCTED UNDER CONVENTIONAL PROCEEDINGS

This section describes the major features of the Commission's hearings conducted under the Conventional Proceedings method as opposed to hearings conducted under Simplified Proceedings. Simplified Proceedings are explained briefly in Section 4 and in a separate guide that should be consulted by those persons interested in that method of hearing cases.

THE COMPLAINT

Within 20 calendar days of receipt of the employer's notice of contest, the Secretary of Labor must file a written complaint with the Commission. A copy must be sent to the employer and any other parties. The complaint sets forth the alleged violation(s), the abatement period and the amount of the proposed penalty. See Appendix 2A for an example of a complaint (see Rule 34).

THE ANSWER

The employer must file a written **answer** to the complaint **with the Commission within 20 calendar days** after receiving the complaint from the Secretary of

Labor. The answer must contain a short, plain statement denying allegations of the complaint that the employer wishes to contest. **Any allegation not denied by the employer is considered to be admitted.** In addition, if the employer has a specific defense it wishes to raise, such as (1) the violation was due to employee error or failure to follow instructions, or (2) compliance with a standard was infeasible, or (3) compliance with a standard posed an even greater hazard, the answer must describe that defense. **If the employer fails to file an answer to the Complaint on time, its Notice of Contest may be dismissed, and the Citation and Penalties may become final.** The Answer must be filed with the Commission by mailing it to:

Executive Secretary
U.S. Occupational Safety and Health
Review Commission
1120 20th Street N.W., 9th Floor
Washington, D.C. 20036-3457

or to the judge, if the case has been assigned to one. A copy of the answer must also be sent to the Secretary of Labor (see Appendix 3, Rule 34).

Discovery

Discovery is a method used whereby one party obtains information from another party or person before a hearing. Discovery techniques in Commission cases include (1) written questions, called interrogatories; (2) oral statements taken under oath, which are depositions; (3) asking a party to admit the truth of certain facts, called requests for admissions; and (4) requests that another party produce certain documents or objects for inspection or copying. In conventional proceedings, any party can use these discovery techniques without the judge's permission, except for depositions, which require that that parties agree to take depositions or that the judge order the taking of depositions after a party files a motion requesting permission to do so (see Rules 51–57).

Scheduling Order or Conference

In conventional cases, discovery takes place after the answer is filed and before the hearing date. After the answer to the complaint is filed, the judge will issue an order setting a schedule for the case and may also hold a conference with the parties to clarify the issues, consider settlement, or discuss other ways to expedite the hearing (see Rule 51).

Withdrawal of Notice of Contest

A party wishing to withdraw its notice of contest to all or parts of a case may do so at any time. The **Notice of Withdrawal** must be served on all affected employees and all other parties. A copy must also be sent to the judge. See example at Appendix 8. The withdrawal terminates the proceedings before the Commission with respect to the citation or citation items covered by the notice of withdrawal (see Rule 102).

SETTLEMENT

The Commission encourages the Settlement of cases. Cases can be settled at any stage. The Secretary of Labor and the employer must agree to the settlement terms, and the affected employees or their union must be shown the settlement before it will be approved.

Any party can also request that a Settlement Judge be appointed to help facilitate a settlement (see Rule 100).

HEARINGS

Hearings are governed by Rules 60–74. The parties will be notified of the time and place of the hearing at least 30 days in advance. The employer must post the hearing notice if there are any employees who do not have a representative and served on all unions representing affected employees. The hearing is usually conducted as near the work place as possible.

At the hearing, a Commission Judge presides. The hearing enables the parties to present evidence on the issues raised in the complaint and answer. Each party to the proceedings may call witnesses, introduce documentary or physical evidence, and cross-examine opposing witnesses. In conventional proceedings, the Commission follows the Federal Rules of Evidence. Under these rules, evidence is only admitted into the record if it meets certain criteria that are designed to assure that the evidence is reliable and relevant.

HEARING TRANSCRIPTS

A transcript of the hearing will be made by a court reporter. A copy may be purchased from the reporter.

POST-HEARING BRIEFS

After the hearing is completed and before the judge reaches a decision, each party is given an opportunity to submit to the judge proposed findings of fact and conclusions of law with reasons why the judge should decide in its favor. Proposed findings of fact are what a party believes actually happened in the circumstances of a case based upon the evidence introduced at the hearing. Proposed conclusions of law are how a party believes the judge should apply the law to the facts of a case. The statement of reasons is known as a **brief** (see Rule 74).

JUDGE'S DECISION AND PETITION FOR DISCRETIONARY REVIEW

After hearing the evidence and considering all arguments, the judge will prepare a decision based upon all of the evidence placed in the hearing record and mail copies of that decision to all parties. The parties then can object to the judge's decision by filing a **Petition for Discretionary Review** (see Appendix 6 for an example). **Instructions for submitting such a petition will be stated in the judge's letter**

transmitting the decision and in a Notice of Docketing of Administrative Law Judge's Decision issued by the Executive Secretary's Office. See Rule 91 for further information on filing **Petitions for Discretionary Review.**

Decisions Final in 30 Days

If a Commissioner does not order review of a judge's decision, it becomes a final order of the Commission 30 days after the decision has been filed. If a Commissioner does direct review, it will ultimately issue its own written decision and that decision becomes the final order of the Commission.

Any party who is adversely affected by a final order of the Commission can appeal to a United States Court of Appeals. However, the courts usually will not hear appeals from parties that have not taken advantage of all possible appeal rights earlier in the case. **Thus, a party who failed to file a petition for review of the judge's decision with the Commission likely will not be able to later appeal that decision to a court of appeals.**

SECTION 4 – SIMPLIFIED PROCEEDINGS – AN OVERVIEW FOR EMPLOYERS AND EMPLOYEES

What are Simplified Proceedings?

Simplified Proceedings are designed to resolve small and relatively simple cases in a less formal, less costly, and less time-consuming manner. **The Commission's Chief Administrative Law Judge ("Chief Judge") or the judge assigned to your case notifies you that your case will be heard under Simplified Proceedings.** Even though the legal process is streamlined, the proceedings are still a trial before an Administrative Law Judge with sworn testimony and witness cross-examination.

Major Features of Simplified Proceedings

Under Simplified Proceedings:

1. Early discussions among the parties and the Administrative Law Judge are required to narrow and define the disputes between the parties.
2. Motions, which are requests asking the judge to order some act to be done, such as having a party produce a document, are discouraged unless the parties try first to resolve the matter among themselves.
3. Disclosure. The Secretary is required to provide the employer with inspection details early in the process. In some cases, the employer will also be required to provide certain documents, such as evidence of their safety program, to the Secretary.
4. Discovery, which is the written exchange of information, documents and questionnaires between the parties before a hearing, is discouraged and permitted only when ordered by the judge.

5. Appeals of actions taken by the judge before the trial and decision, such as asking the Commission to rule on the judge's refusal to allow the introduction of a piece of evidence, called interlocutory appeals, are not permitted.

6. Hearings are less formal. The Federal Rules of Evidence, which govern other trials, do not apply. Each party may present oral argument at the close of the hearing. Post-hearing briefs (written arguments explaining your position in the case), will not be allowed except by order of the judge (see Rule 209(e)). In some instances, the judge will render his or her decision "from the bench," which means the judge will state at the end of the hearing whether the evidence and testimony proved the alleged violations and will state the amount of the penalty the employer must pay, if a violation is found.

CASES ELIGIBLE FOR SIMPLIFIED PROCEEDINGS

It is possible that not all relatively small cases eligible for Simplified Proceedings will be selected (see Rules 202 and 203(a)). **The Chief Judge will assign cases for Simplified Proceedings or, if your case is not selected, you may request that it be chosen.** Cases appropriate for Simplified Proceedings are those with one or more of the following characteristics:

- Relatively simple issues of law or fact with relatively few citation items,
- Total proposed penalty of not more than $30,000,
- A hearing that is expected to take less than two days, or
- A small employer whether appearing with or without an attorney.

Cases having willful or repeated violations or that involve a fatality are not deemed appropriate for Simplified Proceedings.

EMPLOYEE OR UNION PARTICIPATION

Affected employees or their unions who file a notice of contest may also request Simplified Proceedings. Unions or an affected employee (ones exposed to the alleged health or safety hazard) wishing to participate in a dispute may file a notice of contest (see Appendix 1C) challenging the reasonableness of the period of time given to the employer for abating (correcting) an alleged violation. Even if the employer does not contest the citation, unions or affected employees can object to the abatement period. **This must be done in writing within 15 working days of the employer's receipt of the citation.** You might consider Simplified Proceedings if you or your local union wish to avoid the time and expense of a full-blown hearing. You might also participate by electing party status after the employer files a notice of contest, but must do so promptly.

When affected employees or their unions contest the time allowed for abatement, and the employer does not contest the citation, the employer may in turn elect to participate. Once the abatement date has been contested, other employees or unions may likewise elect to participate.

An employee or a union must **mail a written notice of contest to the AD of the OSHA office that issued the citation, not the Commission.** First-class mail will be sufficient for this purpose. The AD's name and address will be listed on the citation. This process is governed by Section 10 of the Act and Commission Rules 20, 22 and 33.

SHOULD YOU ASK FOR SIMPLIFIED PROCEEDINGS?

If you are an employer, have received an OSHA citation, have filed a notice of contest, and the total proposed penalties in the citation are between $20,000 and $30,000, the Chief Judge may designate your case for Simplified Proceedings. If the penalties are $20,000 or less, you may file a request for Simplified Proceedings provided that there is no allegation of willfulness or a repeat violation, and the case does not involve a fatality.

You must file your request within 20 days of docketing of your case by the Executive Secretary's Office. The request must be in writing and it is sufficient if you state: "I request Simplified Proceedings." The Chief Judge or the assigned judge will then rule on your request.

Your case may be appropriate for Simplified Proceedings but that does not necessarily mean that your particular interests are best served by requesting Simplified Proceedings. In addition to considering time and expense, you should base your decision on the facts of your case, the nature of your objections to the citation, what you will try to show the judge at the hearing, the amount of paperwork involved if your case proceeds under conventional proceedings as compared to Simplified Proceedings, and whether you have legal representation.

You should also remember that, in most circumstances, your interests may be best served if you can reach a fair and equitable settlement of your case with OSHA before a hearing. Either way, Simplified Proceedings or conventional, the proceedings are legal and the Secretary of Labor will most likely be represented by an attorney. You have the right to represent yourself or to be represented by an attorney or by anyone of your choosing.

COMPLAINT AND ANSWER

Once your case is selected for Simplified Proceedings, the complaint and answer are not required. However, until an employer is notified that a case has been designated for Simplified Proceedings, conventional procedures should be followed and an answer must be filed (see Rule 205(a)).

BEGINNING SIMPLIFIED PROCEEDINGS

You need not give any reasons for requesting Simplified Proceedings. A letter saying simply "I request Simplified Proceedings," and indicating the Docket Number assigned to your case, is sufficient (see Appendix 4). The letter must be sent to:

Executive Secretary
U.S. Occupational Safety and Health

Review Commission
1120 20th Street, N.W., 9th Floor
Washington, D.C. 20036-3457

NOTIFYING OTHER PARTIES

It is required that a copy of your request for Simplified Proceedings must be sent to the Regional Solicitor of the Department of Labor office for your region. The address is on your Notice of Docketing. All employee representatives, including an employee union, that have elected party status must also be sent a copy of your request for Simplified Proceedings. A brief statement indicating to whom, when, and how your request was served on the parties in the case must be received with the request for Simplified Proceedings. An example of such a "Certificate of Service" follows: (see Rule 203(b)).

Example: I certify that on October 1, 2004, a copy of my request for Simplified Proceedings was sent by first class mail to Jane Doe, Office of the Solicitor, U.S. Department of Labor, 123 Street, City, State Zip Code and to John Doe, President, Local 111, GHI International Union, 456 Street, City, State Zip Code (see Appendix 2B).

OBJECTIONS TO AND DISCONTINUING SIMPLIFIED PROCEEDINGS

Should you decide to object to the Chief Judge's assignment of your case to Simplified Proceedings or another party's request for Simplified Proceedings, all you need to do is file a brief written statement with the judge assigned to your case or, if the case has not been assigned to a judge, with the Chief Judge, explaining why your case is inappropriate for Simplified Proceedings. The judge is required to rule on a request for Simplified Proceedings within 15 days. Therefore, you must file your objections as soon as possible.

If you disagree with another party's request to discontinue Simplified Proceedings and you want your case to continue under Simplified Proceedings rules, you have seven days to file a letter explaining why you disagree (see Rule 204(b)).

If it appears that a case is inappropriate for Simplified Proceedings, the use of this method may be discontinued by the judge at his or her discretion. A party may also request that the judge discontinue Simplified Proceedings. The request must explain why the requesting party believes that the case is inappropriate for Simplified Proceedings. **If you agree with another party's request to discontinue Simplified Proceedings, you should submit a letter saying so**. When all parties agree that a case is inappropriate for Simplified Proceedings, the judge is required to grant the request. If the judge orders that a case be taken out of Simplified Proceedings, the case will proceed under the Commission's conventional procedures.

PRE-HEARING CONFERENCE

Soon after the parties exchange the required information, the judge will hold a pre-hearing conference to either reach settlement in the case or to find out which factual and legal issues the parties agree on. This discussion may be conducted in person but is usually conducted by a telephone conference call. The purpose of the pre-hearing conference is to settle the case or, if settlement is not possible, to determine what areas of dispute must be resolved at a hearing. Even if a settlement of the entire case cannot be reached, the parties are required to attempt agreement on as many facts and issues as possible. The discussion will include the following topics: (see Rule 207).

1. **Narrowing of Issues.** The parties will be expected to discuss all areas in dispute and to resolve as many as possible. Where matters remain unresolved, the judge will list the issues to be resolved at the hearing.
2. **A Statement of Facts.** The parties are expected to agree on as many of the facts as possible. Examples of these facts may include: the size and nature of the business, its safety history, details of the inspection, and the physical nature of the worksite.
3. **A Statement of Defenses.** You will be required to list any specific defenses you might have to the citation. The burden is on the Secretary to establish that each violation occurred. However, you should be prepared to tell the judge all reasons why you believe that the Secretary's allegations are wrong.

You might also have what is called an "affirmative defense." An affirmative defense is a recognized set of circumstances in which an employer will be found not in violation even though the employer did not comply with the cited standard. For example, you may believe that the alleged violation was the result of an employee acting contrary to a work rule that has been effectively communicated and enforced. Or, you may think that compliance with the standard was impossible or infeasible, or would have resulted in a danger to employees that was greater than the danger that the standard was designed to prevent.

You should be aware that **the burden of proving an affirmative defense is on you, the employer.** Therefore, if you argue that the violation was the result of employee misconduct, at the hearing you will have to prove to the judge that you had an effectively communicated and enforced work rule. As will be discussed later, if you raise an affirmative defense, the judge may require you to provide the Secretary of Labor with certain documents before the hearing regarding the defense. For example, if you claim that an employee violated a written work rule, you will probably be required to provide the Secretary with a copy of your company's safety rules.

It is critical that you set forth your defenses at the pre-hearing conference. You may be prohibited from later asserting any defenses not raised at the pre-hearing conference. Remember, even if your defense does not excuse the violation, the judge may find it relevant in determining the penalty amount.

4. **Witnesses and Exhibits.** The parties are expected to list the witnesses they intend to call if there is a hearing, and to list any documents or physical evidence they intend to introduce to support their positions. For example, you should list any photographs that you believe show the existence of a safety device that the Secretary claims you failed to provide.

REVIEW OF THE JUDGE'S DECISION

Any party dissatisfied with the judge's decision may petition the Commission for review of that decision.

No particular form is required for the petition (see Appendix 6). However, it should clearly explain why you believe that the judge's decision is in error on either the facts or the law or both. **Review of a judge's decision is at the discretion of the Commission. It is not a right** (see Rules 91 and 210).

Your petition should be filed no later than 20 days after issuance of the judge's written decision. Under the law, the Commission cannot grant any petition for review more than 30 days after the judge's decision is filed. Therefore, **your petition must be filed as soon as possible to obtain maximum consideration.**

The Commission will notify you whether your petition has been granted (see Appendix 7). If it is granted, your case will then proceed under the Commission's conventional rules.

SECTION 5 – OTHER IMPORTANT THINGS TO KNOW

APPEARANCES IN COMMISSION PROCEDURES

Any employer, employee, or union that initially files a notice of contest is automatically a party to the proceedings. Affected employees or their union may also choose to participate as a party where the employer has filed a notice of contest. Any party may appear in a Commission proceeding either personally, through an attorney, or through another representative (see Rule 22). Such a person need not be an attorney. However, all representatives of parties must either enter an appearance by signing the first document filed on behalf of the party or intervenor, or thereafter by filing an entry of appearance (see Rule 23).

Every party to the case must serve every other party or representative with copies of every document it files with the Commission or judge. Service is made by first class mail, electronic transmission, or personal delivery (see Rule 7(c)).

All notices the Commission sends to the parties will list the name and address of all parties or their representatives (see Rule 22). Parties must do the same.

PENALTIES

OSHA only **proposes** amounts which it believes are appropriate as penalties. These proposals automatically become penalties assessed against the cited employer when the enforcement action is not contested. Once a **citation or proposed penalty** is contested, the amount of the penalty for that citation, if any, will be decided by the Commission or a judge.

When a case goes to hearing before a Review Commission judge, the employer's evidence and argument on what penalty, if any, should be assessed, receives the same consideration as the evidence and argument of the Secretary of Labor.

The four factors that the law requires the Commission to consider in determining the appropriateness of civil penalties are:

- The size of the business of the employer being charged,
- The gravity of the violation,
- The good faith of the employer, and
- The employer's history of previous violations.

The amounts that may be assessed as civil penalties by the Commission under Section 17 of the Act are as follows:

- For a serious or non-serious violation: up to $7,000.00
- For violations committed willfully or repeatedly: up to $70,000.00
- For failure to correct a violation within the period permitted: up to $7,000.00 for each day it remains uncorrected.

PRIVATE (EX PARTE) DISCUSSIONS

Parties to cases before the Commission may not communicate ex parte (without the knowledge or consent of the other parties) with respect to the merits of a case with the judge (except a Settlement Judge), a Commissioner, or any employee of the Commission. In other words, no participant, directly or indirectly, may discuss the case or make any argument about a matter in a case to any of these people unless done in the presence of the other participants who are given an equal opportunity to present their side, or unless it is done in writing and copies are sent to all other parties. Violation of this rule may result in dismissal of the offending party's case before the Commission. This prohibition does not, however, preclude asking questions about the scheduling of a hearing or other matters that deal only with procedures (see Rule 105).

PETITION FOR MODIFICATION OF ABATEMENT

An employer who does not contest a **citation** is required to correct all of the violations within the **abatement period** specified in the **citation**. If the Commission upholds a contested citation, the employer must then correct the violation, with the **abatement period** starting on the date of the Commission's final order. If the employer has made a good faith effort to correct a violation within the **abatement period** but has not been able to do so because of reasons beyond his or her control, the employer may file a **Petition for Modification of Abatement (PMA)**. This petition is filed with the **OSHA** area director and should be filed no later than the end of the next working day following the day on which abatement was to have been completed. It must state why the abatement cannot be completed within the given time. The PMA must be posted in a conspicuous place where all affected employees can see it or near the location where the violation occurred. The PMA must remain posted for 10 days. The Secretary of Labor may not approve a PMA until the expiration of 15 working days from its receipt.

At the end of the 15-day period, if the Secretary of Labor, affected employees, or their union object to the petition, the Secretary of Labor is required to forward the PMA to the Commission. After notice by the Commission to the employer and the objecting parties of its receipt of the PMA, each objecting party has 10 calendar days in which to file a response to the PMA setting out the reasons for opposing it. Proceedings before the Commission are conducted in the same way as notice-of-contest cases, except that they are expedited. The employer must establish that abatement cannot be completed for reasons beyond the employer's control, and has the burden of proving the petition should be granted. In cases of this kind, the employer is called the Petitioner, the Secretary of Labor is called the Respondent (see Rules 37 and 103).

EXPEDITED PROCEEDINGS

In certain situations, time periods allowed for certain procedures are shortened. The Commission's Rules of Procedure provide that an **Expedited Proceeding may** be ordered by the Commission. If an order is made to speed up proceedings, all parties in the case will be specifically notified. All **Petitions for Modification of Abatement and all employee contests** are automatically expedited (see Rule 103). Expedited proceedings are different from Simplified Proceedings (see Rule 103).

MAINTAINING COPIES OF PAPERS FILED WITH THE JUDGE

In order that Affected Employees may have the opportunity to be kept informed of the status of the case, the employer must keep available at some convenient place copies of all pleadings and other documents filed in the case, so they can be read at reasonable times by Affected Employees.

SECTION 6 – DESCRIPTIVE TABLE OF CONVENTIONAL PROCEEDINGS FOR CONTESTING AN OSHA CITATION

EVENTS COMMON TO ALL PROCEEDINGS

- Employer files notice of contest with OSHA office that mailed citation – within 15 working days of receiving the citation.
- Employer receives notification (notice of docketing) from Commission of case, docket number and forms to notify employees.
- Employer posts notification to employees of case in progress.
- Union and/or affected employees may contest reasonableness of abatement period; notice of contest is sent to citing OSHA office within 15 working days of the employer's receipt of the citation.
- If the Chief Administrative Law Judge has not assigned the case for Simplified Proceedings, and if a party has not requested Simplified Proceedings within 20 days of the notice of docketing and the request is not granted, conventional proceedings will be used (see Rule 203).

EVENTS PERTAINING TO CONVENTIONAL PROCEEDINGS

The Employer:

- Receives a complaint from OSHA's attorneys.
- Files an answer to the complaint within 20 calendar days of receiving the complaint.
- Discusses discovery techniques with the judge when applicable.
- Participates in a conference call to discuss issues and a possible settlement.
- Engages in discovery; exchanges interrogatories and depositions.
- Discusses settlement in another conference call with OSHA and judge. If not settled, then:
  - Prepares for and participates in the hearing.
  - May purchase a copy of the hearing transcript and may choose to submit a brief to the judge.
- Judge issues a decision (If dissatisfied, any party may ask for Commission review of the decision.

SECTION 7 – DESCRIPTIVE TABLE OF CONTESTING AN OSHA CITATION AND CHOOSING SIMPLIFIED PROCEEDINGS

EVENTS COMMON TO ALL PROCEEDINGS

- Employer files notice of contest with OSHA office that mailed citation – within 15 working days of receiving the citation.
- Employer receives notification (notice of docketing) from Commission of case, docket number and forms to notify employees.
- Employer posts notification to employees of case in progress.
- Union and/or affected employees may contest reasonableness of abatement period; notice of contest is sent to citing OSHA office within 15 working days of citation's posting at work place.
- If the Chief Administrative Law Judge has assigned the case for Simplified Proceedings, or if a party has requested Simplified Proceedings and the request is granted, Simplified Proceedings will be in effect (see Rule 203).

EVENTS PERTAINING TO SIMPLIFIED PROCEEDINGS

If all disputed issues not resolved at the prehearing conference, then parties:

- List witnesses and exhibits.
- Prepare for and participate in the hearing.
- Present oral arguments at the close of the hearing.
- May purchase a copy of the hearing transcript.
- Decide whether to request permission to file a brief.

Judge issues decision.

- If dissatisfied, any party may ask for Commission review of the decision.

SECTION 8 – DESCRIPTIVE TABLE OF EVENTS
PERTAINING TO REVIEW OF AN ADMINISTRATIVE LAW JUDGE'S DECISION

If an employer is dissatisfied with an administrative law judge's decision and wishes to seek review by the Commission members, the employer:

- Receives judge's decision; dissatisfied with the outcome.
- Files petition for discretionary review of the judge's decision.
- Receives notification from Commission that case is or is not directed for review.

If the case is not directed for review, the judge's decision is a final order of the Commission and the employer may file a petition for review in a Court of Appeals.
  If the case is directed for review, all parties:

- Receive a request from Commission for briefs on review.
- File briefs on review before Commission.
- Receive Commission decision that may supercede the judge's decision and affirm, modify or reverse it. In some cases, the judge's decision may be remanded for further proceedings.
- Files petition for review in Court of Appeals if dissatisfied with Commission decision.

See also Rules 90–96.

Glossary

Abatement Period – Period of time specified in citation for correcting alleged workplace safety or health violation.

Affected Employee – An affected employee is one who has been exposed to or could be exposed to any hazard arising from the cited violations – that is the circumstances, conditions, practices, or operations creating the hazard.

Answer – Written document filed in response to a complaint, consisting of short plain statements denying the allegations in the complaint which the employer contests.

Authorized Employee Representative – A labor organization, such as a union, that has a collective bargaining relationship with the employer and represents affected employees or may be an affected employee(s) in cases where unions do not represent the employees.

Brief – A written document in which a party states what the party believes are the facts of the case and argues how the law should be applied.

Certificate of Service – A document stating the date and manner in which the parties were served (given) a document. See Appendix 2B for sample certificate (Also see definition of "service").

Citation – Written notification from OSHA of alleged workplace violation(s), proposed penalty(ies), and abatement period.

Complaint – Written document filed by the Secretary of Labor detailing the alleged violations contained in a citation.

Conventional Proceedings – Typical Review Commission proceedings, which are similar to, but less formal than, court proceedings.

Discovery – The process by which one party obtains information from another party prior to a hearing.

Exculpatory Evidence – Information that may clear one of a charge or of fault or of guilt; in the context of OSHRC cases, information that might help the employer's case.

Exhibit – Something, e.g. a document, video, etc., that is formally introduced as evidence at a hearing.

File – To send papers to the Commission Executive Secretary, or to the judge assigned to a case, and to give copies of those papers to the other parties in the case.

Interlocutory Appeal – An appeal of a judge's ruling on a preliminary issue in a case that is made before the judge issues a final decision on the full case. These types of appeals are infrequently made and are infrequently allowed. One example of an issue often raised in an interlocutory appeal is whether certain material that a party wants kept confidential, such as an employer's trade secrets or employee medical records, should become part of the public record in a case.

Motion – A request asking that the judge direct some act to be done in favor of the party making the request or motion.

Notice of Appearance – A written letter informing the Review Commission of the name and address of the person or persons who will represent a party (that is, the employer or a union or OSHA) in a case.

Notice of Contest – Written document disagreeing with any part of an OSHA citation.

Notice of Docketing – Written document from the Review Commission's Executive Secretary telling an employer, the Secretary of Labor, and any other parties in a case that the case has been received by the Commission and given an OSHRC docket number.

Notice of Withdrawal – A written document from a party withdrawing its notice of contest or the citation and thus terminating the proceedings before the Commission (see Appendix 8).

Party – The Secretary of Labor, anyone who files a notice of contest, or a union or affected employee(s) that requests party status.

Petition for Discretionary Review – A written request from a party in a case asking the Commission in Washington, DC to review and change the judge's decision. The grounds on which a party may request discretionary review are: (1) it believes the judge made findings of material facts which are not supported by the evidence; (2) it believes that the judge's decision is contrary to law; (3) it believes that a substantial question of law, policy, or abuse of discretion is involved; or (4) it believes that a prejudicial error was committed.

Pro Se – Latin for without an attorney.

Secretary of Labor – The head of the U.S. Department of Labor. OSHA is part of that Department.

Service – Sending by first class mail or personal delivery a copy of documents filed in a case to all parties in the case. See Definition of "Certificate of Service" (see Rule 7).

Settlement – An agreement reached by the parties resolving the disputed issues in a case.

Simplified Proceedings – Review Commission proceedings that are less formal than Conventional Proceedings and designed for smaller and relatively simple cases. A complaint and answer are not required and discovery occurs only if the judge permits it.

Solicitor of Labor – The U.S. Department of Labor's chief lawyer who has offices throughout the country. Lawyers from these offices represent the Secretary of Labor and OSHA in Review Commission cases

Appendixes/Sample Legal Documents

This section is not intended to be a manual of forms, and the sample legal documents here are limited in number. The sample legal documents are intended for illustration to familiarize the reader with the general nature of some of the documents received and issued. Many of the documents received by the Commission, such as those in Appendices 2, 3, and 6 (Complaint, Answer, and Petition for Discretionary Review), vary significantly from case to case.

APPENDIX 1 - NOTICE OF CONTEST

APPENDIX 1A. NOTICE OF CONTEST TO CITATION AND PROPOSED PENALTIES

XYZ Corp.
123 Street
City, State Zip Code
February 26, 2004

ABC, Area Director
Occupational Safety and Health Administration
U.S. Department of Labor, Federal Building
City, State Zip Code

Dear Mr. ABC:

This is to notify you that XYZ Corp. intends to contest all of the items and penalties alleged in the Citation and Proposed Penalty, received February 20, 2004, and dated February 19, 2004 (a copy is attached).

Very truly yours,

XYZ, President

APPENDIX 1B. NOTICE OF CONTEST TO PROPOSED PENALTIES ONLY

XYZ Corp.
123 Street

City, State Zip Code
September 14, 2004

ABC, Area Director
Occupational Safety and Health Administration
U.S. Department of Labor, Federal Building
City, State Zip Code

Dear Mr. ABC:

I wish to contest the amount of the Proposed Penalties of $1,200 issued September 9, 2004, based on the violations cited by you during your recent inspection.

Sincerely,

XYZ, President
General Manager

APPENDIX 1C. NOTICE OF CONTEST BY EMPLOYEE REPRESENTATIVE

GHI International Union
456 Street
City, State Zip Code
June 9, 2004

ABC, Area Director
Occupational Safety and Health Administration
U.S. Department of Labor, Federal Building
City, State Zip Code

Dear Mr. ABC:

We have been authorized by the employee representative, GHI International Union, to file this notice of contest to the OSHA citations issued on June 2, 2004, against the employer, XYZ Co. The abatement dates of June 27, 2004, for Items No. 1 and No. 3 of the non-serious citation, and January 5, 2005, for Item No. 1 of the serious citation, are unreasonable and will continue to expose workers to safety hazards.

Sincerely,

JKL, Director
Safety Department
GHI International Union

APPENDIX 2 - COMPLAINT AND CERTIFICATE OF SERVICE

APPENDIX 2A. COMPLAINT

U. S. Occupational Safety and Health Review Commission
Secretary of Labor,
  Complainant,

  v.   OSHRC Docket No. 99-9999

XYZ Co.,
  Respondent,

COMPLAINT

This action is brought to affirm the Citations and Notifications of penalty issued under the Occupational Safety and Health Act of 1970, 29 U.S.C. § 651, et seq., hereinafter the Act, of violations of §5(a) of the Act and the Safety and Health Regulations promulgated thereunder.

I

Jurisdiction of this action is conferred upon the Commission by §10(a) of the Act.

II

Respondent, XYZ Co., is an employer engaged in a business affecting commerce within the meaning of §3(5) of the Act.

III

The principal place of business of respondent is at 123 Street, City, State, Zip Code, where it was engaged in retail sales as of the date of the alleged violations.

IV

The violations occurred on or about June 9, 2004, at 123 Street, City, State, Zip Code (hereinafter "workplace").

V

As a result of an inspection at said workplace by an authorized representative of the complainant, respondent was issued three Citations and Notifications of Penalty pursuant to §9(a) of the Act.

VI

The Citations and Notifications of Penalty, copies of which are attached hereto and made a part hereof as Exhibits "A," "B," and "C" (consisting of one page each) identify and describe the specific violations alleged, the corresponding abatement dates fixed, and the penalties proposed.

VII

On or about July 29, 2004, by a document dated July 26, 2004, the complainant received notification, pursuant to §10(a) of the Act, of respondent's intention to contest the aforesaid Citations and Notifications of Penalty.

VIII

The penalties proposed, as set forth in Exhibits "A," "B," and "C" are appropriate within the meaning of §17(j) of the Act. The abatement dates fixed were and are reasonable.

WHEREFORE, cause having been show, complainant prays for an Order affirming the Citations and Notifications of Penalty, as aforesaid.

JKL, Attorney
Office of the Solicitor
U.S. Department of Labor, Federal Building
City, State Zip Code

APPENDIX 2B. CERTIFICATE OF SERVICE*

I certify that the foregoing Complaint was served this 19th day of August, 2004, by mailing true copies thereof, by first class mail to:

XYZ
XYZ Corp.
123 Street
City, State Zip Code

PQR
Attorney

*A similar document must accompany all other documents requiring a certificate of service.

APPENDIX 3 - ANSWER

U. S. Occupational Safety and Health Review Commission

Secretary of Labor,
          Complainant,
          v.   OSHRC Docket No. 99-9999
XYZ Corp.,
          Respondent,

ANSWER
I, II, III

Respondent admits Paragraphs I, II and III.

IV

Respondent denies Paragraph IV.

V

Respondent neither admits nor denies the allegations at Paragraph V.

VI

Respondent denies Paragraph VI.

VII

Respondent neither admits nor denies the allegations at Paragraph VII.

VIII

Respondent denies the allegations at Paragraph VIII. The penalties are excessive under § 17(j) of the Act based upon the small size of the employer, which has only twelve employees, and the low gravity of the alleged violations.

IX

Respondent pleads the affirmative defense of "greater hazard." Abatement of the alleged violations will increase the safety risk to employees. Respondent also pleads the affirmative defense of "unpreventable employee misconduct." The alleged conditions were the result of unauthorized actions by certain employees which resulted in the conditions referred to in the alleged violations.

RESPONDENT
By _____
Attorney
XYZ Corp.
123 Street
City, State Zip Code

APPENDIX 4 – REQUEST FOR SIMPLIFIED PROCEEDINGS

XYZ Corp.
123 Street
City, State Zip Code

March 26, 2004

Executive Secretary
U.S. Occupational Safety and Health
Review Commission
1120 20th Street, N.W., 9th Floor
Washington, D.C. 20036-3457

Dear Executive Secretary;

I request Simplified Proceedings. The Review Commission Docket Number assigned to my case is 99-9999.

Very truly yours,

XYZ, President

APPENDIX 5 - NOTICE OF DECISION

Notice of Decision
In Reference To:
Secretary of Labor v. XYZ Corp.
OSHRC Docket No. 99-9999

1. Enclosed is a copy of my decision. It will be submitted to the Commission's Executive Secretary on January 3, 2004. The decision will become the final order of the Commission at the expiration of thirty (30) days from the date of docketing by the Executive Secretary, unless within that time a member of the Commission directs that it be reviewed. All parties will be notified by the Executive Secretary of the date of docketing.

2. Any party that is adversely affected or aggrieved by the decision may file a petition for discretionary review by the Review Commission. A petition may be filed with the Judge within ten (10) days from the date of this notice. Thereafter, any petition must be filed with the Review Commission's Executive Secretary within twenty (20) days from the date of the Executive Secretary's notice of docketing. See Paragraph No. 1. The Executive Secretary's address is as follows:

Executive Secretary
Occupational Safety and Health
Review Commission
1120 20th Street, N.W. - 9th Floor
Washington, D.C. 20036-3457

3. The full text of the rule governing the filing of a petition for discretionary review is 29 C.F.R. 2200.91. It is appended hereto for easy reference, as are related rules prescribing post-hearing procedure.

MNO
Administrative Law Judge

December 1, 2004

APPENDIX 6 - PETITION FOR DISCRETIONARY REVIEW

U.S. Occupational Safety and Health Review Commission
Secretary of Labor,
          Complainant,

          v.   OSHRC Docket No. 99-9999

XYZ Corp.,
          Respondent,

PETITION FOR DISCRETIONARY REVIEW

Comes now Respondent, XYZ Corp., being aggrieved by the Decision and Order of the Administration Law Judge in the above-styled matter, and hereby submits its

Petition for Discretionary Review pursuant to 29 CFR 2200.91-Rule 91, Rules of Procedure of the Occupational Safety and Health Review Commission.

Statement of Portions of the Decision and Order to Which Exception Is Taken

1. XYZ Corp. takes exception to that portion of the Decision and Order wherein the Administrative Law Judge held XYZ Corp. in serious violation of the standard published at 29 CFR 1926.28(a) as alleged in Serious Citation 1, Item 1, in finding that XYZ's employee John Jones was exposed to the alleged violation (Judge's Decision at pp. 8–12).

2. XYZ Corp. takes exception to that portion of the Decision and Order pertaining to Serious Citation 1, Item 1, wherein the Administrative Law Judge held that action of employee John Jones was not unpreventable employee misconduct (Judge's Decision at pp. 13–17).

Statement of Reasons For Which Exceptions Are Taken

1. In his Decision, the Administrative Law Judge failed to follow the test set forth for the Fifth Circuit's Decision in Secretary of Labor v. RPQ Corp. for determining the existence of employee exposure. The testimony at transcript pages 25–45 clearly shows that John Jones was not in the zone of danger because he was on a work break and outside of the definition of the zone.

2. The evidence of record supports XYZ's position that the actions taken by employee John Jones were unpreventable. The Commission has set forth the test for determining unpreventable employee misconduct at Secretary of Labor v. ROM Corp. The testimony of XYZ's employees at transcript pp. 46–59 met all of the requirements of ROM Corp. to prove John Jones's actions were unpreventable.

For the reasons stated herein, XYZ Corp. hereby submits that the Occupational Safety and Health Review Commission should direct review of the Decision and Order of the Administrative Law Judge.

Respectfully submitted,

By _____
Attorney for
XYZ Corp.
123 Street
City, State Zip Code
Tel. No. (999) 999-9999

APPENDIX 7 - DIRECTION FOR REVIEW

U.S. Occupational Safety and Health Review Commission
Secretary of Labor,
        Complainant,

        v.   OSHRC Docket No. 99-9999

XYZ Corp.
        Respondent,

DIRECTION FOR REVIEW

Pursuant to 29 U.S.C. § 66(j) and 29 C.F.R. § 2200.92(a), the report of the Administration Law Judge is directed for review. A briefing order will follow.

COMMISSIONER

Dated:

APPENDIX 8 - NOTICE OF WITHDRAWAL

U.S. Occupational Safety and Health Review Commission

Secretary of Labor,

   Complainant,

   v.   OSHRC Docket No. 99-9999

XYZ Corp,

   Respondent,

Respondent's Withdrawal of Notice of Contest

Respondent, XYZ Corp., by the undersigned representative, hereby withdraws its Notice of Contest in the case with the docket number above, pursuant to 29 CFR 2200.102 of the Rules of Procedure for the Commission.

XYZ

XYZ Corp.

123 Street

City, State Zip Code

March 30, 2004 *

Case Modified for the Purpose of this Text

UNITED STATES OF AMERICA

OCCUPATIONAL SAFETY AND HEALTH REVIEW COMMISSION

1825 K STREET N.W 4TH FLOOR WASHINGTON DC. 20006-1246

SECRETARY OF LABOR – Complainant v. OSHRC Docket STATE SHEET METAL COMPANY, INC., – Respondent.

Nos. 90-1620 and 90-2894

DECISION BEFORE: Chairman, Commissioners. BY THE COMMISSION:

In each of the above cited cases, State Sheet Metal Company ("State") was installing metal roof decking when a compliance officer of the Occupational Safety and Health Administration ("OSHA") inspected the worksites in question. As a result of those inspections, the Secretary of Labor issued two citations, each' alleging that State had failed to comply with various OSHA standards, including the standard at

---

* OSHRC website located at www.oshrc.gov.

29 C.F.R. § 1926.105(a).[*] State contested the citations from both inspections, and a hearing was held in each case before an administrative law judge of this Commission. Decisions have been issued in both cases; in each, the judge found that State had violated section 1926.105(a). State sought review of both decisions, and review was directed pursuant to section 12(j) of the Occupational Safety & Health Act of 1970 ("the Act"), 29 U.S.C. § 661(j). State also sought consolidation of the two cases under Rule 9 of the Commission's Rules of Procedure, 29 C.F.R. § 2200.9.[†] Finding that the parties to both cases are the same and that there are common issues of law and fact, we conclude that consolidation is appropriate. We therefore consolidate Docket Number 90-1620 and Docket Number 90-2894.

The essential facts are largely undisputed. Having carefully reviewed the records in both cases, we conclude that they may be decided without further briefs.

I. BACKGROUND

State installs sheet metal roof decking on new commercial construction. From the records in these cases, it appears that the manufacturer of the metal decking being installed by State normally enters into a contract with the general contractor to supply and install the roof decking and then takes bids from other companies to perform the installation and lets a contract. In both of these cases, the contract was awarded to Nilsen-Smith Sheet Metal Co. ("Nilsen-Smith"), which has the same owners and management as State. Nilsen-Smith, which does not actually install the decking itself, subcontracted the work to State after it was awarded these contracts.

a. Docket Number 90-1620

In Docket Number 90-1620, State was installing sheet metal roof decking in Mount Olive, New Jersey, on a one-story warehouse that would be occupied by United Parcel Service. The warehouse, which was 27 feet high and had 148,000 square feet of floor space, was being constructed in sections, or "bays," 40 feet by 40 feet.

At the time of the inspection, the decking was approximately half completed, with an area 400 feet by 150–200 feet still to be laid. The compliance officer who conducted the Mount Olive inspection saw exposed steel reinforcing bars protruding from the ground below the edge of the completed decking and testified that, because no fall protection was being used, an employee who fell could have been impaled or suffered other serious injury. Mr. Smith, one of the owners of Nilsen-Smith and State, testified that, although it was possible to install nets, it was difficult and expensive. In his opinion, using nets would double

---

[*] That standard provides: § 1926.105 Safety nets.

a. Safety nets shall be provided when workplaces are more than 25 feet above the ground or water surface, or other surfaces where the use of ladders, scaffolds, catch platforms, temporary floors, safety lines, or safety belts is impractical.

[†] That rule provides: 0 2200.9 Consolidation.

Cases may be consolidated on the motion of any party, on the Judge's own motion, or on the Commission's own motion, where there exist parties, common questions of law or fact or in such other circumstances as justice or the administration of the Act require.

the cost of the job, and he could not do the work for his bid price. He does not know what the cost would be either to buy or rent nets, and he has never explored the cost of installing nets or talked to anyone involved in their installation. He had seen nets hung using a power lift, but stated that the floor must be level if a lift' is to be used. He stated that none of his competitors uses nets on a one-story building and that he does not include-the cost of using nets in his bids because none of his competitors does.

b. Docket Number 90-2894

In Docket Number 90-2894, State was installing metal roofing on a one-story. ShopRite Food warehouse in South Brunswick, New Jersey. As a result of the inspection at the South Brunswick worksite, Nilsen-Smith was cited for violating three OSHA standards, and Nilsen-Smith contested the citation.

During the pleadings stage of the case, the Secretary amended the complaint to allege that the correct employer was State, not its sister company Nilsen-Smith; State has admitted that allegation. The Secretary also amended the complaint to allege in the alternative, a violation of 29 C.F.R. 8 1926.10&) or 23 C.F.R. 5 hearing that the warehouse was not a applies only to tiered buildings, it does 1926.750(b)(1)(ii). The parties stipulated at the tiered building. Because section 1926.750(b)(1) not apply to the conditions cited, and the judge therefore adjudicated the allegation that State had violated section 1926.105(a).*

4 The warehouse in South Brunswick was 32 feet, 8 inches high and was designed to have 800,000 square feet of floor space. Its floor space was being divided into 320 bays, each 50 feet by 57 feet. The bays were made up of formed concrete columns supporting large header beams and intermediate bar joists. The compliance officer who performed the South Brunswick inspection testified that he saw employees who were decking the roof step from the edge of the decked portion of the roof onto the 4-inch-wide steel joists. No fall protection was being used to prevent them from falling to the ground 32 feet below. He estimated that the cost of the nets, exclusive of labor, would be $700 per bay or $4000 for enough nets to cover six bays at a time. Mr. Smith and insisted that decking comes in also testified at the hearing in this case. He described the decking process his employees always stood on the decking, not the joists. The metal bundles of 45 sheets. The sheets are three feet wide and come in varying lengths, ranging from 10 feet to

---

* That standard provides: 0 1926,750 Flooring requirements.
...

b. *Temporary flooring–skeleton steel construction in tiered buildings. (1)*
...

ii. On buildings or structures not adaptable to temporary floors, and where scaffolds are not used, safety nets shall be installed and maintained whenever the potential fall distance exceeds two stories or 25 feet. The nets shall be hung with sufficient clearance to prevent contacts with the surface of structures below.

34 feet. At the start of a job, the first bundle of decking is put in place and the bottom sheet becomes the first sheet installed. The employees then take the top sheet of the bundle and, standing on the bundle, they put it in place. They then stand on that sheet while they take the next sheet from the bundle and put it into place, and the work continues in this manner, with the employees standing on the decking at all times. A two-man crew can lay 20,000 square feet of decking a day, and a three-man crew can deck 10 bays a day. Mr. Smith stated that it is physically possible to erect nets and that, while he has never done so himself, he has watched them being put up. He has never seen them used on a one-story building, however, and neither he nor anyone in authority at State had discussed putting up nets on a job like this. In his view, it would not be cost efficient because it would take twice as long to put up the nets as it takes to do the roofing, and the roofing crew could cover more area in a day than a crew could net. Mr. Smith testified that he had bid for this job against five or six other companies who did not include the cost of netting the area in their bids. Mr. Smith said that the ground had not been leveled when the steel framework for this warehouse went up, and it was too bumpy and muddy to operate a lift truck on it. State was not allowed to move earth inside the building itself. He said that, under industry practice, a general contractor might level the ground before the roofing is installed as a favor to the roofing subcontractor, but there is no obligation for it to do so. The concrete floor was not poured until after the roofing was completed. The Secretary called as an expert witness a compliance officer who had not conducted the original inspection but had later visited the South Brunswick worksite. When this compliance officer visited the site, he saw a plumber using a scissor lift to install a sprinkler system. Although there were a few depressions, the compliance officer estimated that 70 percent of the ground was level and that, in general, it was sufficiently level to use a lift truck to install nets. He testified that, because the roofing crew decked six to seven bays per day, it would be necessary to net that many bays at one time. He estimated that it would take four men approximately four hours to erect the nets in one bay, and that the time required might decrease to three hours as they gained experience, but it would take only one hour per bay to take the nets down. It would take approximately two working days to put up nets in seven bays, while the roofing crew could deck seven bays in one day. Although he had never seen netting used to cover several bays on a one-story building like this one, the compliance officer stated that he had seen structural steel erectors net several bays at one time at the Meadowlands. He gave his opinion that, although using nets could make the job cost three to four times as much, it was feasible to do and that it was practical to do so to save a life.

II. THE ELEMENTS OF A VIOLATION

In order to prove that an employer violated an OSHA standard, the Secretary must prove that (1) the standard applies to the working conditions cited; (2)

the terms of the standard were not met; (3) employees had access to the violative conditions; and (4) the employer knew of the violative conditions or could have known with the exercise of reasonable diligence. Kulka Constr. M&t. Cop, 15 BNA OSHC 1870, 1992 CCH OSHD ¶ 29,829 (No. 884167, 1992); Astra Pharmaceutical Prods., Inc., 9 BNA OSHC 2126, 1981 CCH OSHD ¶ 25,578 (No. 78-6247, 1981), aff'd, 681 F.2d 69 (1st Cir. 1982). "A prima facie violation of section 1926.105(a) is established if the Secretary can show that employees were subject to falls of twenty-five feet or more and none of the safety devices listed in the standard were utilized." Cleveland Consol., Inc. v. OSHRC, 649 F.2d 1160, 1165 (5th Cir. Unit B, 1981); Sierra Constr. Corp., 6 BNA OSHC 1278, 1280, 1978 CCH OSHD ¶ 22,506, p. 27,157 (No. 13638, 1978). The essential facts in determining whether a prima facie violation has been established are that both warehouses were more than 25 feet high, the distance specified in section 1926.105(a), and that no fall protection was being used at either site.

a. Applicability of the Standard

State's employees were performing construction work on an untiered building, working more than 25 feet above the ground. We therefore find that the cited standard applies to the cited working conditions.

b. Failure to Comply

State has asserted that it was in compliance because the decking on which its employees were working constituted a temporary floor, which complied with the requirements of section 1926.105(a). In support of this claim, State has cited two decisions involving its sister company, Niken-Smith Roofing & Sheet Metal Co., 80 OSAIRC 13/Cl (No. 77-2735,1980) (ALJ), and Niben-Smith Roofing & Sheet Metal Co., 78 OSAHRC 2O/A9 (No. 16142, 1978) (ALJ). Both of these decisions were issued by the same administrative law judge, and, contrary to State's assertion, both decisions became final orders by operation of law without being directed for review, under section 12(j) of the Act, 29 C.F.R. § 661(j). As unreviewed administrative law judge's decisions, they do not constitute precedent binding on the Commission. Leone Constr. Co., 3 BNA OSHC 1979, 1975-76 CCH OSHD ¶ 20,378 (No. 4090, 1976). More significantly, the full Commission long ago rejected the argument that a roof constituted a temporary floor and has done so consistently. Hamilton Roofing Co., 6 BNA OSHC 1771, 1978 CCH OSHD ¶ 22,856 (No. 14968, 1978); Diamond Roofing Co., 8 BNA OSHC 1080, 1980 CCH OSHD ¶ 24,274 (No. 76.3653,1980); Universal Roofing & Sheet Metal Co., 8 BNA OSHC 1453, 1980 CCH OSHD ¶ 24,503 (No. 77-1756, 1980). The Commission's position has also been adopted by some appellate courts. Corbesco, Inc. v Dole, 926 F.2d 422 (5th Cir. 1991); cf Brock v. Williams Enterp., 832 F.2d 567, 573 (11th Cir. 1987) (temporary floor that does not protect employees from exterior fall does not satisfy section 1926.105(a)). We therefore reject State's assertion that it was in compliance with section 1926.105(a) because its employees were working on a temporary floor. It is well established that a roof is not a floor. Diamond Roo/ij~g Co. v. OSHRC, 528 F.2d 645 (5th Cir. 1976); Langer Roofing & Sheet Metal, Inc. v. Secretuw 4 of Labor, 524 F.2d 1337 (7th Cir. 1975). State argues that it has relied for ten years on the two unreviewed decisions involving its sister company. Because those decisions were not issued by the Commission, however, that reliance was not well founded. The Commission had rejected the rationale on which the Niben-Smith decisions were based, and an employer has a duty to keep itself informed as to the law governing its operations. Corbesco, 926 F.2d at 428. Because State-should have known that the Commission had rejected the rationale on which it was relying, it could not have reasonably relied on the two unreviewed Nikerz-Smith decisions. See Dole v. East Penn Mfg. Co., 894 F.2d 640, 644-46 (3d Cir. 1990). There was no fall protection of any kind to prevent State's employees from falling from the edge of the roof decking or the 4-inch-wide beams to the ground below. We therefore find that the requirements of the standard were not met.

c. Employee Access to the Violative Condition
    The employees were observed working at and near the edge of the metal decking as well as walking on the steel beams on which the decking was being placed. We therefore find that State's employees were exposed to the violative condition, the absence of fall protection.

d. Knowledge of the Violative Condition
    The knowledge element of a violation does not require a showing that the employer was actually aware that it was in violation of an OSHA standard. Rather, it is established if the record shows that the employer knew or should have known of the conditions constituting a violation. Conagra Flour Milling Co., 15 BNA OSHC 1817, 1823, 1992 CCH OSHD ¶ 29,808, p. 40,593 (No. 882572, 1992). State's management officials knew that its employees had to work at the edge of the decking and that no fall protection was being used. We therefore find that State's knowledge of the violative conditions has been established.

By proving, each of these four elements by a preponderance Secretary has established prima facie violations at both worksites. We must therefore determine whether State has proven that it should not be held liable for these violations.

III. STATE'S DEFENSES TO THE CITATIONS
     State presents three arguments that, it claims, establish that compliance with section 1926.105(a) was infeasible and should therefore excuse its failure to comply. It asserts: (1) that it is not the practice in its industry to use nets; (2) that erecting the nets is more dangerous than working without them; and (3) that using nets is impractical. For the reasons given below, we must reject State's infeasibility assertions and find that State was in violation at both sites.

a. Industry Practice
    State argues that one reason it is infeasible to use nets is that it will be placed at a competitive disadvantage because none of its competitors uses nets. The fact that other members of the industry do not use nets is

not dispositive, however. It may be that the reason State's competitors do not use nets is that they comply with the standard by using some other means of fall protection, and State's witnesses did not eliminate this possibility. Furthermore, even if everyone else were leaving their employees unprotected, the fact that State's conduct may have been consistent with the normal practice in its industry is irrelevant if the standard specifically requires a different course of action. William Enterp. Inc., 13 BNA OSHC 1249, 1253, 1986–1987 CCH OSHD ¶ 27,893, p. 36,585 (No. 85-355, 1987); Cleveland Consol., Inc., 13 BNA OSHC 1114, 1117, 1986–1987 CCH OSHD ¶ 27,829, p. 36,428.29 (No. 84-696, 1987); see also Brock v. Williams Enterp., 832 F.2d at 570–71; Brock v. L.R. Willson & Sons., Inc., 773 F.2d 1377, 1386–88 (D.C. Cir. 1985). State cannot use the allure of other members of its industry to comply with the requirements of a standard as a defense to a citation, because an employer cannot be excused from noncompliance on the assumption that everyone else will ignore the law. A.F. Burgess Leather Co., 5 BNA OSHC 1096, 1097 n.2, 1977–1978 CCH OSHD ll21,573, p. 25,887 n.2 (No. 12501, 1977), aff'd, 576 F.2d 948 (1st Cir. 1978).

b.   Greater Hazard

State also argues that it is infeasible to use nets because its employees would have been more exposed to the hazard of falling while erecting the nets than they were while they decked the roof. Although evidence that compliance with a standard will diminish safety or increase it only slightly may be relevant to whether compliance is feasible, the Commission and the courts of appeals have recognized a separate and distinct affirmative defense of greater hazard. To establish the greater hazard affirmative defense, the employer must prove that the hazards caused by complying with 'the standard are greater than those encountered by not complying, that alternative means of protecting employees were either used or were not available, and that application for a variance under section 6(d) of the Act would be inappropriate. See Russ ICaller, Inc., 4 BNA OSHC 1758, 1976–1977 CCH OSHD li 21,152 (No. 11171, 1976). The party raising the affirmative defense has the burden of proof. Dole v. Williams Enterp., 876 F.2d 186, 188–89 (D.C. Cir. 1989). Here, State has not addressed any alternative methods of protection in either case. Although State asserts (without citing us to the source of its support for this claim) that the Secretary agreed that the other means of protection listed in section 1926.105(a) were impractical, that statement, if correct, is irrelevant. Before an employer elects to ignore the requirements of a standard because it believes that compliance creates a greater hazard, the employer must explore all possible alternatives and is not limited to those methods of protection listed in the standard. Additionally, State has presented only the unsubstantiated opinion of its owner, who is hardly a disinterested witness. We are unwilling to accept such conclusory statements without being given any factual basis for them, and State has offered no facts on which this conclusion is based.

While the witness may sincerely believe that his opinion is correct, the courts have recognized that an employer may have an incorrect good-faith belief that compliance creates a greater hazard. Dole v. Williams Enterp., 876 F.2d at n.7; General Elec. Co. v. Secretary of Labor, 576 F.2d 558, 561 (36 Cir. 1978). Furthermore, an employer must prove that there is no possible method of erecting the nets that would not constitute a greater hazard. United States Steel Corp. v. OSHRC, 537 F.2d 780, 783, (3d Cir. 1976). In sum, we find that State has failed to carry its burden of proof as to the greater hazard defense.

c. Infeasibility

When a standard states a specific method of complying, an employer seeking to be excused from liability for its failure to comply with the standard has the burden of demonstrating that the action required by the standard is infeasible under the circumstances. cited. Dun-Par Engd. Form Co., 12 BNA OSHC 1949, 1986–1987 CCH OSHD ll 27,650 (No. 79-2553, 1986), rev'd on other grounds, 843 F.2d 1135 (8th Cir. 1988); Ace Sheeting & Repair Co. v. OSHRC, 555 F.2d 439,441(5th Cir. 1977). In order to carry this burden, an employer who raises the affirmative defense of infeasibility must prove that (1) literal compliance with the requirements of the standard was infeasible-under the circumstances and (2) either an alternative method of protection was used or no alternative means of protection was feasible. Mosser Constr. Co., 15 BNA OSHC 1408, 1416, 1992 CCH OSHD ¶ 29,546, p. 39,907 (No. 89-1027, 1991). Courts that have considered the infeasibility defense have concluded that it encompasses both technological and economic factors. Faultless Div., Bks & Laughlin Indus. v. Secretary, 674 F.2d 1177, 1189 (7th Cir. 1982); Southern Colo. prestress Co. v. OSHRC, 586 F.2d 1342, 1351 (10th Cir. 1978); Atlantic & Gulf Stevedores, Inc. v. OSHRC, 534 F.2d 541 (3d Cir. 1976). In the cases before us, however, the Secretary argued to the administrative law judge that evidence as to the economic impact of compliance was irrelevant. The Secretary is correct that the Commission did generally take that position at one time. See, e.g. StanBest, Inc., 11 BNA OSHC 1222, 123 1, 1983–1984 CCH OSHD ¶ 26,455, p. 33,624 (No. 76-4355, 1983); Research Cottrell, Inc., 9 BNA OSHC 1489, 1498, 1981 CCH OSHD ¶ 25,284, p. 31,264 (No. 11756, 1981). Subsequently, however, the Commission recognized the affirmative defense of infeasibility. See Dun-Par Engd. Form Co., 12 BNA OSHC 1949, 1986–1987 CCH OSHD ll 27,650 (No. 79-2553, 1986), rev'd, 843 F.2d 1135 (8th Cir. 1988) (Dun-Par I). In Dun-Pat Engd. Form Co., 12 BNA OSHC 1962, 1986-87 CCH OSHD ¶ 27,651 (No. 82-928, 1986) (Dun-Par U), the Commission recognized that an infeasibility defense may include economic factors when it found that the employer had not demonstrated that the costs were unreasonable in light of the protection afforded and had not shown what effect, if any, the added costs would have on its contract or on its business as a whole. 12 BNA OSHC at 1966, 1986–1987 CCH OSHD at p. 36,033.2. Accord Walker Towing Corp., 14 BNA OSHC 2072, 2077, 1991 CCH OSHD ¶ 29,239, p. 39,160.61 (No. 87-1359, 1991); see also Atlantic & Gulf Stevedores. The Secretary's argument was therefore incorrect; evidence as to the unreasonable economic impact of compliance with a standard may be relevant to the infeasibility defense. State argued to the judges who heard these cases that the Secretary had the burden of proving that the use of nets was feasible. The cases relied on by State are not apposite because they arose in other contexts. Although the Secretary does have the burden of proving the feasibility of compliance in some circumstances, this is not one of them. When, as here, an employer who has failed to comply with the requirements of an OSHA standard attempts to avoid liability for this noncompliance on the grounds that complying would be infeasible, the employer has the burden of proving that affirmative defense. Walker Towing, 14 BNA OSHC at 2075–77, 1991 CCH OSHD at pp. 39,158.61; see also Quality Stamping Prod. v. OSHRC, 709 F.2d 1093, 1099 (6th Cir. 1983); Arkansas-Best Freight Sys., Inc. v. OSHRC, 529 F.2d 649, 65.4 (8th Cir. 1976). We therefore reject State's argument that the Secretary must prove that nets are feasible. State argues that, if it must use safety nets it will be forced out of business because none of its competitors uses nets and they will therefore be able to submit lower bids. Thus, according to State, it will never get any more business. If State were the only company in its industry required to comply with the standard, State probably could not compete. We cannot vacate the citation on that basis, however, because an employer cannot be excused from compliance on the assumption that everyone else will ignore the law. A.F. Burgess Leather Co., 5 BNA OSHC 1096, 1097 n.2, 1977–1978 CCH OSHD ¶ 21,573, p. 25,887 n.2 (No. 12501, 1977), aff'd, 576 F.2d 948 (1st Cir. 1978). A primary goal of the Act was to eliminate any competitive disadvantage that a safety-conscious employer might suffer by requiring that every employer comply with tke applicable OSHA standards. American Textile Mfrs. Inst. v+ Donovan, 452 U.S. 490, 521 n.38 (1981). Although State may plausibly argue that the Secretary could be more vigorous in informing the sheet metal roof-decking industry about the requirements of section 1926105(a) and in enforcing those requirements, we cannot accept "everybody else was ignoring the law, too," as an excuse for an employer's failure to obey the requirements of the law. On the evidence in these combined records, we find that State has failed to carry that burden of showing that compliance with section 1926.105(a) was unreasonable in light of the protection afforded. Although Mr. Smith expressed the opinion that it was not practical to use nets, such an opinion, unsupported by underlying facts, is not enough. Even the admission by the compliance officer who testified for the Secretary as a safety expert that using nets could triple or quadruple the cost of installing the roof decking is not sufficient because it does not address whether such costs would have a severe adverse economic effect on State. 1 In addition, to prove the infeasibility affirmative defense, an employer seeking to avoid liability for its noncompliance must show that alternative forms of protection were used or that no alternative form of protection was available, just as it must do to prove the greater hazard affirmative defense. Trinity Indus., 15 BNA OSHC 1985, 1987, 1992 CCH OSHD ¶ 29,889, p. 40,787 (No. 892316, 1992). As noted in our discussion of State's greater hazard defense, before an employer will be excused from ignoring a standard's requirements and leaving its employees unprotected, it must show that it has explored all possible alternate forms of protection. Having searched both records here, we find that State has failed to mention any alternative means of protection, much less show that they could not be used. State has therefore failed to prove that element of its affirmative defense. State asserts that requiring the use of nets will have a devastating effect on the roofing industry. While that assertion may or may not be true, it is not supported by the evidence in these records. More importantly, it misconstrues the effect of our holding. We want to make it clear that we are not saying State or other members of its industry must use nets; all we are holding is that the standard requires that some form of fall protection be used. Because of the wording of section 1926.105(a), it has often been misunderstood. Under the terms of that standard, nets are the least-preferred means of protecting employees. If one of the other methods specified can be used, it should be used. We are familiar from past cases with various methods of protection that might be effective to protect the employees laying the roof decking. In some cases, employers have erected static lines to which a lanyard connected to a safety belt can be attached. In places where the ground was level enough, a catch platform on a mobile scaffold has been used. Given the evidence in the record as to the time and expense involved in erecting safety nets, we assume that State and its competitors will use their ingenuity to find methods of compliance other than nets. We want to emphasize that State is being found in violation for using to fall protection at all and that State could have avoided being found in violation by using any effective means of protection. Nets are merely one means of complying with section 1926.105(a), and the least-favored means at that.

IV. CHARACTERIZATION OF THE VIOLATION

The judges both found that the violations were serious. Under section 17(k) of the Act, 29 U.K. 0 666(k), a violation is serious if there is a substantial probability that death or serious physical harm could result. This statement does not mean that the occurrence of an accident must be a substantially probable result of the violative condition but, rather, that a serious injury is the likely result should an accident occur. Super Excavators, Inc., 15 BNA OSHC 1313,1315,1991 CCH OSHD 9 29,498, p. 39,804 (No. 89.2253,1991); Natkin & Co., 1 BNA OSHC 1204, 1205, 1971–1973 CCH OSHD ll 15,679, pp. 20,967.68 (No. 401, 1973). It is clear that the consequences of State's failure to use safety nets could result in serious harm. We therefore find that the violations were serious.

V PENALTY

Section 17(j) of the Act provides that the Commission shall assess an appropriate penalty for each violation, giving due consideration to the size of the employer, the gravity of the violation, the good faith of the employer, and the employer's history of previous violations. 29 U.S.C. § 666(j). The most significant factor to be considered in assessing an appropriate penalty, however, is gravity. Natkin, 1 BNA OSHC at 1205, 1971-73 CCH OSHD at p. 20,968. We will not reduce the penalty proposed when the violation is of high gravity. See Kus-Tum Builders, Inc., 10 BNA OSHC 1128, 1981 CCH OSHD ¶ 25,738 (No. 76-2644, 1981). The Secretary proposed a penalty of $810 for the violation in Docket Number 90-1620, and the judge found a penalty of $100 to be appropriate for the violation and assessed that amount. The Secretary also proposed a penalty of $810 for the violation in Docket Number 90-2894. The judge in that case also found $100 to be an appropriate penalty for that violation and assessed a penalty of $100. The Secretary has not challenged the findings of either judge on this issue. HaSving considered the information in the record regarding the four penalty factors and the Secretary's failure to object, we consider the penalties assessed by the judges to be appropriate in each case.

VI CONCLUSION

Accordingly, we find that the administrative law judges did not err in finding, in each of these cases, that State had committed a serious violation of 29 C.F.R. 6 1926.105(a), and we assess a penalty of $100 for each violation. Dated: April 27, 1993

12 OSHA Defenses

Do not follow where the path may lead. Go instead where there is no path and leave a trail.

Ralph Waldo Emerson

To acquire knowledge, one must study; but to acquire wisdom, one must observe.

Marilyn Vos Savant

STUDENT LEARNING OBJECTIVES

1. Analyze the types of possible defenses.
2. Analyze and assess procedural defenses.
3. Analyze and assess possible factual defenses.
4. Understand when and how to utilize defenses to an Occupational Safety and Health Administration (OSHA) violation.

Safety professionals should begin to prepare their defenses far in advance of an OSHA compliance inspection. Although it is far better not to have any violations, if a violation and proposed penalty should arise, the safety professional should be prepared to search his/her index of possible defenses to ascertain if one or more defenses fit the facts and circumstances of the situation as well as can be supported by the evidence. Safety professionals should remember that the burden of proof is on OSHA for any citation or proposed penalty. Thus, the safety professional at informal conference or as part of the legal team on appeal is attempting to disprove what the compliance officer identified as a citable violation. Additionally, it is important to review each and every element of the alleged violation (identified in the OSHA Field Manual) to ensure that OSHA can prove all elements as well as the categorization and proposed monetary penalties.

As identified in Chapter 1 of this text, the safety professional, as well as the company, possesses rights under the United States Constitution. Although most, if not all of the constitutional challenges to the Occupational Safety and Health (OSH) Act were addressed in the early days of the Act, if a constitutional right has been infringed upon as part of the compliance inspection, constitutional challenges remain and can be utilized depending on the circumstances.

The other categories of identifiable defenses which have been used before the OSHRC fall in the categories of procedural defenses and factual defenses. Safety professionals should be aware that once OSHA has established a prima facie case that the citation issued to the employer is supported by the evidence, the employer has the burden to rebut OSHA's prima facie case and may present contrary evidence or establish affirmative defenses to justify noncompliance with the particular standard.

Under the category of procedural defenses, these defenses address the method through which OSHA conducted the inspection or required procedures as well as jurisdictional issues. These defenses can include the Statute of Limitation defense, Lack of Reasonable Promptness defense, Failure to Timely Forward Notice of Contest Defense, and Improper Service Defense. These defenses are very specific to a specific time requirement for OSHA to have completed some task. Additionally, under the category of procedural defenses, issues involving OSHA's jurisdiction to conduct the inspection and issue citations are addressed. These defenses include Lack of Commerce Clause jurisdiction defense, Preemption by another Federal Agency, and State Plan coverage. Under these defenses, another entity possessed jurisdiction over the particular workplace and thus OSHA did not possess the authority to conduct the inspection and issue citations.

Procedural defenses also encompass the required employer–employee relationship request under the OSH Act, as well as challenges to the standard itself. Defenses challenging the employer–employee relationship address construction sites, loaded employees, and related areas where OSHA may assume an employer–employee relationship. Safety professionals should also refer to the Multi-Employer Worksite Rule. Challenges to the standard itself can include the standard was not properly promulgated (for new standards), the standard lacks particularity, the standard was improperly amended, and the standard is arbitrarily vague. Correlating defenses in the area of lack of due process may also be available.

Factual defenses are the primary area of defenses utilized by safety professionals today. The availability of the below listed factual defenses will depend solely on the specific facts of the situation. The recognized factual defenses include the following:

1. A Greater Hazard in Compliance Defense:

    This defense is based on the theory that compliance with the OSH Act or a specific standard would create a greater hazard for employees than noncompliance with the standard. For example, the ALJ in *Ashland Oil, Inc.* vacated a citation of the standard requiring a guardrail around the open sides of a platform which was four or more feet above the ground. The judge found that the risk of injury increased with the installation of the guardrail and the guardrail created a risk which did not exist.[*]

2. Lack of Employer's Knowledge Defense:

    Although the employer's knowledge or lack thereof is an element which OSHA is required to prove as part of their prima facie case, safety professionals have often utilized this as a defense to an appropriate violation. In essence, when analyzing the definition of a "serious violation," the OSH Act includes the statement "unless the employer did not, or could not with the exercise of reasonable diligence, know of the presence of the violation."[†] Thus, with a serious violation, employer knowledge is a required element of proof. Other categories of violations do not appear to possess this specific requirement for employer knowledge. Safety professionals should note that the Lack

---

[*] 1 OSHC 3246 (ALJ, 1973).
[†] OSH Act Section 17(k); 29 USC Section 666(j).

of Employer's Knowledge defense is closely related to the Isolated Incident Defense discussed below. However, safety professionals should note that the Isolated Incident defense is an affirmative defense which shifts the burden of proof to the employer, wherein the Lack of Employer's defense maintains the burden on OSHA and is an element of the OSHA violation. The absence of prior incidents may bolster this defense; however, the existence of prior violations or incidents may undermine the use of this defense.

3. The Machine is Not in Use Defense:

The Machine is Not in Use defense is also an affirmative defense. This defense is based on the theory that the equipment which the compliance officer cited was not in use at the time it was viewed by the compliance officer and thus could not create a hazard. Safety professionals should be prepared to prove that the particular machine or operation was not in use with substantial supporting evidence.

> Stupidity is not a valid defense for us.
>
> **Raul Ilarsi Merjer**

4. Isolated Incident Defense:

Safety professionals should be aware that, to prove the isolated incident affirmative defense, the safety professional must be able to demonstrate the following: (A) the violation identified resulted exclusively from the employee's conduct; (B) the violation was not participated in, observed by, or performed with the knowledge and/or consent of any supervisory or management personnel; (C) the employee's conduct contravened a well-established company policy or work rule which was in effect at the time, well-published to employees, and actively enforced through disciplinary action or other appropriate procedures.[*] Additionally, the safety professional must have a specific and verifiable safety program in place for instructing employees in safe work practices.[†]

It should be noted that the Isolated Incident defense is an affirmative defense; thus, this defense must be raised "affirmatively during the formation of the issues of the case."[‡] Safety professionals can also raise this defense at informal conference with supporting evidence. However, safety professionals should ensure that appropriate and compelling evidence for each of the elements is readily available as well as a viable and operational safety program with appropriate and documented training provided to employees.

5. Impossibility of Compliance Defense:

The Impossibility of Compliance defense involves the theory that compliance with a specific OSHA standard is impossible because of the nature of the specific work being performed. In essence, the safety professional is admitting that the work being performed is not in compliance but is impossible to achieve or maintain compliance with the standard. Safety professionals should exercise caution in that any admission or implied admission that compliance is possible can result in the defense failing.[§]

---

[*] Bill Turpin Painting, Inc. 5 OSHC 1576 (1977)
[†] OSHA Field Operations Manual at Section X-€(1).
[‡] See, for example, Otis Elevator Co., 5 OSHC 1514(1977).
[§] See, Taylor Building Associates, 5 OSHC 1083 (1977).

6. Employee Has No Exposure to the Hazard:

OSHA possesses the burden of proving that at least one employee was exposed to, or had access to, the alleged condition(s) for which OSHA cited the employer. Safety professionals should review the facts and evidence and if no employees were exposed to the hazard and can prove this fact, this defense may be available. The safety professional must be able to prove that no employees were exposed to the hazard identified by the compliance officer.

Although safety professionals have addressed this defense through several approaches including demonstration of engineering and administrative controls that there is no feasible methods to achieve compliance with the specific requirements of the standard and to demonstrate the impossibility to perform the necessary work if compliance with the standard is met. Safety professionals should be aware that the employer has the burden to prove or demonstrate the applicability of this defense.

7. Employee Misconduct Defense:

The theory of this defense is that the employer with a good safety and health program should not be penalized for a condition or hazard created by a trained employee. Additionally, it would be unfair to the employer and the hazard created by the employee through his/her misconduct is unpreventable by the employer. Safety professionals should be aware that, in order to establish this defense, the safety professional must demonstrate the following: (A) the violation identified by the compliance officer resulted exclusively from the employee's misconduct; (B) the violation was not participated in, observed by, or performed with the knowledge and/or consent of any supervisory or management personnel; and (C) the employee's misconduct contravened a well-established company policy or work rule which was in effect at the time, well-publicized to the employees, and actively enforced through disciplinary action or other appropriate procedures. Additionally, the safety professional must prove through documentation or other sources that the employee was appropriately trained and instructed in safe work practices. For this defense, the safety professional should be aware that the burden is on the employer to prove and establish that the safety program exists and is uniformly enforced.

8. No Hazard Defense:

When OSHA promulgates a standard, there is a presumption that a hazard exists. In situations where the employer has been previously inspected by a compliance officer and the compliance officer indicated that the particular situation or condition was not a violation, safety professionals may be able to argue that the current alleged violation is not a recognizable hazard and only the subjective opinion on the compliance officer. Safety professionals should be aware that OSHA compliance officer possess different backgrounds and different opinions with regards to hazards. No opinion by an OSHA compliance officer is binding on OSHA or the OSHRC.

Safety professionals should be aware that, although the factual defenses identified are recognized defenses, other potential defenses can be argued by creative practitioners. Depending on the facts and circumstances, new and creative challenges can be made by safety professionals at informal conference as well as before the OSRRC. Safety professionals are encourages to review and utilize the OSHA Field Operations Manual to "reverse engineer" the citation and alleged violations providing special focus on the categorization of the penalties and standard(s) cited. Safety professionals should remember that OSHA possesses the burden of proof and safety professionals should "turn over every stone" to find applicable defenses if the facts and circumstances support the defense. In the event that the safety professional possesses no defense(s), good faith and immediately addressing and eliminating the hazard can go a long way in reducing the penalties through settlement.

THE BEST DEFENSE IS TO ACHIEVE AND MAINTAIN COMPLIANCE WITH THE OSHA STANDARDS!!

Questions

1. What is a procedural defense and when can it be used?
2. What is a No Hazard defense and when can it be used?
3. What elements must be proved in an Employee Misconduct defense?
4. What should a safety professional do if there is no defense to the citation/ violation?
5. What are the required elements which OSHA must prove for a willful violation?

Selected Case Study

Case modified for the purpose of this text.
United States of America
OCCUPATIONAL SAFETY AND HEALTH REVIEW COMMISSION
OSHRC Docket No. 94-1374
SECRETARY OF LABOR, Complainant, v. DAYTON TIRE,
BRIDGESTONE/FIRESTONE,
Respondent, UNITED STEEL WORKERS OF AMERICA, LOCAL 998,
Authorized Employee Representative.

DECISION AND ORDER

Before: ROGERS, Chairman; ATTWOOD, Commissioner. BY THE COMMISSION: In a September 10, 2010 Decision and Order, the Commission affirmed ninety-nine violations of the general industry lockout/tagout ("LOTO") standard, 29 C.F.R. § 1910.147, alleged in a citation issued to Dayton Tire, Bridgestone/Firestone ("Dayton") under the OSH Act, 29 U.S.C. §§ 651-678. Dayton Tire, 23 BNA OSHC 1247, 2010 CCH OSHD ¶ 33,098 (No. 94-1374, 2010). The Commission characterized all of the affirmed violations as willful and assessed a total penalty of $1,975,000.

Dayton filed a petition for review with the U.S. Court of Appeals for the D.C. Circuit, challenging, inter alia, the Commission's willful characterization of these violations. The D.C. Circuit vacated this portion of the Commission's order, holding that there was insufficient evidence to support a finding that any of Dayton's ninety-nine violations were willful, and "remand[ed] for the Commission to reassess the nature of Dayton's violations and recalculate the appropriate penalty." Dayton Tire v. Sec'y of Labor, 671 F.3d 1249, 1257 (D.C. Cir. 2012).

Under the OSH Act, a violation is characterized as serious if "there is a substantial probability that death or serious physical harm could result." 29 U.S.C. § 666(k). Based on the record evidence described in our previous decision, we find that a "substantial probability" of "death or serious physical harm" could have resulted from the servicing and maintenance activities performed by Dayton employees on the machines and equipment at issue, and that compliance with the cited LOTO provisions would have minimized or eliminated these hazards. Dayton Tire, 23 BNA OSHC at 1252, 2010 CCH OSHD at p. 54,816. We therefore affirm all ninety-nine LOTO standard violations as serious. See Burkes Mech., Inc., 21 BNA OSHC 2136, 2141, 2004-09 CCH OSHD ¶ 32,922, p. 53,564 (No. 04-1475, 2007) (affirming LOTO violation as serious based on record evidence). The penalties for these serious violations are considered in light of the OSH Act's statutory factors, which require the Commission to give "due consideration to the appropriateness of the penalty with respect to the size of the business of the employer being charged, the gravity of the violation, the good faith of the employer, and the history of previous violations." 29 U.S.C. § 666(j). In our previous decision, we concluded that no reductions were warranted for business size or good faith, but that a reduction was warranted for history. Dayton Tire, 23 BNA OSHC at 1266-67, 2010 CCH OSHD at p. 54,829. We also concluded that the gravity of each violation was high. Id. at 1267, 2010 CCH OSHD at p. 54,829. On remand, our analysis of business size, history, and gravity remain the same. With respect to good faith, however, we have taken into account the D.C. Circuit's findings regarding Dayton's efforts to comply with the LOTO standard – particularly that Dayton's safety manager "made some effort to ensure Dayton's LOTO compliance," but she "may not have displayed the kind of initiative [one] would expect when lives and limbs are at stake." Dayton Tire, 671 F.3d at 1257.Given the foregoing analysis, we assess the following penalty amounts, totaling $197,500, for the affirmed items: Items 1 through 6 - $2,500 each; Item 7 - $1,500; Items 8a and 8b - $1,000 (grouped); and Items 9 through 12, 14 through 17, 20 through 30, 32 through 48, 50 through 83, 86, 87, 89 through 98, 100 through 106, and 108 – $2,000 each.
SO ORDERED.

13 Evidence and OSHA's Variances

There's no harm in hoping for the best, as long as you're prepared for the worst.

Stephen King

Maturity includes the recognition that no one is going to see anything in us that we don't see in ourselves. Stop waiting for a producer. Produce yourself.

Marianne Williamson

STUDENT LEARNING OBJECTIVES

1. Analyze and assess the requirements for a compliance program.
2. Analyze and assess the need for a written compliance program.
3. Analyze and assess the Occupational Safety and Health Administration's (OSHA) Variance Program
4. Analyze and understand the utilization of an OSHA's variance.

Safety professionals should be aware that their written compliance programs as well as training documents, disciplinary actions, and all documentation generated within the safety function can be utilized as evidence, whether as part of the employer's defense or subpoenaed by OSHA or a third party. Written compliance programs that adhere to all of the specific OSHA standard requirements as well as being customized to the specific operations within the company are an essential component to any safety and health program. Written compliance programs are utilized not only for consistency and uniformity but also to ensure that employees are provided the proper and correct information to ensure their safety and health in the workplace. Although there are many positive reasons for safety professionals to develop written compliance programs that are customized to their workplace (and not purchased on the internet), the primary purpose within this legal arena is "proof": proof that the safety professional possessed the written safety and health program meeting the minimum requirements of the specific standard; proof that authorized or affected employees were properly trained and educated in accordance with the standard requirements; and proof that the compliance program was in effect and operational, as well as being enforced. Without written compliance programs, training documentation, and other related written documents, the safety professional possesses no proof that he/she actually performed the safety and health activities when presented with inquiries by a compliance officer or a court of law.

Safety professionals should be aware that there is "no one right way" to develop a written compliance program so long as all elements of the standard, at a minimum, are appropriately addressed. There are no page requirements or usually no specific ways of implementation of your program. The same compliance program (such as Control of Hazardous Energy or Lockout/Tagout) may require 5 pages to achieve compliance for a small employer while achieving compliance for a large employer may require 300 pages. The safety professional must make this judgment in full knowledge that he/she may be "second guessed" during a compliance inspection. Additionally, often companies possess a specific format in which safety and health programs, as well as policies or procedures, must comply. Safety professionals should be aware that OSHA possesses vertical standards which are usually industry specific and horizontal standards which usually cross industries. It is up to the safety professional to identify which standards are applicable to his/her workplace. Failure to identify an applicable OSHA standard is not a defense when the compliance officer identified the need for compliance with a specific standard. And safety professionals should recognize that new standards are being promulgated, old standards are being revised and modified, and state plan standards may be different that of federal standards. It is the safety professional function to be able to identify the applicable standards and develop written compliance programs to address each and every applicable OSHA standard.

So, where does a safety professional start when developing a new written compliance program? Below, please find a step-by-step process:

Step 1: Identify the applicable OSHA standard. Read and re-read the standard. Identify the major elements required to achieve compliance with the standard.

Step 2: Draft the written compliance program. Visualize your written program in action. Identify additional elements (such as a disciplinary component) that are required in order for your compliance program to operate efficiently and effectively.

Step 3: Finalize your written compliance program. Acquire all levels of approvals and funding required within your company. (Note: Unionized operations may also require negotiations with the labor organization.)

Step 4: Acquire all necessary equipment, PPE, etc., necessary to implement the compliance program. Please remember to involve your employees in equipment selection and other aspects of the decision-making process.

Step 5: Implement your program and complete and document all required training. Adjust your written program as necessary to adhere to modifications identified during implementation.

Step 6: Review your written program at least on an annual basis and update and modify as necessary.

After completion and implementation, safety professionals should remember that your compliance programs must be strictly enforced. Safety professionals should educate and direct supervisory personnel and management team members on the disciplinary requirements required within the compliance program and hold the management team responsible for the initiation of fair and appropriate disciplinary actions for noncompliance within the company's disciplinary policies. Safety professionals should be managers and directors of the safety and health function and not the "safety police" issuing disciplinary action personally to offending employees.

Safety professionals should be aware that other documentation, such as documents related to training and disciplinary action, are often utilized as evidence within the OSHA appeal structure. Safety professionals must prove that an employee was provided the required training and also is often called upon to prove that the employee understood such training. Additionally, it is often not sufficient to simply identify that employees have been disciplined for violation of safety rules and requirements. Safety professionals should document all disciplinary actions from verbal warnings through termination and maintain this documentation for possible future use. Documentation of all facets of the safety function is essential for today's safety professional. Appropriate documentation is proof of the specific safety event or activities as well as the employee's participation, understanding, and adherence to the specified safety requirements.

> **Simple Compliance with the OSHA standards does not make an effective and efficient safety and health program.**

Safety professionals should be aware that simply achieving compliance with the OSHA standards does not make an effective and efficient safety and health program. Compliance with the OSHA standards is the "bare bones" minimum that is required by law; however, safety professionals should strive to develop a comprehensive safety and health programs that goes far above the minimum requirements. Safety professionals should strive to write and develop their compliance programs in a matter that ensure transparency as well as complete understanding as well as writing in a way that is defensible in a court of law. As noted above, written compliance programs are often the focal point and proof of required compliance during and after a compliance inspection. Safety professionals should strive to develop written compliance programs that he/she would be proud to present to a compliance officer, at informal conference or at hearing before the OSHRC or court of law. If the safety professional has taken the time and effort to develop, implement, and appropriately enforce the written compliance program, this document can serve not only as the basis for the overall program but also the proof needed to avoid and address possible citations and penalties.

OSHA'S VARIANCE PROGRAM

One proactive tool that safety professionals often overlook is that of OSHA's Variance Program. "A variance is a regulatory action that permits an employer to deviate from the requirements of an OSHA standard under specified conditions. A variance does not provide an outright exemption from a standard, except in cases involving national defense as described below. Sections 6 and 16 of the Occupational Safety and Health Act of 1970 (OSH Act), and the implementing rules contained in the Code of Federal Regulations (29 CFR 1905 and 1904.38), authorized variances from the OSHA standards. An employer or class of employers may request a variance for any specific workplaces. Employers can request a variance for many reasons, including not being able to fully comply on time with a new safety or health standard because of a shortage of personnel, materials, or equipment. Employers may prefer to use methods, equipment, or facilities that they believe protect workers as well as, or better than, OSHA standards."*

Safety professionals should be aware that achieving compliance with a standard is not always a simple application of the standard to the equipment, worksite, or personnel. Safety professionals should be aware that some state plan states offer free consultation services and federal OSHA offers the Variance Program to assist in addressing unique situations where compliance with the standard is not feasible; however, there are possible alternatives outside of the standard which creates a safe and healthful work environment for employees. Safety professionals should be aware that significant time and effort are required to pursue a variance and there are different kinds of variances.

Types of Variances

Permanent

Section 6(d) of the Occupational Safety and Health (OSH) Act of 1970 (29 U.S.C. 651 et seq.) authorizes permanent variances from OSHA standards. An employer may apply for a permanent variance by following the regulatory requirements specified by 29 CFR 1905.11. An employer (or class or group of employers*) may request a permanent variance for a specific workplace(s). A permanent variance authorizes the employer(s) to use an alternative means to comply with the requirements of a standard when they can prove that their proposed methods, conditions, practices, operations, or processes provide workplaces that are at least as safe and healthful as the workplaces provided by the OSHA standards from which they are seeking the permanent variance. In the application, the employer must demonstrate, by a preponderance of the evidence, that the proposed alternative means of compliance provides its workers with safety and health protection that is equal to, or greater than, the protection afforded to them by compliance with the standard(s) from which they are seeking the variance. In addition, the employer must notify employees of the variance application and of their right to participate in the variance process. ***Inability to afford the cost of complying with the standard is not a valid reason for requesting a permanent variance.***

Temporary

Section 6(b)6(A) of the OSH Act of 1970 (29 U.S.C. 651 et seq.) authorizes temporary variances from OSHA standards. Employers may apply for a temporary variance by following the regulatory requirements specified by 29 CFR 1905.10. An employer (or class or group of employers*) may request a temporary variance for a specific workplace(s). A temporary variance authorizes an employer short-term (i.e. limited time) relief from a standard when the employer cannot comply with newly published OSHA requirements by the date the standard becomes effective because they cannot complete the necessary construction or alteration of the facility in time, or when technical personnel, materials, or equipment are temporarily

---

* OSHA website located at www.osha.gov.

unavailable. *(Note: The employer must submit the application for a temporary variance to OSHA prior to the effective date of the standard.)* To be eligible for a temporary variance, an employer must implement an effective compliance program as quickly as possible. In the meantime, the employer must demonstrate to OSHA that it is taking all available steps to safeguard workers. *Inability to afford the cost of complying with the standard is not a valid reason for requesting a temporary variance*. In addition, the employer must notify employees of the variance application and of their right to participate in the variance process.

Experimental

Section 6(b)6(C) of the OSH Act of 1970 (29 U.S.C. 651 et seq.) authorizes experimental variances from OSHA standards. An employer (or class or group of employers*) may request an experimental variance for a specific workplace(s). An experimental variance authorizes the employer(s) to demonstrate or validate new or improved safety and health techniques when they can prove that their proposed experimental methods, conditions, practices, operations, or processes provide workplaces that are at least as safe and healthful as the workplaces provided by the OSHA standards from which they are seeking the experimental variance. In the application, the employer must describe in detail the proposed experimental design and demonstrate how performing the experiment will provide workers with safety and health protection that is at least equal to the protection afforded by compliance with the standard(s). In addition, the employer must do the following: obtain a written statement signed by each worker who agrees to participate in the proposed experiment that he/she does so knowingly, willingly, and voluntarily; and provide certification that the employer informed the volunteer workers of the plan of the proposed experiment, its attendant risk, and the right to terminate participation in the experiment.

National Defense

Section 16 of the OSH Act of 1970 (29 U.S.C. 651 et seq.) authorizes national defense variances granting reasonable variations, tolerances, and exemptions from OSHA standards to avoid serious impairment of the national defense. If a national defense variance is in effect for more than six months, employers seeking the variance must notify their workers, and employees must be afforded an opportunity for a public hearing on the issues involved. An employer may apply for a national defense variance by following the regulatory requirements specified by 29 CFR 1905.12. Only Federal OSHA may grant national defense variances. An employer (or class or group of employers*) may request a national defense variance for a specific workplace(s). A national defense variance authorizes the employer(s) reasonable variations, tolerances, and exemptions from compliance with the requirements of a standard when they can show that the proposed variance is necessary and proper to avoid serious impairment to the national defense. In addition, the employer must notify employees of the variance application and of their right to petition OSHA for a hearing.

Interim Order

When employers apply for a temporary or permanent variance, OSHA can, upon request, grant them an interim order allowing them to use the proposed alternative means of compliance while OSHA is reviewing their variance application. However, for permanent variances, OSHA will grant an interim order only after it determines that the interim order will protect workers at least as effectively as the standard from which the employer is seeking the variance. If OSHA grants the interim order on a temporary or permanent variance, employers must inform workers of the order using the same means of notification used to inform employees of the variance application.

Recordkeeping Variance

This variance allows employers to use an alternative recordkeeping procedure to comply with OSHA's occupational injury and illness recordkeeping regulation at 29 CFR Part 1904 ("Recording and Reporting Occupational Injuries and Illnesses"). Alternate recordkeeping procedures must meet the purposes of the OSH Act, must not otherwise interfere with the administration of the OSH Act, and must provide the same information as the Part 1904 regulations provide. For details on the information required in the application for a recordkeeping variance, see *29 CFR 1904.38*.[*]

How to Apply for a Variance

OSHA developed four variance application forms and four corresponding application checklists. Use of the forms can significantly reduce the burden of wading through the complexity of federal standards in order to interpret and understand the information requirements associated with applying for a variance. When used together with the appropriate application forms the checklists can prevent common errors likely to occur in completing variance applications. The forms are based on the *Occupational Safety and Health (OSH) Act* and the implementing rules (for further information and links, see Variance Application Checklists and Forms below).

As the regulations do not specify a format, the application also can be prepared and submitted in the form of a letter including the following information:

- An explicit request for a variance.
- The specific standard from which the employer is seeking the variance.
- Whether the employer is applying for a *permanent, temporary, experimental, national defense, or recordkeeping variance, and an interim order.* (If the application is for a temporary variance, state when the employer will be able to comply with the OSHA standard.)
- A statement of the alternative means of compliance with the standard from which the applicant is seeking the variance. The statement must contain sufficient details to support, by a preponderance of the evidence, a conclusion that the employer's proposed alternate methods, conditions, practices, operations, or processes would provide workers with protection that is at least equivalent to the protection afforded to them by the standard from which the employer is seeking the variance (National defense variances do not require such a statement, and the statement submitted by an employer applying for a temporary variance

---

[*] Id.

must demonstrate that the employer is taking all available steps to safe-guard workers).
- The employer's address, as well as the site location(s) that the variance will cover.
- A certification that the employer notified employees using the methods specified in the appropriate variance regulation.

Submit the original of the completed application, as well as other relevant documents, to:
  By regular mail:

  Assistant Secretary for Occupational Safety and Health
  Director Office of Technical Programs and Coordination Activities
  Occupational Safety and Health Administration
  U.S. Department of Labor
  Room N3655
  200 Constitution Avenue, NW
  Washington, DC 20210

  By facsimile:
  202 693-1644
  Electronic (email):
  *VarianceProgram@dol.gov**

Safety professionals should be aware that pursuit of a variance is not a simple activity and can take substantial time and effort in completing the application, as well as the potential site assessment. Depending on the complexity of the situation, site assessment scheduling, availability of technical experts, publication in *Federal Register*, and other factors, this process may take a substantial period of time. Additionally, safety professionals should be aware that there is a probability that the variance application/petition can be denied. Safety professionals should be aware that Variance Applications are often denied because of the following:

- Employer requested a variance to avoid or resolve an existing citation while contesting the citation (29 CFR 1905.5);
- Employer requested a variance without offering a proposed alternate means of protection (i.e. requested an exemption or waiver from the applicable standard) (29 CFR 1905.11);
- Employer failed to demonstrate that the proposed alternate means of protection was at least as effective as the protection afforded by the standard from which the applicant is seeking a variance (see, for example, 29 CFR 1905.11);
- Employer requested a variance from a standard where OSHA previously issued an interpretation (in a letter of interpretation, for example) indicating that the proposed alternate means of protection is permitted under the standard, or an enforcement policy stating that it would not issue citations

---
* Id.

in connection with violations of the standard if the employer followed the proposed alternate means of protection. In such cases, the granting of a variance would be unnecessary;

- Employer requested a variance for an establishment(s) located solely in a state that operates its own OSHA-approved occupational safety and health plan. In such situations, applicants must follow procedures specified by the applicable State Plans (29 CFR 1952);
- Employer requested OSHA approval of a product or product design. It is OSHA's policy not to approve or endorse products or product designs (see, for example, Dec. 30, 1983 letter of interpretation);
- Employer requested a variance from a proposed standard that has not been published as a final rule and is subject to possible alteration and revision; or
- Employer requested a variance from a performance standard or definition, which does not describe a specific safety practice for meeting its hazard control requirements, and therefore leaves open-ended or unspecified the means and methods for meeting its safety requirements.[*]

When faced with unique situations where compliance with the standard is not feasible, safety professionals may wish to explore the potential of a variance in order to address the issues and offer protection to their company against future violations. Variance petitions/applications should be another tool in the tool belt of the safety professional to protect their employer from potential liability while safeguarding employees through alternative methods of achieving and maintaining compliance.

Questions

1. When could a request for permanent variance be utilized?
2. What are the benefits of a written compliance program?
3. What are the steps in developing a written compliance program?
4. Please develop a written variance application.
5. Please identify one OSHA horizontal standard and outline a written compliance program.

[*] Id

14 Workers' Compensation

Common sense is an uncommon degree of what the world calls wisdom.

Samuel Taylor Coleridge

The law does not generate justice, the law is nothing but a declaration and application of what is already just.

P.J. Proudhon

STUDENT LEARNING OBJECTIVES

1. Assess and understand the concepts of state workers' compensation systems.
2. Analyze and assess "arising out of and in the course of employment."
3. Analyze and assess medical, time loss, and permanency benefit levels.
4. Analyze and assess the differences between Occupational Safety and Health Administration (OSHA) recordkeeping requirement and workers' compensation requirements.
5. Analyze and assess the differences between OSHA requirements and state workers' compensation requirements.

As safety professionals are aware, the safety and health function is primarily proactive in our attempts to prevent injuries and illnesses from happening. Workers' compensation is reactive and provides a method of monetary payment to employees who are injured or killed on the job. Although some employers believe these important functions are one in the same (and often combine the job functions), there is a distinct difference between the proactive safety and the reactive workers' compensation functions. If our safety and health function is effective, there is no injury or illness. Where our safety and health efforts fail, there is often an injury or illness incurred by our employees. Work-related injuries and illnesses, in addition to the pain and suffering by the injured or ill employee, cost the organization money. The goal of the safety and health professional is to eliminate or minimize the potential risks in the workplace in order to avoid the potential hazards which can result in workplace injuries and illnesses. The reason most organizations employ a safety and health professional is primarily and fundamentally because work-related injuries and illnesses cost the organization money. If there was no monetary cost correlation with work-related injuries and illnesses, many organizations would simply marginalize the compliance and related requirements and align safety and health responsibilities within another organizational function.

When an employee is injured on the job, safety professionals should be aware that each individual state possesses its own workers' compensation administrative system with individual state law governing every aspect of workers' compensation within the state. Unlike OSHA, there is no overriding federal oversight for state workers' compensation programs. Generally, most workers' compensation systems have been designed to provide payment for medical, work time loss, and a monetary value on the loss of function or appendage to the injured employee. Each state established the values and the workers' compensation system is funded by employers and state revenues. Each state possesses their individual required forms, documents, and procedures.

Workers' compensation evolved as a compromised method to eliminate the burden on the court systems and to provide certainty for both the employee and the employer. For the injured employee, the benefits of workers' compensation include payment of all medical costs, a quick payment of time loss benefits, monetary payment for permanent losses, and relative ease. These loss and benefits can be acquired almost automatically through the completion of the appropriate and required forms. For the employer who is usually required to participate in the state workers' compensation system, the major benefits are that (1) injured employees would be barred from pursuing legal action that could result in higher costs; and (2) the certainty of the cost as established by the individual state workers' compensation laws. For the courts, the volume of workers' compensation cases would be managed through the established administrative system and most avoid the court system altogether. Generally, the negative aspects of workers' compensation for injured workers include reduced benefits, such as 66 percent of their average weekly wage for time loss benefits, a fixed schedule for permanent or total disability and often the bureaucracy of the workers' compensation system. For employers, the primary issue often involved the increasing costs of workers' compensation, usually established by state legislatures, as well as the management of the workers' compensation claims. Although the workers' compensation systems in most states have all but eliminated the need for the courts to be involved in workers' compensation claims, new theories and legislation has created inroads wherein certain claims or actions would be permitted to be heard before the state court system.

For safety professionals, the required workers' compensation coverage acquired by employers can take different administrative forms including self-insurance, self-insured with outside administration or traditional coverage. If self-insured, the cost of the workers' compensation claim is paid directly by the employer and often large bonds are required by the state workers' compensation agency to ensure against default. This option is usually utilized by very large organizations and the claims management can be internal or through a third party. Traditional coverage can be through a third part or often through a quasi-governmental entity who manages the claims. Under this type of system, there is often a 3–5 year mode system where improvements in safety and health programs with the correlating reduction in claims is evaluated on a 3–5 year period of time.

With individual states establishing and effectively managing their workers' compensation system, safety professionals should be aware that there are many similarities, however, also many differences among and between individual state workers' compensation systems. Without a system to preside over workers' compensation in the United States, an expanding scope of inequities has developed among and between state programs. For example, the benefit levels for time loss and permanent partial disability for identical injuries in different states would result in substantially different monetary payments to the injured employee. Safety and health profession-als should be aware of the differences among and between the various state workers' compensation systems in which their operations are located and be aware that the systems are not "apples to apples" when comparing costs for work-related injury and illness claims. Safety and health professionals should also be cognizant that any and all work-related injury or illness will generate a claim which is the mechanism through which to pay the medical providers and other benefits. A claim = costs.

Under the recordkeeping requirements established by OSHA and adopted by vir-tually all of the state plan states, the work-related injury or illness is required to be recorded on the OSHA provided forms. However, safety professionals should be aware that the criteria through which a work-related injury or illness becomes "recordable" is substantially narrower than that of a workers' compensation claim. A work-related workers' compensation claim in which monies are spent by the employer may not meet the criteria to become an OSHA recordable case. Thus, given the dif-ferent criteria between workers' compensation and OSHA, the same injury or illness could potentially be a difference depending on which system is being evaluated.

"How do I decide whether a particular injury or illness is recordable?" The decision tree for recording work-related injuries and illnesses below shows the steps involved in making this determination.[*]

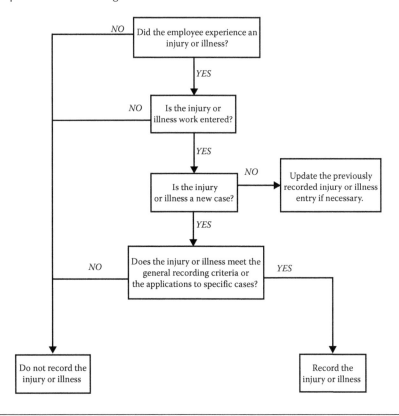

---

[*] 29 C.F.R. 1904.4 (b)(2).

For new safety professionals, this can be a bit confusing. The same work-related injury or illness in operations in different states will generate a claim; however, the monetary cost and results of the claims can be substantially different. The same work-related injury or illnesses could not meet the threshold and criteria to be recordable under the OSHA recordkeeping system and thus may not be identified under the OSHA system. Additionally, the OSHA recordkeeping standard placed the burden upon the employer to ensure accuracy with the criteria, however subjective, wherein the workers' compensation system is self-regulating, given the demand for payment for medical services rendered by the health care provider. For example, if an employee goes to the emergency room for treatment, one of the first questions the health care provider asks is whether this is work-related. If the answer is "yes," the claim is generated so the emergency room can acquire payment for their services. There is a cost to the employer or organization. Conversely, the employee may have generated a claim and has been treated by the emergency room; however, the diagnosis does not meet the recordkeeping criteria and thus would not be a "recordable" injury or illness under OSHA recordkeeping criteria. There would still be a cost to the company or organization due to the filing of the claim and subsequent medical treatment.

Safety professionals should be aware that the recording time for OSH and state workers' compensation claims can also cause confusion. OSHA recordkeeping required the injuries and illnesses to be maintain in the required log for a period from January 1 to December 31 for each year and the "slate is wiped clean" for the new year. With most state workers' compensation laws, there is an extended period of many years in which the claim could remain open. Safety professionals with workers' compensation responsibilities, this is an area of possible confusion and a way of losing track of an employee collecting workers' compensation benefits. For example, Employee X incurs a severe injury requiring an extended period of time away from work in December. The safety professional will record the injury and identify days off through December 31 of the year and post the data as required in April of the following year. However, the OSHA log would start anew on January 1 for the subsequent year. However, Employee X has been and will continue to receive medical and time loss benefits until released by his/her attending physician. Given the fact that Employee X is not at work, not on the OSHA log, and not on the safety professional's "radar screen," if the safety professional is responsible for managing Employee X's workers' compensation claim, there is a probability that Employee X would continue to collect workers' compensation benefits automatically with no oversight by the safety professional. Safety professionals with both safety and workers' compensation responsibilities should know the laws, regulations, and standards of both OSHA and the individual state workers' compensation laws inside out as well as the significant differences within the systems. Safety professionals with operations in multiple states should know the nuisances and differences among and between the individual state workers' compensation systems.

In general, most if not all state workers' compensation systems provide no fault coverage to employees whose injury or illness arises "out of or in the course of employment" or, in essence, on the job. Virtually every state possesses claim and other forms that are required to be completed by the injured employee, the employer, and/ or the medical provider, or all. Upon initiation of a claim, most states provide full and complete coverage for all medical costs for as long as the claim remains open. Many states have a maximum number of weeks or years the claim can remain open. The second area of coverage is time loss or temporary total disability payments. Often, based upon the employee's wage, with a minimum requirement and a maximum cap, the employee usually received between 65 percent and 70 percent of his/her wages often after an initial waiting period (3–7 days). The last category of benefits is often a percentage of permanent disability or loss (often referred to as "PPD"). Depending on the state, a panel of individual physicians would evaluate the injured employee when he/she reaches maximum medical recovers and determine a percentage of loss. This percentage is converted to a monetary amount which the employee receives for the loss.

WC = Medical + Time Loss + Permanency.

Safety professionals should be aware that it is relatively easy for an employee to file a claim and, in most state systems, everything is to be liberally construed in favor of the claimant. However, the trade-off for employers is the fact that, in most states, employees are prohibited from bringing a legal action against the employer for the injury or illness. Although many employers may disagree, the benefit levels under most state workers' compensation systems are relatively low in comparison with a jury award of compensatory and possibly punitive damages. Additionally, our already overloaded current court system would not be able to handle the deluge of workers' compensation cases. In some states, safety professionals should be aware that employees injured as a result of the willful negligence of the employer may be provided an avenue to pursue the injury claim in a court of law. Other states have provided increased monetary benefits if the employer's safety program is found to be deficient. Conversely, in some states, employees injured while under the influence of alcohol or controlled substances may have their benefits reduced or even terminated.

Safety professionals with workers' compensation responsibilities often encounter situations where their boss(es) want to deny the claim for injury or illness arguing that the injury or illness was not work related. Safety professionals should exercise caution when pursuing a denial of a workers' compensation claim. Depending on the state workers' compensation laws, the administrative law judge hearing the case and many other factors, it is often very difficult to overcome the liberal bias in favor of the injured or ill employee. Often the employer spends more in investigating and preparing the case than to simply pay the claim. However, there are cases in which the employer prevails in denying a claim when the evidence can clearly show that the injury or illness was not work related.

In summation, safety professionals should make a clear distinction as to the proactive safety requirement and the reactive state workers' compensation laws. Although these laws and regulations may converge as a result of a work-related injury or illness, the requirements, dates, and many other aspects of the two distinct systems should be maintained separate, and the safety professional should acquire a thorough knowledge of each system. Although safety and workers' compensation may be housed within the corporate hierarchy in one office or with one person, these are two distinctly different systems with separate laws and regulations and separate requirements.

Questions

1. Identify and explain at least 3 differences between OSHA compliance and state workers' compensation.
2. What is an OSHA "recordable" case?
3. What are time loss benefits and how are they calculated?
4. How is permanent, partial, or total disability calculated in your state?
5. What is the difference between an OSHA recordable case and a worker's compensation claim?
6. Explain the difference between safety and workers' compensation?
7. Explain how time loss benefits are calculated in your state?
8. What is the difference between a recordable injury and a worker's compensation claim?
9. What does it mean if a company is "self-insured"?
10. What are your state's workers' compensation benefit levels?

Case Modified for the Purposes of this Text

386 F.Supp.2d 442
United States District Court,
S.D. New York.
Stanley WOJCIK, Plaintiff,
v.
42ND STREET DEVELOPMENT PROJECT, INC. and Turner
Construction Co., Defendants.
No. 02 Civ. 7019(CSH).
Aug. 26, 2005.

SYNOPSIS

Background: Ironworker who was employed by subcontractor and was injured while working at construction site sued property owner and general contractor, asserting claims under state workplace safety statutes and for common-law negligence. After action was removed, defendants moved for summary judgment.

Holdings: The District Court, Senior District Judge, held that:

1. Factual issues precluded summary judgment for owner and contractor on claim under scaffold law;
2. Factual issues precluded summary judgment for owner and contractor on claim alleging violation of New York safe workplace statute for construction, excavation, and demolition work;
3. Owner was not liable under general workplace safety statute or under common-law negligence for ironworker's injuries; and

4. Contractor was not liable under common-law negligence or New York's general workplace safety statute for ironworker's injuries.

Motion granted in part and denied in part.

SENIOR DISTRICT JUDGE

This diversity case removed from a state court is now before this Court on the motion of defendants 42nd Street Development Project, Inc. and Turner Construction Co., ("defendants") for summary judgment on plaintiff Stanley Wojcik's *447 claims based upon New York Labor Law §§ 240(1), 241(6), 200, and common law negligence. For the reasons explained herein, I deny defendants' motion as to plaintiff's Labor Law § 240(1) and § 241(6) claims, but grant their motion as to plaintiff's Labor Law § 200 and common law negligence claims.

I. PRELIMINARY

Before I proceed to a recitation of the circumstances underlying this action, I address a preliminary issue. Plaintiff, represented by counsel, has wholly failed to submit a statement complying with Local Rule 56.1 statement. The consequences of that failure must be considered.

District courts have the discretion to adopt local rules which they deem necessary to carry out the conduct of their business. *Frazier v. Heebe,* 482 U.S. 641, 645, 107 S.Ct. 2607, 96 L.Ed.2d 557 (1987) (citing 28 U.S.C. §§ 1654, 2071; Fed. R. Civ. Pro. 83). Pursuant to Local Civil Rule 56.1(a) adopted in this District, a motion for summary judgment must have annexed to it a short and concise statement, in numbered paragraphs, of the material facts as to which the moving party contends there is no issue to be tried. Local Civil Rule 56.1(a). Here, defendants, as the moving party, included such a statement with their motion for summary judgment. Defendants' statement contains eighty-two separate paragraphs with citations to the record.

In addition, Rule 56.1(b) imposes a parallel mandate on the party opposing summary judgment. "The papers opposing a motion for summary judgment *shall* include a correspondingly numbered paragraph responding to each numbered paragraph in the statement of the moving party." Local Civil Rule 56.1(b) (emphasis added). Counsel for plaintiff has filed an affidavit in opposition (the "Sacks Affidavit") which contains a desultory assortment of factual allegations. But these allegations— contained in thirty-three numbered paragraphs—merely recite the asserted facts underlying plaintiff's case. Counsel for plaintiff has not submitted the statement in opposition required by Rule 56.1(b). In that circumstance, Local Rule 56.1(c) provides as follows:

Each numbered paragraph in the statement of material facts set forth in the statement required to be served by the moving party *will* be deemed to be admitted for purposes of the motion unless *448 specifically controverted by a correspondingly numbered paragraph in the statement required to be served by the opposing party.

Local Civil Rule 56.1(c) (emphasis added); *Giannullo v. City of New York,* 322 F.3d 139, 140 (2d Cir.2003). ("If the opposing party then fails to controvert a fact so set forth in the moving party's Rule 56.1 statement, that fact will be deemed admitted."); *Gubitosi v. Kapica,* 154 F.3d 30, 31 (2d Cir.1998) (same).

However, "[t]he local rule does not absolve the party seeking summary judgment of the burden of showing that it is entitled to judgment as a matter of law, and a Local Rule 56.1(a) statement is not itself a vehicle for making factual assertions that are otherwise unsupported in the record." *Holtz v. Rockefeller & Co., Inc.,* 258 F.3d 62, 74 (2d Cir.2001). Further, Rule 56.1(b) allows the opposing party to "include ... additional paragraphs containing a separate short and concise statement of additional material facts as to which it is contended that there exists a genuine fact to be tried." Local Civil Rule 56.1(b). As described above, the Sacks Affidavit does contain various factual allegations, many of which expressly dispute the allegations in defendants' 56.1 Statement. Although neither short nor concise, insofar as plaintiff's allegations contained in the affidavit are properly supported by citations to the record, I will consider the Sacks Affidavit as proffering additional material facts as to which plaintiff contends that there exists a genuine fact to be tried.

Based upon the foregoing, and for the purpose of adjudicating defendants' motion for summary judgment, I will be guided by two principles. First, any fact alleged in defendants' Rule 56.1 statement, supported in fact by the record, and not specifically and expressly contradicted by properly supported allegations in the Sacks Affidavit, will be deemed admitted by plaintiff. Second, any fact alleged in defendants' Rule 56.1 statement, supported in fact by the record, but which is specifically and expressly controverted by facts contained in the Sacks Affidavit which are supported in the record, will not be deemed admitted by plaintiff.

II. BACKGROUND

This action is the result of a construction accident which occurred on June 28, 2002 at the Times Square Tower Project at Seven Times Square in New York (the "project"), a property in which defendant 42nd Street Development Project, Inc. ("42nd St. Development") has an ownership interest. Defendants' 56.1 Statement, ¶¶ 1–3. Plaintiff was an ironworker employed by Canron Construction Corp. ("Canron"), a subcontractor of defendant Turner Construction Co. ("Turner"), which was hired to provide steel erection services to the project. *Id.* at ¶ 6.

Plaintiff began working at the project site in April 2002 and was part of a detail gang which assisted in a variety of different construction tasks. Wojcik Aff., pp. 25–26 *in* Sparling Aff., Ex. C. The foreman of plaintiff's detail gang was Canron employee Michael O'Donnell. Defendants' 56.1 Statement, ¶ 39. According to the plaintiff, on the morning of the accident he was initially working in a subbasement at ground level when he was instructed by O'Donnell to move to a higher level to ***449*** remove part of the Q-deck floor—a form of temporary flooring—in order to create a hole through which elevator motors could be lowered. Sacks Aff., ¶ 5; Defendants' 56.1 Statement, ¶ 43. While removing the Q-deck, plaintiff fell approximately thirteen feet through the hole in the floor which he had created, onto the concrete floor below, injuring himself. Sparling Aff., Ex. AA; Defendants' 56.1 Statement, ¶ 64; Wojcik Aff., p. 70 *in* Sparling Aff., Ex. C.

Plaintiff contends that his request, prior to his fall, that scaffolding be erected under his new work site was denied by O'Donnell. Sacks Aff., ¶ 5. Moreover, he claims that the working conditions on C–1 were openly dangerous: to wit, the decking was wet and strewn with debris and the lighting was poor. Sacks Aff., Ex. C., pp. 34–37; Sacks Aff., ¶¶ 5–7. Plaintiff asserts that he was not provided with a safety harness, referred to as a "Personal Fall Arrest System" or "PFAS," and that no PFAS was available to him in Canron's "gang box" which contained the equipment. Sacks Aff., ¶ 5. Moreover, plaintiff claims that because no safety lines were erected in the area of his fall, even if he had been given a PFAS, he would not have had any place to tie-off. Wojcik Aff., ¶ 10 *in* Sacks Aff., Ex. A.

Defendants respond that "Canron provided every ironworker at the Seven Times Square Tower Project with a PFAS," as well as instructions on how to use the PFAS, and weekly reminders to use it. Defendant's 56.1 Statement, ¶¶ 17, 24. In fact, according to defendants, plaintiff received exactly such a reminder less than one hour before his accident. *Id.* at ¶ 38. Defendants further contend that the accident and eyewitness reports demonstrate that when plaintiff fell, he was actually wearing the PFAS, though he had not "tied off to an adequate anchorage point," *Id.* at ¶ 77 (quoting Scuola Aff., ¶ 7), despite the presence of two such points which were readily available to him. *Id.* at ¶¶ 56–61.

On July 24, 2002, plaintiff commenced this action in the Supreme Court of New York, New York County. Plaintiff's complaint alleges violations of New York Labor Law §§ 200, 240(1), 241(6) (and concomitant Industrial Code violations), common law negligence, and violation of OSHA standards, and requests damages in the amount of $20 million. The case was removed by the defendants to this Court on September 4, 2002. Defendants now move for summary judgment pursuant to Rule 56 of the Federal Rules of Civil Procedure.

Defendants claim that they are entitled to summary judgment on plaintiff's Labor Law § 240(1) claim on two grounds: (i) plaintiff's conduct was the sole proximate cause of his injuries, and (ii) plaintiff was a "recalcitrant worker" as that term is defined by the New York courts. Defendants claim that they are entitled to summary judgment on plaintiff's Labor Law § 241(6) claim because plaintiff's cannot allege any violation of the New York Industrial Code. Finally, defendants claim that they are entitled to summary judgment on plaintiff's Labor Law § 200 and common law negligence claims on three grounds: (i) defendants did not supervise or control plaintiff's work; (ii) defendants did not have notice of the alleged unsafe condition; and (iii) the hole in the flooring *450 was an open and obvious condition, created by the plaintiff himself.

For the reasons that follow, I deny defendants' summary judgment motion in part and grant it in part.

III. DISCUSSION

A. STANDARD OF REVIEW ON MOTION FOR SUMMARY JUDGMENT PURSUANT TO RULE 56

Rule 56 of the Federal Rules of Civil Procedure provides that a court shall grant a motion for summary judgment "if the pleadings, depositions, answers to interrogatories, and admissions on file, together with the affidavits, if any, show that there is no genuine issue of material fact and that the moving party is entitled to a judgment as a matter of law." Fed.R.Civ.P. 56(c); *see also Celotex Corp. v. Catrett, 477 U.S. 317, 106 S.Ct. 2548, 91 L.Ed.2d 265 (1986).* "The party seeking summary judgment bears the burden of establishing that no genuine issue of material fact exists and that the undisputed facts establish her right to judgment as a matter of law." *Rodriguez v. City of New York,* 72 F.3d 1051, 1060–61 (2d Cir.1995). The substantive law governing the case will identify those facts which are material and "only disputes over facts that might affect the outcome of the suit under governing law will properly preclude the entry of summary judgment." *Anderson v. Liberty Lobby, Inc.,* 477 U.S. 242, 248, 106 S.Ct. 2505, 91 L.Ed.2d 202 (1986). In the case at bar, the parties agree that New York law governs.

In determining whether a genuine issue of material fact exists, a court must resolve all ambiguities and draw all reasonable inferences against the moving party. *Matsushita Elec. Indus. Co. v. Zenith Radio Corp.,* 475 U.S. 574, 587, 106 S.Ct. 1348, 89 L.Ed.2d 538 (1986). "If, as to the issue on which summary judgment is sought, there is any evidence in the record from any source from which a reasonable inference could be drawn in favor of the non-moving party, summary judgment is improper." *Chambers v. TRM Copy Centers Corp.,* 43 F.3d 29, 37 (2d. Cir.1994).

B. PLAINTIFF'S LABOR LAW § 240(1) CLAIM

567For 120 years Labor Law § 240(1)—commonly known as the scaffold law—has provided legal recourse to workers injured while engaging in construction at heights. *Blake v. Neighborhood Hous. Servs. of N.Y. City, Inc.,* 1 N.Y.3d 280, 284–85, 771 N.Y.S.2d 484, 803 N.E.2d 757 (2003). Section § 240(1) states, in relevant part:

All contractors and owners and their agents … in the erection … repairing, [or] altering … of a building or structure shall furnish or erect, or cause to be furnished or erected for the performance of such labor, scaffolding, hoists, stays, ladders, slings, hangers, blocks, pulleys, braces, irons, ropes, and other devices which shall be so constructed, placed and operated as to give proper protection to a person so employed.

N.Y. Labor Law § 240(1) (McKinney 2002). In order to prevail under § 240(1), an injured plaintiff must prove (1) that a violation of the statute, (2) is the proximate cause of his injury. *Id.* at 287, 771 N.Y.S.2d 484, 803 N.E.2d 757; *Davidson v. Ambrozewicz,* 12 A.D.3d 902, 785 N.Y.S.2d 149 (3rd Dep't 2004); *Meade v. Rock–McGraw, Inc.,* 307 A.D.2d 156, 159, 760 N.Y.S.2d 39 (1st Dep't 2003). Once a plaintiff makes these two showings, the defendant is subject to absolute liability. **451 Koenig v. Patrick Const. Corp.,* 298 N.Y. 313, 316–17, 83 N.E.2d 133 (1948).

8910In order to demonstrate a violation of the statute, plaintiff must prove that he was not provided proper protection in the form of scaffolding, hoists, stays, ladders, slings, hangers, blocks, pulleys, braces, irons, ropes, or other devices. Section 240(1) "is to be construed as liberally as may be for the accomplishment of the purpose for which it was framed, however, this principle operates to impose absolute liability only *after* a violation of the statute has been established." *Narducci v. Manhasset Bay Associates,* 96 N.Y.2d 259, 267, 727 N.Y.S.2d 37, 750 N.E.2d 1085 (2001) (internal citations and quotations omitted).

At no time, however, did the Court or the Legislature ever suggest that a defendant should be treated as an insurer after having furnished a safe workplace. The point of Labor Law § 240(1) is to compel contractors and owners to comply with the law, not to penalize them when they have done so.

Blake, 1 N.Y.3d at 286, 771 N.Y.S.2d 484, 803 N.E.2d 757. Once an injured plaintiff proves a violation of § 240(1), he must then demonstrate that the statutory violation proximately caused his injury. "Violation of the statute alone is not enough; plaintiff [is] obligated to show that the violation was a contributing cause of his fall." *Duda v. John W. Rouse Const. Corp.,* 32 N.Y.2d 405, 410, 345 N.Y.S.2d 524, 298 N.E.2d 667 (1973); *see also Ross v. Curtis–Palmer Hydro–Electric Company et al., 81 N.Y.2d 494, 501, 601 N.Y.S.2d 49, 618 N.E.2d 82 (1993).* ("Labor Law § 240(1) was designed to prevent those types of accidents in which the scaffold, hoist, stay, ladder or other protective device proved inadequate to shield the injured worker *from harm directly flowing from the application of the force of gravity to an object or person."*) (emphasis in original).

111213In *Smith v. Hooker Chems. & Plastic Corp.*—a case which the Court of Appeals of New York has repeatedly and expressly cited with approval—the First Department elucidated what has come to be known as the "recalcitrant worker" defense. 89 A.D.2d 361, 365–66, 455 N.Y.S.2d 446 (1st Dep't 1982). "While the Legislature has sensibly acted to protect workers from a failure by owners or contractors **452* to supply equipment or for supplying faulty equipment, the statutory protection does not extend to workers who have adequate and safe equipment available to them but refuse to use it." *Id.* at 366, 455 N.Y.S.2d 446 (emphasis added). An owner or contractor who has provided appropriate safety devices to workers and properly instructed workers in their use will not be held liable for failing to "insist that a recalcitrant worker use the devices." *Id.* at 365, 455 N.Y.S.2d 446. Furthermore, a defendant need not show that plaintiff disregarded *immediate* instruction to use a safety harness. The Court of Appeals has held that instructions to the plaintiff to use the safety device given weeks before the accident were a sufficient basis for defendant's recalcitrant worker defense. *Cahill v. Triborough Bridge and Tunnel Authority,* 4 N.Y.3d 35, 39, 790 N.Y.S.2d 74, 823 N.E.2d 439 (2004).

14In order to prevail on their motion for summary judgment on plaintiff's Labor Law § 240(1) claim, defendants must demonstrate that there is no genuine issue of material fact that (i) there was no violation of the statute because plaintiff was provided with appropriate safety devices and properly instructed in their use, or (ii) that any violation which occurred did not proximately cause plaintiff's injury. Because there is a genuine issue of material fact as to whether defendants violated § 240(1)—that is to say, whether defendants provided plaintiff with a PFAS and an appropriate tie-off point—I deny their motion for summary judgment on plaintiff's Labor Law § 240(1) claim.

Defendant asserts that all ironworkers employed by Canron, including plaintiff, were provided with a brand new PFAS. Defendants' Rule 56.1 Statement, ¶¶ 17–18; Kraham Aff., p. 22 *in* Sparling Aff., Ex. E ("Q. Did Stan Wojcik get fall protection on this job site? A. Fall protection equipment? Q. Equipment? A. Yes, everybody did."). In fact, defendants present evidence that at the time of his fall, plaintiff was actually wearing a safety harness, albeit one that was not tied-off. Defendants' Rule 56.1 Statement, ¶¶ 56–61, 77. Defendants further claim that plaintiff had multiple appropriate tie-off points. "Plaintiff had two readily available, convenient nearby locations to tie-off … [t]here was an elevator column and safety fence post installed by Canron in the immediate vicinity of Plaintiff's work location." Defendants' Rule 56.1 Statement, ¶¶ 56–57. However, plaintiff also presents evidence—in the form of an affidavit by the plaintiff, and deposition testimony by plaintiff's co-worker, Basil Nicholson, and his foreman, Michael O'Donnell. These deponents testified that a PFAS was not provided to plaintiff and none were contained in the Canron gang boxes on the morning of the accident. Sacks Aff., ¶¶ 6–8; Wojcik Aff., ¶¶ 5, 8, 10 *in* Sacks Aff., Ex. A; Nicholson Deposition, pp. 75–80, 83–84 *in* Sacks Aff., Ex. B; O'Donnell Deposition, pp. 81–83 *in* Sacks Aff., Ex. D. *453* Moreover, plaintiff alleges, and defendant does not dispute, that no safety lines had been erected in the vicinity of plaintiff's accident. Sacks Aff., ¶¶ 5, 6, 8; Plaintiff's Aff., ¶¶ 6, 10 *in* Sacks Aff., Ex. A. In addition, plaintiff disputes defendants' assertion that the elevator column or safety fence post were proper tie-off points, claiming that "in my career as an ironworker I have never been instructed to tie off to an elevator post or a barricade." Wojcik Aff., ¶ 10 *in* Sacks Aff., Ex. A; see also Kraham Aff., pp. 105–06 *in* Sacks Aff., Ex. D (same); O'Donnell Aff., pp. 59–61 *in* Sacks Aff., Ex. C. (same). In fact, plaintiff claims that the safety fence post was not present on the morning of his fall, and was actually installed after the accident. Sacks Aff., ¶ 16.

Because the issues of whether defendants properly furnished a PFAS and, since there were no safety lines in place, whether the two purported tie-off points were proper, are genuine issues of material fact, I deny defendants motion for summary judgment on plaintiff's Labor Law § 240(1) claim.

C. PLAINTIFF'S LABOR LAW § 241(6) CLAIM

15161718Section 241(6) of the Labor Law empowers the Commissioner of the Department of Labor to promulgate regulations to promote the safety of workers engaged in construction, excavation and demolition, and provides that the violation of certain of those regulations by an owner or contractor constitutes a breach of § 241(6). *Ross,* 81 N.Y.2d at 501–02, 601 N.Y.S.2d 49, 618 N.E.2d 82. The law provides in pertinent part:

All areas in which construction, excavation or demolition work is being performed shall be so constructed, shored, equipped, guarded, arranged, operated and conducted as to provide reasonable and adequate protection and safety to the persons employed therein…. The commissioner may make rules to carry into effect the provisions of this subdivision, and the owners and contractors and their agents … shall comply therewith.

N.Y. Labor Law § 241(6) (McKinney 2002). Section 241(6) was written "to place the 'ultimate responsibility for safety practices at building construction jobs where such responsibility actually belongs, on the owner and general contractor.'" *Rizzuto v. L.A. Wenger Contracting Co., Inc.,* 91 N.Y.2d 343, 348, 670 N.Y.S.2d 816, 693 N.E.2d 1068 (1998) (quoting 1969 N.Y. Legis. Ann., 407–08). Thus, like § 240(1), § 241(6) is nondelegable, so a plaintiff "need not show that defendants exercised supervision or control over his worksite in order to establish his right of recovery." *Ross,* 81 N.Y.2d at 502, 601 N.Y.S.2d 49, 618 N.E.2d 82; *see supra* n. 8.

***454** 19But not all violations of regulations are actionable under § 241(6). "[A] distinction must be drawn between provisions of the Industrial Code mandating compliance with concrete specifications and those that establish general safety standards by invoking ... general descriptive terms.... The former give rise to a nondelegable duty, while the latter do not." *Ross,* 81 N.Y.2d at 505, 601 N.Y.S.2d 49, 618 N.E.2d 82. Hence, only the violation of those provisions of the Industrial Code which mandate compliance with concrete specifications can form the basis of a § 241(6) action. *Compare* 12 NYCRR § 23–1.7(b)(1)(i) ("Every hazardous opening into which a person may step or fall shall be guarded by a substantial cover fastened in place or by a safety railing constructed and installed in compliance with this Part (rule).") *with* 12 NYCRR § 23–1.4[a] (requiring the provision of materials and equipment "of such kind and quality as a reasonable and prudent [person] experienced in construction ... operations would require in order to provide safe working conditions").

20In the case at bar, plaintiff claims that defendant violated an assortment of provisions of Rule 23 of the Industrial Code of the State of New York, including §§ 1.7, 1.8, 1.15, 1.16, 1.17, 1.21, 1.32, 2.2, 2.3, 2.4, and 5. Compl., ¶ 10. Because there are genuine issues of material fact as to whether defendants violated § 1.7(b)(1)(i), I deny defendants' motion for summary judgment on plaintiff's § 241(6)claim.

Section 1.7(b)(1)(i) provides that "[e]very hazardous opening into which a person may step or fall shall be guarded by a ... a safety railing constructed and installed in compliance with this Part." This regulation has been held sufficient to support a § 241(6) cause of action. *See, e.g., Dorrian v. Caldor Corp., 152 F.3d 917, 1998 WL 279429 (2d Cir.1998); Reinoso v. Ornstein Layton Management, Inc.,* 19 A.D.3d 678, 798 N.Y.S.2d 95 (2nd Dep't 2005). Defendants do not dispute that no safety railing had been constructed around the opening through which plaintiff fell. Defendants' Memorandum, p. 15.

2122The interpretation of an Industrial Code regulation and the determination ***455** as to whether a particular condition is within the scope of the regulation both present questions of law for the court. *Messina,* 300 A.D.2d at 123, 752 N.Y.S.2d 608; *see also Penta v. Related Companies, L.P., 286 A.D.2d 674, 675, 730 N.Y.S.2d 140 (2d Dep't 2001); Millard v. City of Ogdensburg,* 274 A.D.2d 953, 710 N.Y.S.2d 507 (4th Dep't 2000). The cases addressing § 1.7 make it abundantly clear that in the case at bar, the hole through which plaintiff fell is a "hazardous opening" as that term is used in § 1.7(b)(1)(i). *See Ryan v. Freidman Decorating Co., 2005 WL 1802861, at *18 (S.D.N.Y. Jul.28, 2005)* (citing *Wells v. British American Dev. Corp.,* 2 A.D.3d 1141, 770 N.Y.S.2d 161 (3d Dep't 2003) (holding that elevator pit into which employee fell was sufficiently large to support violation of regulation); *but c.f. Rice v. Board of Ed., 302 A.D.2d 578, 755 N.Y.S.2d 419 (2d Dep't 2003)* (holding the regulation inapplicable where worker's leg fell into one-foot deep hole in rear of flat-bed truck); *Plump v. Wyoming County*, 298 A.D.2d 886, 748 N.Y.S.2d 195 (4th Dep't 2002) (holding the regulation inapplicable to worker's four-and-one-half-foot fall from flatbed of delivery truck at construction site); *Sopha v. Combustion Eng'g, Inc.*, 261 A.D.2d 911, 690 N.Y.S.2d 813 (4th Dep't 1999) (holding that worker who fell while climbing through window did not fall through "hazardous opening"); *Bennion v. Goodyear Tire & Rubber Co.*, 229 A.D.2d 1003, 645 N.Y.S.2d 195 (4th Dep't 1996) (holding the regulation inapplicable where worker fell three to four feet from rafter to the floor); *DeLong v. State St. Assocs.*, 211 A.D.2d 891, 621 N.Y.S.2d 172 (3d Dep't 1995) (holding that four to five feet foot fall down slope of hill was not an "opening")). The hole in the Q-deck floor through which plaintiff fell was apparently about thirteen feet above the concrete floor upon which he landed. Sparling Aff., Ex. AA; Wojcik Aff., p. 70 *in* Sparling Aff., Ex. C. For the purposes of defendants' motion, then, I hold that the hole through which plaintiff fell constitutes the type of "hazardous opening" contemplated by § 1.7(b)(1)(i).

Defendants argue, without citing any cases, that because the plaintiff created the hole he subsequently fell through, it would have been "impossible to have placed any protective material around the opening," and hence § 1.7(b)(1)(i) cannot apply. Defendants' Memorandum, p. 15. But there is no basis for defendants' conclusion that solely because plaintiff created the hole, defendants are absolved as a matter of law from the responsibility of adhering to the mandates of § 1.7(b)(1)(i), particularly where it appears to be undisputed that defendants directed plaintiff to create the hole for the purpose of lowering elevator motors through it, in furtherance of the project. Whether defendants were required to install protective material around that opening pursuant to § 1.7(b)(1)(i), whether they violated that regulation, and whether and to what degree plaintiff's own negligence contributed to his injury, are disputed issues of material fact which should be resolved after each party has had a full opportunity to present its evidence. In these circumstances, I deny defendants' motion for summary judgment on plaintiff's Labor Law § 241(6) claim.

D. PLAINTIFF'S LABOR LAW § 200 AND COMMON LAW NEGLIGENCE CLAIMS

23Labor Law § 200 codifies landowners' and general contractors' common law duty to maintain a safe workplace. ***456** Ross,* 81 N.Y.2d at 505, 601 N.Y.S.2d 49, 618 N.E.2d 82. The law provides in pertinent part:

All places to which this chapter applies shall be so constructed, equipped, arranged, operated and conducted as to provide reasonable and adequate protection to the lives, health and safety of all persons employed therein or lawfully frequenting such places. All machinery, equipment, and devices in such places shall be so placed, operated, guarded, and lighted as to provide reasonable and adequate protection to all such persons.

N.Y. Labor Law § 200(1) (McKinney's 2002).

24Unlike claims arising under § 240(1) and § 241(6), however, Labor Law § 200 requires plaintiff to prove that defendant "exercised some supervisory control over the operation." *Ross,* 81 N.Y.2d at 505, 601 N.Y.S.2d 49, 618 N.E.2d 82. This rule is consistent with the common law principle that "an owner or general contractor could not be held responsible for the negligent acts of others over whom he had no direction or control." *Allen v. Cloutier Const. Corp.,* 44 N.Y.2d 290, 299, 405 N.Y.S.2d 630, 376 N.E.2d 1276 (1978).

25 The prerequisite that the owner or general contractor must possess some meaningful supervisory control over the operation which led to plaintiff's injury is not a mere technicality. In fact, owners and general contractors can maintain a significant presence at a worksite without incurring § 200 liability. "[A]n owner or general contractor's retention of general supervisory control, presence at the worksite or authority to enforce general safety standards is insufficient to establish the necessary control" for a § 200 claim. *Soshinsky v. Cornell University,* 268 A.D.2d 947, 947, 703 N.Y.S.2d 550 (3rd Dep't 2000); *see also Poulin v. E.I. Dupont DeNemours and Co., 883 F.Supp. 894, 899 (W.D.N.Y.1994)* ("[A]n owner or employer does not supervise or control the performance of the work for the purposes of Labor Law § 200 merely by presenting ideas and suggestions, making observations and inquiries, and inspecting the work.") (internal quotations omitted); *Comes v. New York State Elec. and Gas Corp.,* 82 N.Y.2d 876, 877, 609 N.Y.S.2d 168, 631 N.E.2d 110 (1993)(upholding dismissal of § 200 claim despite the presence of defendant's inspector at job site, because "there [wa]s no evidence that defendant exercised supervisory control or had any input into how the steel beam [that caused plaintiff's injury] was moved"); *Cooper v. Sonwil Distribution Center, Inc.,* 15 A.D.3d 878, 879, 789 N.Y.S.2d 583 (4th Dep't 2005) ("The daily presence of defendant's construction manager at the work site to check on the progress of the work does not constitute the control or supervision necessary to establish liability under section 200 or for common-law negligence.") (internal quotations omitted).

26 The *sine qua non* of a § 200 action against an owner or general contractor is that the defendant maintained supervisory control over the method employed by the subcontractor in accomplishing a specific task, operation or activity. *See *457 Palen v. ITW Mortgage Investments III, Inc.,* 2003 WL 1907980, at *5–6 (S.D.N.Y. Apr.17, 2003) ("Where a claim under section 200 'arises out of alleged defects or dangers arising from a *subcontractor's methods* or materials, recovery against the owner or general contractor cannot be had unless it is shown that the party to be charged exercised some supervisory control over *the operation.'")* (citing *Bailey v. Bethlehem Steel Corp.,* 1994 WL 586944, at *7 (W.D.N.Y. Oct.4, 1994) (emphasis added)); *Sainato v. City of Albany,* 285 A.D.2d 708, 709, 727 N.Y.S.2d 741 (3rd Dep't 2001) (granting summary judgment to defendant because "it did not exercise any direct control over the contractor's employees or *manner* in which the work was performed") (emphasis added); *Riley v. John W. Stickl Const. Co., Inc.,* 242 A.D.2d 936, 937, 662 N.Y.S.2d 660 (4th Dep't 1997) (granting summary judgment to defendant landowner because "the defect or dangerous condition [wa]s created by the contractor's own *methods* of work") (emphasis added); *Merkle v. Weibrecht,* 234 A.D.2d 696, 698, 650 N.Y.S.2d 471 (3rd Dep't 1996) ("[B]ecause the dangerous condition that existed was a result of the *manner* in which plaintiff elected to gain entrance to the lift station, liability cannot be imposed absent a showing, not made here, that defendants or their employees supervised or controlled *that aspect* of his work") (emphasis added); *Persichilli v. Triborough Bridge and Tunnel Authority,* 16 N.Y.2d 136, 145, 262 N.Y.S.2d 476, 209 N.E.2d 802 (1965) ("[T]he duty to provide a safe

place to work is not breached when the injury arises out of a defect *in the subcon-tractor's own ... methods,* or through negligent acts of the subcontractor *occurring as a detail of the work.*") (emphasis added). If an owner or general contractor does not exercise supervisory control over the means or methods employed by the subcon-tractor to accomplish a task, it will not incur liability pursuant to § 200.

27Finally, neither an owner nor a general contractor has a duty to protect work-ers from open and obvious hazards. *Shandraw v. Tops Markets, Inc.,* 244 A.D.2d 997, 998, 665 N.Y.S.2d 486 (4th Dep't 1997) ("[A] party potentially liable under Labor Law § 200 or for common-law negligence 'has no duty to protect workers against a condition that may be readily observed.'") (internal quotations omitted); *Merkle,* 234 A.D.2d at 698, 650 N.Y.S.2d 471 ("The duty to protect prescribed by section 200 does not extend to hazards, such as that at issue here, that are read-ily apparent, taking into consideration the age, intelligence and experience of the worker").

Defendants claim that they are entitled to summary judgment on plaintiff's § 200 claim for three reasons: (i) defendants did not supervise or control plaintiff's work; (ii) defendants did not have specific notice of the alleged unsafe condition; and (iii) **458* because the condition was open and obvious. Defendants' Memorandum of Law, p. 19. Because I find no genuine issue of fact exists as to whether either defen-dant supervised plaintiff's work, I grant defendants' motion as to plaintiff's Labor Law § 200 and common law negligence claims.

1.   Defendant/Owner 42nd Street Development Project, Inc.

2829Although neither party apparently sees fit to distinguish between plaintiff's § 200 claims against the two defendants, for obvious reasons independent analysis for each is warranted. "It is settled law that where the alleged defect or dangerous con-dition arises from the contractor's methods and the owner exercises no supervisory control over the operation, no liability attaches to the owner ... under section 200 of the Labor Law." *Lombardi v. Stout,* 80 N.Y.2d 290, 295, 590 N.Y.S.2d 55, 604 N.E.2d 117 (1992); *Yong Ju Kim v. Herbert Constr. Co.,* 275 A.D.2d 709, 712, 713 N.Y.S.2d 190 (2nd Dep't 2000). Plaintiff has not proffered a single piece of evidence to show that the landowner, 42nd St. Development, had any supervisory control over plain-tiff's work. In fact, neither his Affidavit in Opposition—which I have treated as "additional material facts as to which it is contended that there exists a genuine fact to be tried," pursuant to Local Civil Rule 56.1(b)—nor his papers in opposition to defendants' summary judgment motion even mention 42nd St. Development's role at the project site. *See, e.g.,* Plaintiff's Memorandum of Law in Opposition, p. 20 (containing the section challenging defendants' motion for summary judgment on plaintiff's § 200 and negligence claim entitled: "There Are Clearly Issues of Fact that Require a Trial as to *Turner Construction's* Negligence Under Labor Law § 200") (emphasis added).

Even drawing all reasonable inferences in plaintiff's favor, there is no genuine issue of material fact that defendant 42nd St. Development did not supervise plain-tiff's work and hence cannot be liable under § 200 and the common law. 42nd St. Development's motion for summary judgment as to these claims is granted.

2. Defendant/General Contractor Turner Construction Co.

30Plaintiff makes a variety of assertions regarding defendant Turner's responsibilities at the project site, which he contends are sufficient to demonstrate that Turner
supervised the plaintiff's work such that it should be liable under § 200 and ***459***
common law negligence. I disagree. Even drawing all reasonable inferences in plaintiff's favor, there is no genuine issue of material fact: Turner, as the general contractor, did not exercise meaningful supervisory control over the activity which led to
plaintiff's injury.

31According to plaintiff, a Turner employee informed a Canron supervisor,
Steve Dawson, that he wanted the Q-deck flooring removed in order to create a hole
through which the elevator motors could be lowered. *Id.* at ¶¶ 7, 29. The morning
of the accident, Dawson informed plaintiff's foreman, Michael O'Donnell, another
Canron employee, that O'Donnell should move his crew to remove the Q-deck.
Sacks Aff., ¶ 7. O'Donnell then gave plaintiff the instructions to remove the Q-deck
flooring and directed the method to be used by plaintiff. Defendants' 56.1 Statement,
¶ 43; Plaintiff's Aff., ¶ 3 ("Michael O'Donnell came down to the work areas and
instructed us to remove corrugated decking.... We were instructed by our foreman
[O'Donnell] to cut out and burn out tack welds in order to remove the deck."). "As
foreman, Michael O'Donnell gave all instructions and was plaintiff's sole supervisor
at the time of the accident." Sacks Aff., ¶ 5; Plaintiff's Aff., ¶ 3 ("Michael O'Donnell
was my sole supervisor at the time of the accident and the individual who gave me
my instructions on a daily basis."). Plaintiff also asserts that he "requested that a
scaffold be set up underneath the opening. This request was denied by his foreman
[O'Donnell]." Sacks Aff., ¶ 5.

Plaintiff also makes general assertions concerning Turner's role at the project
site. Plaintiff states that Turner "retained the subcontractors … and coordinated
the work." Sacks Aff., ¶ 29. Plaintiff continues that "[d]espite the fact that Turner
had site safety superintendents walking the site on a daily basis, they failed to erect
any protection around the opening in question." *Id.* Plaintiff also contends that
"Turner held a safety meeting … stating it was [sic] *mandatory to provide* personal
protective equipment for fall protection to all workers" and required that the safety
cable be ½ inch. *Id.* at 31. Plaintiff concludes that Turner's negligence in its "overall supervision of the job site" provides a proper foundation for liability under §
200. These assertions are insufficient on their face to preclude summary judgment.

32In addition, the uncontroverted allegations contained in defendants' ***460*** Rule
56.1 Statement make plain that Turner did not meaningfully supervise the plaintiff.
It was Canron and the Local 40 Ironworkers' Union that provided instruction in the
proper use of PFAS. Defendants' Rule 56.1 Statement ¶¶ 10, 14. Canron actually
provided the PFAS to its ironworkers. *Id.* at ¶ 17. When plaintiff did have access to a
PFAS, it was contained in Canron's gang boxes. Reminders that that use of a PFAS
was mandatory when working at heights were made during weekly safety meetings
conducted by Canron's ironworker steward. *Id.* at ¶¶ 24–29. Moreover, and more
importantly, as I observed above, it was a Canron employee, Dawson, who instructed
plaintiff's foreman, O'Donnell, another Canron employee, to remove the Q-deck
and it was O'Donnell, exclusively, who instructed plaintiff which decking should be

removed, how much decking shouled be removed, and how to remove the decking. *Id.* at ¶ 49; *see also* ¶¶ 43–44, 46; Saks Aff., Ex. C., pp. 65–68.

In sum, there is no evidence that Turner exercised supervisory control or had any input into how plaintiff removed the Q-deck flooring, the activity that caused plaintiff's injury. Based upon the foregoing, even resolving all ambiguities and drawing all reasonable inferences against Turner, there is no genuine issue of material fact and Turner's motion for summary judgment on plaintiff's Labor Law § 200 and common law negligence claims is granted.

IV. CONCLUSION

In these circumstances, and based upon the foregoing:

1. Defendants' motion for summary judgment on plaintiff's New York Labor Law § 241(6) claim is denied.
2. Defendants' motion for summary judgment on plaintiff's New York Labor Law § 240(1) claim is denied.
3. Defendants' motion for summary judgment on plaintiff's New York Labor Law § 200 and common law negligence claims are granted.

In the light of these rulings, counsel for the parties are directed to send letters to the Court, with copies to each other, not later than September 19, 2005, advising (1) whether any further pretrial discovery is required; (2) if so, the nature and extent of that discovery; and (3) if the case is now trial ready, the estimated time each party will require for the presentation of its case in chief. In the latter eventuality, the Court will then enter its final pretrial order and schedule the case for trial.

It is SO ORDERED.

15 Americans with Disabilities Act

Conformity is the jailer of freedom and the enemy of growth.

John F. Kennedy

In our work and in our living, we must recognize that difference is a reason for celebration and growth, rather than a reason for destruction.

Audre Lorde

STUDENT LEARNING OBJECTIVES

1. Analyze and assess the requirements under the five titles under ADA.
2. Analyze and assess the requirements for a qualified Individual with a Disability.
3. Analyze and understand how ADA impacts the safety function.

Safety professionals do not work in a vacuum. On a daily basis, safety professionals are impacted by other laws and regulations which may not directly impact their job function, however, may impact other departments or entities within the organization. However, because the safety function touches virtually every aspect within the organization, safety becomes involved, either directly or indirectly, and the safety professional's actions or inactions can impact other functions or the overall organization. One of the laws which is more human resource department-related, however, impacts the safety function is the ADA.

The ADA is an extensive law which can have a definite impact on the safety and health function. Safety professionals should also be aware that many states also possess state laws which can parallel the ADA. In short, the ADA prohibits discriminating against qualified individuals with physical or mental disabilities in all employment settings. For safety professionals, the areas of workers' compensation, restricted duty programs, facility modifications, training, and other safety functions are often areas where safety and health and the ADA may intersect and create duties and responsibilities for the safety professional as well as potential liabilities for the company or organization.

Safety professionals should keep in mind that the ADA is an extensive law and there are interpretations and decisions being made in the courts and agencies (primarily the Equal Employment Opportunity Commission or EEOC) virtually every day. A prudent safety professional does not need to be an "expert" in the ADA; however, he/she should be aware and cognizant of the requirements of the ADA and be able to recognize when the ADA is applicable to the safety situation.

It is important that safety professionals possess a base-level knowledge of the ADA as well as key areas in which the ADA and safety function may intersect in order to be able to recognize when the ADA may be applicable to the situation. The agency responsible for enforcement is the EEOC on the federal level and information can be found on their website located at www.eeoc.gov. Safety professionals should also be aware that individual states may also possess laws which parallel or are more stringent that the federal ADA. Additionally, it is vital that the safety and health professional acquires all of the facts before making a decision which may violate a qualified individual with a disability's rights under the ADA. Prudent safety professionals should gather all of the facts, document all aspects of the interaction, acquire assistance from human resources, EEO or legal counsel and review thoroughly prior to making any decisions involving the ADA. If the issue possesses possible ADA implications, safety professionals should direct the matter to the appropriate department and avoid making any statements or hasty decisions. By simply asking, "How can I help you?" the safety professional can usually gather sufficient information to direct the individual to Human Resources or other appropriate departments.

From a broad prospective, the ADA is divided into five titles, and all titles possess the potential of substantially impacting the safety and health function in covered public or private sector organizations.

Title I contains the employment provisions that protect all individuals with disabilities who are in the United States, regardless of their national origin or immigration status. Title II prohibits discriminating against qualified individuals with disabilities or excluding them from the services, programs, or activities provided by public entities. Title II contains the transportation provisions of the Act. Title III, entitled "Public Accommodations," requires that goods, services, privileges, advantages, and facilities of any public place be offered "in the most integrated setting appropriate to the needs of the individual."*

Title IV also covers transportation offered by private entities and addresses telecommunications. Title IV requires that telephone companies provide telecommunication relay services and that public service television announcements that are produced or funded with federal money include closed caption. Title V includes the miscellaneous provisions. This Title notes that the ADA does not limit or invalidate other federal and state laws providing equal or greater protection for the rights of individuals with disabilities, and addresses related insurance, alternate dispute, and congressional coverage issues.

Title I also prohibits covered employers from discriminating against a "qualified individual with a disability" with regard to job applications, hiring, advancement, discharge, compensation, training, and other terms, conditions, and privileges of employment.†

---

* ADA Section 305.
† ADA Section 102(a); 42 U.S.C. Section 12112.

Section 101 (8) defines a "qualified individual with a disability" as any person who, with or without reasonable accommodation, can perform the essential functions of the employment position that such individual holds or desires ... consideration shall be given to the employer's judgment as to what functions of a job are essential, and if an employer has prepared a written description before advertising or interviewing applicants for the job, this description shall be considered evidence of the essential function of the job.[*]

The EEOC provides additional clarification of this definition by stating, "an individual with a disability who satisfies the requisite skill, experience and educational requirements of the employment position such individual holds or desires, and who, with or without reasonable accommodation, can perform the essential functions of such position."[†]

Congress did not provide a specific list of disabilities covered under the ADA because "of the difficulty of ensuring the comprehensiveness of such a list."[‡] Under the ADA, an individual has a disability if he or she possesses:

- A physical or mental impairment that substantially limits one or more of the major life activities of such individual;
- A record of such an impairment; or
- Is regarded as having such an impairment.[§]

For an individual to be considered "disabled" under the ADA, the physical or mental impairment must limit one or more "major life activities." Under the U.S. Justice Department's regulation issued for section 504 of the Rehabilitation Act, "major life activities" are defined as, "functions such as caring for one's self, performing manual tasks, walking, seeing, hearing, speaking, breathing, learning and working."[¶] Congress clearly intended to have the term "disability" broadly construed. However, this definition does not include simple physical characteristics, nor limitations based on environmental, cultural, or economic disadvantages.[**]

The second prong of this definition is "a record of such an impairment disability." The Senate Report and the House Judiciary Committee Report each stated:

> This provision is included in the definition in part to protect individuals who have recovered from a physical or mental impairment which previously limited them in a major life activity. Discrimination on the basis of such a past impairment would be prohibited under this legislation. Frequently occurring examples of the first group (i.e. those who have a history of an impairment) are people with histories of mental or emotional illness, heart disease or cancer; examples of the second group (i.e. those who have been misclassified as having an impairment) are people who have been misclassified as mentally retarded.[††]

---

[*] ADA Section 101 (8).

[†] EEOC Interpretive Rules, 56 Fed. Reg. 35 (July 26, 1991).

[‡] 42 Fed. Reg. 22686(May 4, 1977); S. Rep. 101-116; H Rep. 101-485, Part 2, 51.

[§] Subtitle A, § 3(2). The ADA departed from the Rehabilitation Act of 1973 and other legislation is using the term "disability" rather than "handicap."

[¶] 28 C.F.R. § 41.31. This provision is adopted by and reiterated in the Senate Report at page 22.

[**] See *Jasany v. U.S. Postal Service*, 755 F.2d 1244 (6th Cir. 1985).

[††] S. Rep. 101-116, 23; H. Rep. 101-485, Part 2, 52–53.

The third prong of the statutory definition of a disability extends coverage to individuals who are "being regarded as having a disability." The ADA has adopted the same "regarded as" test that is used in section 504 of the Rehabilitation Act:

> "Is regarded as having an impairment" means (A) has a physical or mental impairment that does not substantially limit major life activities but is treated ... as constituting such a limitation; (B) has a physical or mental impairment that substantially limits major life activities only as a result of the attitudes of others toward such impairment; (C) has none of the impairments defined (in the impairment paragraph of the Department of Justice regulations) but is treated ... as having such an impairment.[*]

Under the EEOC's regulations, this third prong covers three classes of individuals:

1. Persons who have physical or mental impairments that do not limit a major life activity but who are nevertheless perceived by covered entities (employers, places of public accommodation) as having such limitations. (For example, an employee with controlled high blood pressure that is not, in fact, substantially limited, is reassigned to less strenuous work because of his employer's unsubstantiated fear that the individual will suffer a heart attack if he continues to perform strenuous work. Such a person would be "regarded" as disabled.)[†]
2. Persons who have physical or mental impairments that substantially limit a major life activity only because of a perception that the impairment causes such a limitation. (For example, an employee has a condition that periodically causes an involuntary jerk of the head, but no limitations on his major life activities. If his employer discriminates against him because of the negative reaction of customers, the employer would be regarding him as disabled and acting on the basis of that perceived disability.)[‡]
3. Persons who do not have a physical or mental impairment, but are treated as having a substantially limiting impairment. (For example, a company discharges an employee based on a rumor that the employee is HIV-positive. Even though the rumor is totally false and the employee has no impairment, the company would nevertheless be in violation of the ADA.)[§]

Thus, a "qualified individual with a disability" under the ADA is any individual who can perform the essential or vital functions of a particular job with or without the employer accommodating the particular disability. The employer is provided the opportunity to determine the "essential functions" of the particular job before offering the position through the development of a written job description. This written job description will be considered evidence to which functions of the particular job are essential and which are peripheral. In deciding the "essential functions" of a

---

[*] 45 C.F.R. 84.3(j)(2)(iv), quoted from H. Rep. 101-485, Part 3, 29; S. Rep. 101-116, 23; H. Rep. 101-485, Part 2, 53; Also see *School Board of Nassau County, Florida v. Arline*, 107 S. Ct. 1123 (1987) (leading case).

[†] EEOC Interpretive Guidelines, 56 Fed. Reg. 35,742 (July 26, 1991).

[‡] S. Comm. on Lab. and Hum. Resources Rep. at 24; H. Comm. on Educ. and Lab. Rep. at 53; H. Comm. on Jud. Rep. at 30–31.

[§] 29 C.F.R. § 1630.2(l).

particular position, the EEOC will consider the employer's judgment, whether the written job description was developed prior to advertising or beginning the interview process, the amount of time spent performing the job, the past and current experience of the individual to be hired, relevant collective bargaining agreements, and other factors.*

The EEOC defines the term "essential function" of a job as meaning "primary job duties that are intrinsic to the employment position the individual holds or desires" and precludes any marginal or peripheral functions which may be incidental to the primary job function.† The factors provided by the EEOC in evaluating the "essential functions" of a particular job include the reason that the position exists, the number of employees available, and the degree of specialization required to perform the job.‡ This determination is especially important to safety and health professionals who may be required to develop the written job descriptions or to determine the "essential functions" of a given position.

Safety and health professionals should recognize the important and pertinent issue of "direct threat" to the safety and health of the individual or others. Safety and health professionals should recognize this situation when the treatment of the disabled individual, who, as a matter of fact or due to prejudice, is believed to be a direct threat to the safety and health of themselves or others in the workplace. This sensitive issue often places the burden directly on the shoulders of the safety and health professional to evaluate and render a decision which will not only impact the individual with a disability but also the company or organization. To address this issue, the ADA provides that any individual who poses a direct threat to the health and safety of others that cannot be eliminated by reasonable accommodation may be disqualified from the particular job.§ The term "direct threat" to others is defined by the EEOC as creating "a significant risk of substantial harm to the health and safety of the individual or others that cannot be eliminated by reasonable accommodation."¶ The determining factors that safety and health professionals should consider in making this determination include the duration of the risk, the nature and severity of the potential harm, and the likelihood that the potential harm will occur.**

Additionally, safety professionals should consider the EEOC's Interpretive Guidelines, which state:

> [If] an individual poses a direct threat as a result of a disability, the employer must determine whether a reasonable accommodation would either eliminate the risk or reduce it to an acceptable level. If no accommodation exists that would either eliminate the risk or reduce the risk, the employer may refuse to hire an applicant or may discharge an employee who poses a direct threat.††

---

* ADA, Title I, Section 101(8).
† EEOC Interpretive Rules, supra, note 11.
‡ Id.
§ ADA, Section 103(b).
¶ EEOC Interpretive Guidelines, supra Note 11.
** Id.
†† 56 Fed. Reg. 35,745 (July 26, 1991); Also see *Davis v. Meese*, 692 F. Supp. 505 (E.D. Pa. 1988) (Rehabilitation Act decision).

Safety professionals should also note that Title I additionally provides that if an employer does not make reasonable accommodations for the known limitations of a qualified individual with disabilities, it is considered to be discrimination. Only if the employer can prove that providing the accommodation would place an undue hardship on the operation of the employer's business can discrimination be disproved. Section 101(9) defines a "reasonable accommodation" as:

> (a) making existing facilities used by employees readily accessible to and usable by the qualified individual with a disability and includes:
>
> (b) job restriction, part-time or modified work schedules, reassignment to a vacant position, acquisition or modification of equipment or devices, appropriate adjustments or modification of examinations, training materials, or policies, the provisions of qualified readers or interpreters and other similar accommodations for ... the QID (qualified individual with a disability).*

The EEOC further defines "reasonable accommodation" as:

1. Any modification or adjustment to a job application process that enables a qualified individual with a disability to be considered for the position such qualified individual with a disability desires, and which will not impose an undue hardship on the ... business; or
2. Any modification or adjustment to the work environment, or to the manner or circumstances which the position held or desired is customarily performed, that enables the qualified individual with a disability to perform the essential functions of that position and which will not impose an undue hardship on the ... business; or
3. Any modification or adjustment that enables the qualified individual with a disability to enjoy the same benefits and privileges of employment that other employees enjoy and does not impose an undue hardship on the ... business.†

Safety professionals should be aware that the company or organization would be required to make "reasonable accommodations" for any/all known physical or mental limitations of the qualified individual with a disability, unless the employer can demonstrate that the accommodations would impose an "undue hardship" on the business, or that the particular disability directly affects the safety and health of that individual or others. Safety professionals should also be aware that included under this section is the prohibition against the use of qualification standards, employment tests, and other selection criteria that can be used to screen out individuals with disabilities, unless the employer can demonstrate that the procedure is directly related to the job function. In addition to the modifications to facilities, work schedules, equipment, and training programs, the company or organization is required to initiate an "informal interactive (communication) process" with the qualified individual to promote voluntary disclosure of his or her specific limitations and restrictions to

---

* ADA Section 101(9).
† EEOC Interpretive Guidelines, supra Note 11.

enable the employer to make appropriate accommodations that will compensate for the limitation.*

Safety professionals should be aware that Section 101(10)(a) defines "undue hardship" as "an action requiring significant difficulty or expense," when considered in light of the following factors:

- The nature and cost of the accommodation;
- The overall financial resources and work force of the facility involved;
- The overall financial resources, number of employees, and structure of the parent entity; and
- The type of operation, including the composition and function of the work force, the administration, and the fiscal relationship between the entity and the parent. †

Of particular importance to safety professionals is Section 102(c)(1) of the ADA. This section prohibits discrimination through medical screening, employment inquiries, and similar scrutiny. Safety professionals should be aware that underlying this section was Congress's conclusion that information obtained from employment applications and interviews "was often used to exclude individuals with disabilities—particularly those with so-called hidden disabilities such as epilepsy, diabetes, emotional illness, heart disease and cancer—before their ability to perform the job was even evaluated."‡

Additionally, under Section 102(c)(2), safety and health professionals should be aware that conducting pre-employment physical examinations of applicants and asking prospective employees if they are qualified individuals with disabilities is prohibited. Employers are further prohibited from inquiring as to the nature or severity of the disability, even if the disability is visible or obvious. Safety and health professionals should be aware that individuals may ask whether any candidates for transfer or promotion who have a known disability can perform the required tasks of the new position if the tasks are job-related and consistent with business necessity. An employer is also permitted to inquire about the applicant's ability to perform the essential job functions prior to employment. The employer should use the written job description as evidence of the essential functions of the position.§

Safety professionals may require medical examinations of employees only if the medical examination is specifically job related and is consistent with business necessity. Medical examinations are permitted only after the applicant with a disability has been offered the job position. The medical examination may be given before the applicant starts the particular job, and the job offer may be contingent upon the results of the medical examination if all employees are subject to the medical examinations and information obtained from the medical examination is maintained in separate, confidential medical files. Employers are permitted to conduct voluntary

---

* Id.
† See *Gruegging v. Burke*, 48 Fair Empl. Prac. Cas. (BNA) 140 (D.D.C. 1987); *Bento v. ITO Corp.*, 599 F. Supp. 731 (D.R.I. 1984).
‡ S. Comm. on Lab. and Hum. Resources Rep. at 38; H. Comm. on Jud. Rep. at 42.
§ ADA. Title I, Section 102(c)(2).

medical examinations for current employees as part of an ongoing medical health program, but again, the medical files must be maintained separately and in a confidential manner.* The ADA does not prohibit safety professionals or their medical staff from making inquiries or requiring medical or "fit for duty" examinations when there is a need to determine whether or not an employee is still able to perform the essential functions of the job, or where periodic physical examinations are required by medical standards or federal, state, or local law.†

Another area of particular importance for safety and health professionals is the area of controlled substance testing. Under the ADA, the employer is permitted to test job applicants for alcohol and controlled substances prior to an offer of employment under section 104(d). The testing procedure for alcohol and illegal drug use is not considered a medical examination as defined under the ADA. Employers may additionally prohibit the use of alcohol and illegal drugs in the workplace and may require that employees not be under the influence while on the job. Employers are permitted to test current employees for alcohol and controlled substance use in the workplace to the limits permitted by current federal and state law. The ADA requires all employers to conform to the requirements of the Drug-Free Workplace Act of 1988. Thus, safety and health professionals should be aware that most existing pre-employment and postemployment alcohol and controlled substance programs which are not part of the pre-employment medical examination or ongoing medical screening program will be permitted in their current form.‡ Individual employees who choose to use alcohol and illegal drugs are afforded no protection under the ADA. However, employees who have successfully completed a supervised rehabilitation program and are no longer using or addicted are offered the protection of a qualified individual with a disability under the ADA.§

Title II of the ADA is designed to prohibit discrimination against disabled individuals by public entities. This title covers the provision of services, programs, activities, and employment by public entities. A public entity under Title II includes:

- A state or local government.
- Any department, agency, special purpose district, or other instrumentality of a state or local government.
- The National Railroad Passenger Corporation (Amtrak), and any commuter authority as this term is defined in section 103(8) of the Rail Passenger Service Act.¶

Although limited in the applicability for public sector safety and health professionals, Title II of the ADA prohibits discrimination in the area of ground transportation, including buses, taxis, trains, and limousines. Air transportation is excluded from the

---

* ADA Section 102(c)(2)(A).
† EEOC Interpretive Guidelines, 56 Fed. Reg. 35,751 (July 26, 1991). Federally mandated periodic examinations include such laws as the Rehabilitation Act, Occupational Safety and Health Act, Federal Coal Mine Health Act, and numerous transportation laws.
‡ ADA Section 102©.
§ ADA Section 511(b).
¶ ADA Section 201(1).

ADA but is covered under the Air Carriers Access Act. Covered organizations may be affected in the purchasing or leasing of new vehicles and in other areas such as the transfer of disabled individuals to the hospital or other facilities. Title II requires covered public entities to make sure that new vehicles are accessible to and usable by the qualified individual, including individuals in wheelchairs. Thus, vehicles must be equipped with lifts, ramps, wheelchair space, and other modifications unless the covered public entity can justify that such equipment is unavailable despite a good faith effort to purchase or acquire this equipment. Covered organizations may want to consider alternative methods to accommodate the qualified individual, such as use of ambulance services or other alternatives.

Title III of the ADA builds upon the foundation establishing by the Architectural Barriers Act and the Rehabilitation Act. This title basically extends the prohibitions that currently exist against the prohibition discrimination to apply to all privately operated public accommodations. Title III focuses on the accommodations in public facilities, including such covered entities as retail stores, law offices, medical facilities, and other public areas. This section requires that goods, services, and facilities of any public place provide "the most integrated setting appropriate to the needs of the (qualified individual with a disability)" except where that individual may pose a direct threat to the safety and health of others that cannot be eliminated through modification of company procedures, practices, or policies. Prohibited discrimination under this section includes prejudice or bias against the individual with a disability in the "full and equal enjoyment" of these services and facilities.[*]

The ADA makes it unlawful for public accommodations not to remove architectural and communication barriers from existing facilities or transportation barriers from vehicles "where such removal is readily achievable."[†] This statutory language is defined as "easily accomplished and able to be carried out without much difficulty or expense,"[‡] for example, moving shelves to widen an aisle, lowering shelves to permit access, etc. The ADA also requires that when a commercial facility or other public accommodation is undergoing a modification that affects the access to a primary function area, specific alterations must be made to afford accessibility to the qualified individual with a disability.

Title III also requires that "auxiliary aids and services" be provided for the qualified individual with a disability including, but not limited to, interpreters, readers, amplifiers, and other devices (not limited or specified under the ADA) to provide that individual with an equal opportunity for employment, promotion, etc.[§] Congress did, however, provide that auxiliary aids and services do not need to be offered to customers, clients, and other members of the public if the auxiliary aid or service creates an undue hardship on the business. Safety and loss prevention professionals may want to consider alternative methods of accommodating the qualified individual with a disability. This section also addresses the modification of existing facilities to provide access to the individual and requires that all new facilities be readily accessible and usable by the individual.

---

[*] ADA Section 302.
[†] ADA Section 302(b)(2)(A)(iv).
[‡] ADA Section 301(9).
[§] ADA Section 3(1).

Safety professionals should be aware of **Title IV**; however, there is limited applicability for most private sector safety professionals. Title IV requires all telephone companies to provide a "telecommunications relay service" to aid the hearing and speech impaired individuals. The Federal Communication Commission has issued a regulation requiring the implementation of this requirement by July 26, 1992 and has also established guidelines for compliance. This section also requires that all public service programs and announcements funded with federal monies be equipped with closed caption for the hearing impaired.[*]

Safety professionals should be aware that Title V assures that the ADA does not limit or invalidate other federal or state laws that provide equal or greater protection for the rights of individuals with disabilities. Thus, safety and health professionals should also be aware of any individual state laws or regulations addressing the same or similar areas as the ADA.

When enacting the ADA, safety professionals should be aware that Congress expressed its concern that sexual preferences could be perceived as a protected characteristic under the ADA or that the courts could expand ADA's coverage beyond Congress's intent. Accordingly, Congress included section 511(b), which contains an expansive list of conditions that are not to be considered within the ADA's definition of disability. This list includes individuals such as transvestites, homosexuals, and bisexuals. Additionally, the conditions of transsexualism; pedophilia; exhibitionism; voyeurism; gender identity disorders not resulting from physical impairment; and other sexual behavior disorders are not considered as a qualified disability under the ADA. Compulsive gambling, kleptomania, pyromania, and psychoactive substance use disorders (from current illegal drug use) are also not afforded protection under the ADA.[†]

Safety professionals should be aware that all individuals associated with or having a relationship to the qualified individual with a disability are extended protection under this section of the ADA. This inclusion is unlimited in nature, including family members, individuals living together, and an unspecified number of others.[‡] The ADA extends coverage to all "individuals," legal or illegal, documented or undocumented, living within the boundaries of the United States, regardless of their status.[§] Under section 102(b)(4), unlawful discrimination includes "excluding or otherwise denying equal jobs or benefits to a qualified individual because of the known disability of the individual with whom the qualified individual is known to have a relationship or association."[¶] Therefore, the protections afforded under this section are not limited to only familial relationships. There appears to be no limits regarding the kinds of relationships or associations that are afforded protection. Of particular

---

[*] Report of the House Committee on Energy and Commerce on the Americans With Disabilities Act of 1990, H.R. Rep. No. 485, 101st Cong., 2d Sess. (1990) (hereinafter cited as H. Comm. on Energy and Comm. Rep.); H. Comm. on Educ. and Lab. Rep., supra; S. Comm. on Lab. and Hum. Resources Rep.

[†] ADA §§ 511(a), (b); 508. There is some indication that many of the conditions excluded from the disability classification under the ADA may be considered a covered handicap under the Rehabilitation Act. See Rezza v. Dept. of Justice, 46 Fair Empl. Prac. Cas. (BNA) 1336 (E.D. Pa. 1988) (compulsive gambling); Fields v. Lyng, 48 Fair Empl. Prac. Cas. (BNA) 1037 (D. Md. 1988) (kleptomania).

[‡] ADA Sections 102 and 302.

[§] H. Rep. 101-485, Part 2, 51.

[¶] ADA Section 102.

note is the inclusion of unmarried partners of persons with AIDS or other qualified disabilities.[*]

As with the OSH Act, the ADA requires that employers post notices of the pertinent provisions of the ADA in an accessible format in a conspicuous location within the employer's facilities. A prudent safety professional may wish to provide additional notification on job applications and other pertinent documents.[†]

Under the ADA, safety professionals should be aware that it is unlawful for an employer to "discriminate on the basis of disability against a qualified individual with a disability" in all areas, including the following:

- Recruitment, advertising, and job application procedures.
- Hiring, upgrading, promoting, awarding tenure, demotion, transfer, layoff, termination, the right to return from layoff, and rehiring.
- Rate of pay or other forms of compensation and changes in compensation.
- Job assignments, job classifications, organization structures, position descriptions, lines of progression, and seniority lists.
- Leaves of absence, sick leave, or other leaves.
- Fringe benefits available by virtue of employment, whether or not administered by the employer.
- Selection and financial support for training, including apprenticeships, professional meetings, conferences and other related activities, and selection for leave of absence to pursue training.
- Activities sponsored by the employer, including social and recreational programs.
- Any other term, condition, or privilege of employment. [‡]

The EEOC has also noted that it is "unlawful … to participate in a contractual or other arrangement or relationship that has the effect of subjecting the covered entity's own qualified applicant or employee with a disability to discrimination." This prohibition includes referral agencies, labor unions (including collective bargaining agreements), insurance companies and others providing fringe benefits, and organizations providing training and apprenticeships.[§]

Safety professionals should be aware that the ADA has the same enforcement and remedy scheme as Title VII of the Civil Rights Act of 1964, as amended by the Civil Rights Act of 1991. Compensatory and punitive damages (with upper limits) have been added as remedies in cases of intentional discrimination, and there is also a correlative right to a jury trial. Unlike Title VII, there is an exception when there is a good faith effort at reasonable accommodation.[¶]

Safety professionals should be aware that the governing federal agency for the ADA is the EEOC. Enforcement of the ADA is also permitted by the attorney general or by private lawsuit. Remedies under these titles included the ordered modification of a

---

[*] H. Rep. 101-485, Part 2, 61-62, 38-39.
[†] ADA Section 105.
[‡] EEOC Interpretive Guidelines, EEOC, 1994.
[§] Id.
[¶] Civil Rights Act of 1992, Section 102.

facility, and civil penalties of up to $50,000.00 for the first violation and $100,000.00 for any subsequent violations. Section 505 permits reasonable attorney fees and litigation costs for the prevailing party in an ADA action but, under section 513, Congress encourages the use of arbitration to resolve disputes arising under the ADA.*

With the passage of the Civil Rights Act of 1991, the remedies provided under the ADA were modified. Employment discrimination (whether intentional or by practice) that has a discriminatory effect on qualified individuals may include hiring, reinstatement, promotion, back pay, front pay, reasonable accommodation, or other actions that will make an individual "whole." Payment of attorney fees, expert witness fees, and court fees are still permitted, and jury trials also allowed.

Compensatory and punitive damages were also made available if intentional discrimination is found. Damages may be available to compensate for actual monetary losses, future monetary losses, mental anguish, and inconvenience. Punitive damages are also available if an employer acted with malice or reckless indifference. The total amount of punitive and compensatory damages for future monetary loss and emotional injury for each individual is limited and is based upon the size of the employer.

Although safety professionals are not expected to be "ADA experts," it is important that safety professionals possess a grasp of the general requirements of the ADA, as well as issues which may impact the safety and health function. It is important for safety professionals to listen to their employees in order to identify potential ADA issues and acquire the appropriate guidance from human resources, legal counsel or your company's ADA professionals.

Questions

1. Identify and explain a minimum of two areas or issues in which the ADA impacts the safety function.
2. How does an individual qualify for protection under the ADA?
3. What is a "reasonable accommodation"?
4. What are the potential penalties for violation under the ADA?
5. What federal agency is responsible for the enforcement of the ADA?

SELECTED CASE SUMMARY

Case modified for the purposes of this text.
1 F.Supp.2d 635
United States District Court,
N.D. Texas,
Dallas Division.
EQUAL EMPLOYMENT
OPPORTUNITY COMMISSION – Plaintiff

---

* ADA Sections 505 and 513.

v.

EXXON CORPORATION – Defendant.

Civil Action Nos. 3:95–CV–1311–H, 3:95–CV–2537–H.

|

April 10, 1998.

The EEOC sued an oil company, claiming that the company's policy of barring rehabilitated substance abusers from safety-sensitive positions violated the Americans with
Disabilities Act (ADA). The EEOC moved to strike affirmative defenses asserted by the
oil company in its answer. The District Court, Sanders, Senior District Judge, adopting
the findings, conclusions and recommendation of Boyle, United States Magistrate
Judge, held that: (1) the oil company was required to show that rehabilitated abusers
posed a direct threat to the health or safety of others; (2) the EEOC was entitled to
summary judgment as to purported nonsafety concerns motivating the adoption of the
policy; (3) the EEOC was not judicially estopped from challenging the regulation by
the position of the government in earlier litigation involving a large oil spill, in which
the company was criticized for allowing a person with a history of alcohol abuse to
navigate a tanker that ran aground; and (4) the oil company could argue that its refusal
to place rehabilitated substance abusers in safety-sensitive positions was in furtherance of a bona fide occupational requirement only to the extent of claiming that it was
impossible or impracticable to individually assess individuals affected by its policy.

Motions granted in part, denied in part.

A qualification standard may also include a requirement that an individual not
pose a direct threat to the health or safety of other individuals in the workplace....

In order to determine whether an individual poses a direct threat to the health
and safety of other individuals in the workplace, the Committee intends to use the
same standard as articulated by the Supreme Court in *School Board of Nassau
County v. Arline.*While the *Arline* case involved a contagious disease, tuberculosis,
the reasoning in that case is applicable to other circumstances. A person with a
disability must not be excluded, or found to be unqualified, based on stereotypes or
fear. Nor may a decision be based on speculation about the risk of harm to others.
Decisions are not permitted to be based on generalizations about the disability, but
rather must be based on the facts of an individual's case. ... the purpose of creating
the "direct threat" standards, is to eliminate exclusions which are not based on
objective evidence about the individual involved. ***644** H.R.Rep. No. 485, 101st
Cong., 2d Sess., (III), at 45 (1990), reprinted in 1990 U.S.C.C.A.N. at 468. By adopting *Arline's* significant risk standard, this text from legislative history of the ADA
manifests a clear Congressional intent to apply a stringent standard to safety-based
qualification safety standards that tend to screen out the disabled based on specula-
tive risks of harm. This, in turn, supports the position set forth in the EEOC's regulations that when an employer imposes qualification standards bearing on safety
concerns, that the *Arline* generated direct threat test provides the exclusive means
of defense.

Other portions of the legislative history of the ADA suggest that it is safety-based
qualification standards as opposed to other types of qualification standards that are
most susceptible to employer speculation and stereotyping and, thus, most in need of

exacting review. For example, in addressing qualification standards in general, the House Report contains the following statement:

> Under this [ADA] legislation, an employer may still devise physical and other job criteria and tests for a job so long as the criteria or tests are job-related and *consistent with business necessity.* Thus for example, an employer can adopt a physical criterion that an applicant be able to lift 50 pounds, *if that ability is necessary to an individual's ability to perform the essential functions of the job in question.* Or, for example, security concerns may constitute valid job criteria. For example, jewelry stores often employ security officers because of the frequency of "snatch and run" thefts.

Mobility and dexterity may be essential job criteria functions in such jobs....

It is also acceptable to deny employment to an applicant or to fire an employee with a disability on the basis that the individual poses a direct threat to the health or safety of others or poses a direct threat to property. H.R.Rep. No. 485, 101st Cong., 2d Sess., (II), at 56 (1990) reprinted in 1990 U.S.C.C.A.N. 303 (emphasis added).

The House Report advises that job criteria tied to concrete functions of the job – mobility and dexterity for jewelry store security officers are consistent with business necessity if the ability to perform such tasks is necessary to carry out the essential functions of the job. As compared to safety-based qualification standards, determining business necessity under these circumstances appears to be a much more straightforward undertaking because the qualification standard is directly tied to the tasks necessary to do the job. Safety-based qualification standards, on the other hand, are not directly tied to the performance of a concrete function of the job, rather, they are based upon concerns about the *safe* performance of the essential functions of the job. Because these standards are not directly measured against the tasks necessary to complete the job, they are particularly susceptible to employer speculation and stereotyping precisely what the authors of the ADA's legislative history through the adoption of *Arline* sought to prevent. In other words, because safety-based qualification standards are, by their nature, more susceptible to employer speculation than qualification standards directly tied to the essential functions of the job, the direct threat test appears the appropriate standard by which carry out the principles embodied in the legislative history and *Arline.*

In sum, the legislative history of the ADA, by adopting *Arline* and through its discussion of qualification standards in general, supports a finding that the EEOC's construction of the statute is firmly rooted in its.

In determining the purpose behind the creation of the ADA, one need only look to the statute itself. Section 12101(b) of the Act lists its statutory aims. 42 U.S.C.A. § 12101(b). Among the ADA's goals, is to "provide clear, strong, consistent, enforceable standards addressing discrimination against individuals with disabilities." 42 U.S.C.A. § 12101(b)(2). As the driving force behind its stated objectives, the ADA sets out a litany of Congressional findings on the plight ***645** of the disabled in America. Included in the findings is a recognition that the disabled have historically been subjected to stereotypical assumptions and prejudice.

With the foregoing statutory goals and findings as a backdrop, the undersigned finds again that the EEOC's view of safety standards, as set forth in its regulations, constitutes a reasonable interpretation of the Act. Limiting the defense of safety-based qualification standards to the direct threat test is consistent with the aim of the Act to prevent stereotyping and prejudice against the disabled. In sum, because the purpose of the ADA is furthered by the EEOC's construction of the statute regarding safety standards, the Court finds an additional basis upon which to find that the EEOC's view of the ADA is a permissible one.

C. BUSINESS NECESSITY DEFENSE–CONCLUSION

In conclusion, despite the lack of case authority or explicit guidance in the ADA itself, the Court finds that Exxon's business necessity defense is subject to the direct threat standard. As stated above, the statutory scheme of the ADA, its legislative history and stated purpose support a finding that safety-based qualification standards which screen out the disabled can only be justified by meeting the direct threat test. Consequently, Exxon's reliance on potential civil and criminal liability, concerns about the environment and its corporate citizenship will not suffice to justify its policy as a business necessity. 9 Accordingly, this Court recommends that the EEOC's motion for summary judgment be granted in favor of the EEOC as to Exxon's affirmative defenses set forth in paragraphs 14 and 15 of its First Amended Answer to the extent those paragraphs rely on factors other than the direct threat standard.

2. EQUITABLE DEFENSES

The EEOC next seeks to bar Exxon from asserting its equitable defenses of judicial estoppel, unclean hands and ratification. The Court turns first to Exxon's judicial estoppel defense.

A. JUDICIAL ESTOPPEL

The EEOC takes issue with Exxon's judicial estoppel defense contending that it would be inappropriate to apply judicial estoppel in this case because if Exxon prevails on that defense, the EEOC will be estopped from enforcing the ADA as Congress intended. The EEOC argues that the effect of applying judicial estoppel to the Government in this case would be to grant Exxon a "perpetual license to violate the ADA." Further, the EEOC asserts that the case authority demonstrates that it is rarely appropriate to apply estoppel doctrines to the government. Before addressing the merits of this argument, the general principles of judicial estoppel must be reviewed. Judicial estoppel is a common law doctrine by which a party may be estopped from asserting a position in a legal proceeding that is inconsistent with a position previously taken in the same or an earlier proceeding. *Ergo Science, Inc., v. Martin,* 73 F.3d 595, 598 (5th Cir.1996). The judicial estoppel doctrine's purpose is to "to prevent parties from playing fast and loose with the courts to suit the exigencies of self interest." *Brandon v. Interfirst Corp.,* 858 F.2d 266, 268 (5th Cir.1988). Judicial estoppel serves a different purpose than equitable estoppel and therefore, at least one Circuit has held, in some cases, "may apply against the Government when equitable estoppel would not." *United States v. Owens,* 54 F.3d 271, 275 (6th Cir.), *cert. dismissed,* 516 U.S. 983, 116 S.Ct. 492, 133 L.Ed.2d 418 (1995). However, as is the case with equitable estoppel, courts construe the doctrine of judicial estoppel narrowly when applied against the Government.

Although the United States Supreme Court has never applied estoppel against the Government, it has declined to adopt an absolute rule that estoppel may never run against the Government. However, to date, the Supreme Court has reversed every case it has reviewed in which a federal court of appeals has applied estoppel against the Government. The Supreme Court has explained that it is seldom appropriate to apply estoppel doctrines to the Government because [w]hen the Government is unable to enforce the law because the conduct of its agents has given rise to an estoppel, the interest of the citizenry as a whole in obedience to the rule of law is undermined. It is for this reason that it is well settled that the Government may not be estopped on the same terms as any other litigant.

It is recommended that summary judgment be granted in favor of the EEOC as to Exxon's ***649** affirmative defense set forth in paragraphs 25 and 26 of its First Amended Answer to the extent that those paragraphs rely upon the doctrine of judicial estoppel.

B. UNCLEAN HANDS AND RATIFICATION

C

The EEOC also seeks to prevent Exxon from presenting its defenses of unclean hands and ratification. With regard to Exxon's unclean hands defense, specifically set forth in paragraph 26 of its First Amended Answer, the EEOC's states simply that "Exxon has not and cannot prove any fraudulent or dishonest conduct on the part of the Government rendering its hands unclean." These conclusory assertions by the EEOC are not sufficient to establish that they are entitled to summary judgment under Fed.R.Civ.P. 56. Exxon's ratification theory is also pled in paragraph 26 of Exxon's First Amended Answer. However, other than to state its challenge to this theory of defense, the EEOC has failed to provide the Court with any legal basis upon which this defense should be subject to summary judgment. Consequently, the EEOC's motion for summary judgment on the unclean hands and ratification defenses must be denied.

3. BFOQ

Finally, the EEOC challenges Exxon's affirmative defense that its policy is "an implementation of a bona fide occupational qualification." The EEOC takes issue with this defense because, it argues, the ADA does not contain the defense of bona fide occupational qualification ("BFOQ"). Both Title VII and the Age and Discrimination Employment Act of 1967 ("ADEA") contain BFOQ provisions. Under these statutes, the BFOQ provisions permit an employer to discriminate on the basis of "religion, sex, or national origin [or age] in those certain instances where religion, sex, or national origin [or age] is a bona fide occupational qualification reasonably necessary to the normal operation of that particular business or enterprise," The BFOQ provisions of these statutes are narrowly drawn and sparingly applied defenses.

As contrasted with Title VII and the ADEA, the ADA does not contain a BFOQ defense. In urging this defense, Exxon relies upon language used by the undersigned in previous findings suggesting the permissibility of a "BFOQ-type impossibility defense under the ADA". While this Court did suggest the plausibility of a BFOQ type defense under the ADA, it was in the context of a discussion on the validity of Exxon's blanket policy and whether or not Exxon's failure to conduct individualized assessments rendered their policy *per se* unlawful under the ADA. In finding that Exxon's policy was not *per se* invalid, this court relied, in part, on cases under Title VII and the ADEA in which, under the BFOQ provisions of those statutes, blanket policies were found permissible. This Court also relied on cases permitting blanket policies decided under the Rehabilitation Act which contains no BFOQ provision. Id. at 60–61. The Court did not recommend that a BFOQ defense be incorporated into the ADA. Rather, it was the reasoning upon which the courts had relied in the past—under BFOQ and non-BFOQ statutes alike—to uphold blanket policies, that was the focus of the analysis. Based, in part, on these cases, this court found that Exxon's policy was not facially invalid and that the company should be permitted to establish that it was "impossible or impractical" to individually assess each safety-sensitive job applicant.

In sum, the ADA contains no BFOQ provision. Under this Court's and the District Court's previous holdings, Exxon is, however, permitted to attempt to establish that it is impossible or impractical to individually assess individual affected by its policy. To the extent that this defense resembles a BFOQ defense, it is not subject to summary judgment for the reasons stated in this court's and the District Court's previous opinions. However, in all other respects, Exxon's attempt to assert a BFOQ defense under the ADA fails and summary judgment must be granted. Accordingly, to the extent Exxon seeks to assert a BFOQ defense beyond what has been permitted by the District Court with regard to its impossibility defense, this Court recommends that summary judgment be granted as to its defense.

CONCLUSION

In conclusion, this Court recommends that the Plaintiff's Motion to Strike the Defendant's Affirmative Defenses, and the Plaintiff EEOC's Supplemental Brief in Support of its Motion to Strike

Defendant's Affirmative Defenses, filed January 8, 1998, be **GRANTED** in part, and **DENIED** in part, as follows: It is **RECOMMENDED** that summary judgment be granted as to Exxon's affirmative defense of business necessity, set forth in paragraphs 14 and 15 of its First Amended Answer, to the extent those paragraphs rely on factors other than the direct threat standard. It is further **RECOMMENDED** that summary judgment be granted as to Exxon's affirmative defense of judicial estoppel as set forth in paragraphs 25 and 26 of its First Amended Answer. As to Exxon's affirmative defenses of unclean hands and ratification set forth in paragraphs 25 and 26 of its First Amended Answer, it is **RECOMMENDED** that summary judgment be denied. It is further **RECOMMENDED** that summary judgment be granted on Exxon's affirmative defense that its policy is justified as a Exxon's BFOQ as set forth in paragraph 24 of its First Amended Answer.

So Recommended,

Appendix A: Occupational Safety And Health Act Of 1970

Public Law 91-596
84 STAT. 1590
91st Congress, S.2193
December 29, 1970,
as amended through January 1, 2004.*

AN ACT

To assure safe and healthful working conditions for working men and women; by authorizing enforcement of the standards developed under the Act; by assisting and encouraging the States in their efforts to assure safe and healthful working conditions; by providing for research, information, education, and training in the field of occupational safety and health; and for other purposes.

Be it enacted by the Senate and House of Representatives of the United States of America in Congress assembled, **That this Act may be cited as the "Occupational Safety and Health Act of 1970."**

SEC. 2.   CONGRESSIONAL FINDINGS AND PURPOSE

a. The Congress finds that personal injuries and illnesses arising out of work situations impose a substantial burden upon, and are a hindrance to, interstate commerce in terms of lost production, wage loss, medical expenses, and disability compensation payments.

   29 USC 651

b. The Congress declares it to be its purpose and policy, through the exercise of its powers to regulate commerce among the several States and with foreign nations and to provide for the general welfare, to assure so far as possible every working man and woman in the Nation safe and healthful working conditions and to preserve our human resources—

   1. By encouraging employers and employees in their efforts to reduce the number of occupational safety and health hazards at their places of employment, and to stimulate employers and employees to institute new and to perfect existing programs for providing safe and healthful working conditions;

---

* See Historical notes at the end of this document for changes and amendments affecting the OSH Act since its passage in 1970 through January 1, 2004.

2. By providing that employers and employees have separate but dependent responsibilities and rights with respect to achieving safe and healthful working conditions;

3. By authorizing the Secretary of Labor to set mandatory occupational safety and health standards applicable to businesses affecting interstate commerce, and by creating an Occupational Safety and Health Review Commission for carrying out adjudicatory functions under the Act;

4. By building upon advances already made through employer and employee initiative for providing safe and healthful working conditions;

5. By providing for research in the field of occupational safety and health, including the psychological factors involved, and by developing innovative methods, techniques, and approaches for dealing with occupational safety and health problems;

6. By exploring ways to discover latent diseases, establishing causal connections between diseases and work in environmental conditions, and conducting other research relating to health problems, in recognition of the fact that occupational health standards present problems often different from those involved in occupational safety;

7. By providing medical criteria which will assure insofar as practicable that no employee will suffer diminished health, functional capacity, or life expectancy as a result of his work experience;

8. By providing for training programs to increase the number and competence of personnel engaged in the field of occupational safety and health; affecting the OSH Act since its passage in 1970 through January 1, 2004.

9. By providing for the development and promulgation of occupational safety and health standards;

10. By providing an effective enforcement program which shall include a prohibition against giving advance notice of any inspection and sanctions for any individual violating this prohibition;

11. By encouraging the States to assume the fullest responsibility for the administration and enforcement of their occupational safety and health laws by providing grants to the States to assist in identifying their needs and responsibilities in the area of occupational safety and health, to develop plans in accordance with the provisions of this Act, to improve the administration and enforcement of State occupational safety and health laws, and to conduct experimental and demonstration projects in connection therewith;

12. By providing for appropriate reporting procedures with respect to occupational safety and health which procedures will help achieve the objectives of this Act and accurately describe the nature of the occupational safety and health problem;

13. By encouraging joint labor-management efforts to reduce injuries and disease arising out of employment.

SEC. 3.   DEFINITIONS

For the purposes of this Act —
29 USC 652

1. The term "Secretary" means the Secretary of Labor.
2. The term "Commission" means the Occupational Safety and Health Review Commission established under this Act.
3. The term "commerce" means trade, traffic, commerce, transportation, or communication among the several States, or between a State and any place outside thereof, or within the District of Columbia, or a possession of the United States (other than the Trust Territory of the Pacific Islands), or between points in the same State but through a point outside thereof.

   For Trust Territory coverage, including the Northern Mariana Islands, *see Historical notes*
4. The term "person" means one or more individuals, partnerships, associations, corporations, business trusts, legal representatives, or any organized group of persons.
5. The term "employer" means a person engaged in a business affecting commerce who has employees, but does not include the United States (not including the United States Postal Service) or any State or political subdivision of a State.

   Pub. L. 105-241 United States Postal Service is an employer subject to the Act. *See Historical notes.*
6. The term "employee" means an employee of an employer who is employed in a business of his employer which affects commerce.
7. The term "State" includes a State of the United States, the District of Columbia, Puerto Rico, the Virgin Islands, American Samoa, Guam, and the Trust Territory of the Pacific Islands.
8. The term "occupational safety and health standard" means a standard which requires conditions, or the adoption or use of one or more practices, means, methods, operations, or processes, reasonably necessary or appropriate to provide safe or healthful employment and places of employment.
9. The term "national consensus standard" means any occupational safety and health standard or modification thereof which (1), has been adopted and promulgated by a nationally recognized standards-producing organization under procedures whereby it can be determined by the Secretary that persons interested and affected by the scope or provisions of the standard have reached substantial agreement on its adoption, (2) was formulated in a manner which afforded an opportunity for diverse views to be considered and (3) has been designated as such a standard by the Secretary, after consultation with other appropriate Federal agencies.
10. The term "established Federal standard" means any operative occupational safety and health standard established by any agency of the United States and presently in effect, or contained in any Act of Congress in force on the date of enactment of this Act.

11. The term "Committee" means the National Advisory Committee on Occupational Safety and Health established under this Act.
12. The term "Director" means the Director of the National Institute for Occupational Safety and Health.
13. The term "Institute" means the National Institute for Occupational Safety and Health established under this Act.
14. The term "Workmen's Compensation Commission" means the National Commission on State Workmen's Compensation Laws established under this Act.

SEC. 4.   APPLICABILITY OF THIS ACT

a. This Act shall apply with respect to employment performed in a workplace in a State, the District of Columbia, the Commonwealth of Puerto Rico, the Virgin Islands, American Samoa, Guam, the Trust Territory of the Pacific Islands, Wake Island, Outer Continental Shelf Lands defined in the Outer Continental Shelf Lands Act, Johnston Island, and the Canal Zone. The Secretary of the Interior shall, by regulation, provide for judicial enforcement of this Act by the courts established for areas in which there are no United States district courts having jurisdiction.

   29 USC 653

   For Canal Zone and Trust Territory coverage, including the Northern Mariana Islands, *see Historical notes.*

b.
   1. Nothing in this Act shall apply to working conditions of employees with respect to which other Federal agencies, and State agencies acting under Section 274 of the Atomic Energy Act of 1954, as amended (42 U.S.C. 2021), exercise statutory authority to prescribe or enforce standards or regulations affecting occupational safety or health.
   2. The safety and health standards promulgated under the Act of June 30, 1936, commonly known as the Walsh-Healey Act (41 U.S.C. 35 et seq.), the Service Contract Act of 1965 (41 U.S.C. 351 et seq.), Public Law 91-54, Act of August 9, 1969 (40 U.S.C. 333), Public Law 85-742, Act of August 23, 1958 (33 U.S.C. 941), and the National Foundation on Arts and Humanities Act (20 U.S.C. 951 et seq.) are superseded on the effective date of corresponding standards, promulgated under this Act, which are determined by the Secretary to be more effective. Standards issued under the laws listed in this paragraph and in effect on or after the effective date of this Act shall be deemed to be occupational safety and health standards issued under this Act, as well as under such other Acts.
   3. The Secretary shall, within three years after the effective date of this Act, report to the Congress his recommendations for legislation to avoid unnecessary duplication and to achieve coordination between this Act and other Federal laws.

4. Nothing in this Act shall be construed to supersede or in any manner affect any workmen's compensation law or to enlarge or diminish or affect in any other manner the common law or statutory rights, duties, or liabilities of employers and employees under any law with respect to injuries, diseases, or death of employees arising out of, or in the course of, employment.

SEC. 5.   DUTIES

a. Each employer —
1. Shall furnish to each of his employees employment and a place of employment which are free from recognized hazards that are causing or are likely to cause death or serious physical harm to his employees;
    29 USC 654
2. Shall comply with occupational safety and health standards promulgated under this Act.
b. Each employee shall comply with occupational safety and health standards and all rules, regulations, and orders issued pursuant to this Act which are applicable to his own actions and conduct.

6.   OCCUPATIONAL SAFETY AND HEALTH STANDARDS

a. Without regard to Chapter 5 of title 5, United States Code, or to the other subsections of this section, the Secretary shall, as soon as practicable during the period beginning with the effective date of this Act and ending two years after such date, by rule promulgate as an occupational safety or health standard any national consensus standard, and any established Federal standard, unless he determines that the promulgation of such a standard would not result in improved safety or health for specifically designated employees. In the event of conflict among any such standards, the Secretary shall promulgate the standard which assures the greatest protection of the safety or health of the affected employees.
    29 USC 655
b. The Secretary may by rule promulgate, modify, or revoke any occupational safety or health standard in the following manner:
1. Whenever the Secretary, upon the basis of information submitted to him in writing by an interested person, a representative of any organization of employers or employees, a nationally recognized standards-producing organization, the Secretary of Health and Human Services, the National Institute for Occupational Safety and Health, or a State or political subdivision, or on the basis of information developed by the Secretary or otherwise available to him, determines that a rule should be promulgated in order to serve the objectives of this Act, the Secretary may request the recommendations of an advisory committee appointed under Section 7 of this Act. The Secretary shall

provide such an advisory committee with any proposals of his own or of the Secretary of Health and Human Services, together with all pertinent factual information developed by the Secretary or the Secretary of Health and Human Services, or otherwise available, including the results of research, demonstrations, and experiments. An advisory committee shall submit to the Secretary its recommendations regarding the rule to be promulgated within ninety days from the date of its appointment or within such longer or shorter period as may be prescribed by the Secretary, but in no event for a period which is longer than two hundred and seventy days.

2. The Secretary shall publish a proposed rule promulgating, modifying, or revoking an occupational safety or health standard in the Federal Register and shall afford interested persons a period of thirty days after publication to submit written data or comments. Where an advisory committee is appointed and the Secretary determines that a rule should be issued, he shall publish the proposed rule within sixty days after the submission of the advisory committee's recommendations or the expiration of the period prescribed by the Secretary for such submission.

3. On or before the last day of the period provided for the submission of written data or comments under paragraph (2), any interested person may file with the Secretary written objections to the proposed rule, stating the grounds therefor and requesting a public hearing on such objections. Within thirty days after the last day for filing such objections, the Secretary shall publish in the Federal Register a notice specifying the occupational safety or health standard to which objections have been filed and a hearing requested, and specifying a time and place for such hearing.

4. Within sixty days after the expiration of the period provided for the submission of written data or comments under paragraph (2), or within sixty days after the completion of any hearing held under paragraph (3), the Secretary shall issue a rule promulgating, modifying, or revoking an occupational safety or health standard or make a determination that a rule should not be issued. Such a rule may contain a provision delaying its effective date for such period (not in excess of ninety days) as the Secretary determines may be necessary to insure that affected employers and employees will be informed of the existence of the standard and of its terms and that employers affected are given an opportunity to familiarize themselves and their employees with the existence of the requirements of the standard.

5. The Secretary, in promulgating standards dealing with toxic materials or harmful physical agents under this subsection, shall set the standard which most adequately assures, to the extent feasible, on the basis of the best available evidence, that no employee will suffer material impairment of health or functional capacity even if such employee has regular exposure to the hazard dealt with by such standard for the period of his working life. Development of standards under this subsection shall be based

upon research, demonstrations, experiments, and such other information as may be appropriate. In addition to the attainment of the highest degree of health and safety protection for the employee, other considerations shall be the latest available scientific data in the field, the feasibility of the standards, and experience gained under this and other health and safety laws. Whenever practicable, the standard promulgated shall be expressed in terms of objective criteria and of the performance desired.

6.

  A. Any employer may apply to the Secretary for a temporary order granting a variance from a standard or any provision thereof promulgated under this section. Such temporary order shall be granted only if the employer files an application which meets the requirements of clause (B) and establishes that —

    i. He is unable to comply with a standard by its effective date because of unavailability of professional or technical personnel or of materials and equipment needed to come into compliance with the standard or because necessary construction or alteration of facilities cannot be completed by the effective date,

    ii. He is taking all available steps to safeguard his employees against the hazards covered by the standard, and

    iii. He has an effective program for coming into compliance with the standard as quickly as practicable.

      Any temporary order issued under this paragraph shall prescribe the practices, means, methods, operations, and processes which the employer must adopt and use while the order is in effect and state in detail his program for coming into compliance with the standard. Such a temporary order may be granted only after notice to employees and an opportunity for a hearing: *Provided,* That the Secretary may issue one interim order to be effective until a decision is made on the basis of the hearing. No temporary order may be in effect for longer than the period needed by the employer to achieve compliance with the standard or one year, whichever is shorter, except that such an order may be renewed not more that twice (I) so long as the requirements of this paragraph are met and (II) if an application for renewal is filed at least 90 days prior to the expiration date of the order. No interim renewal of an order may remain in effect for longer than 180 days.

  B. An application for temporary order under this paragraph (6) shall contain:

    i. A specification of the standard or portion thereof from which the employer seeks a variance,

    ii. A representation by the employer, supported by representations from qualified persons having firsthand knowledge of the facts represented, that he is unable to comply with the standard or portion thereof and a detailed statement of the reasons therefor,

        iii.   A statement of the steps he has taken and will take (with specific dates) to protect employees against the hazard covered by the standard,

        iv.   A statement of when he expects to be able to comply with the standard and what steps he has taken and what steps he will take (with dates specified) to come into compliance with the standard, and

        v.   A certification that he has informed his employees of the application by giving a copy thereof to their authorized representative, posting a statement giving a summary of the application and specifying where a copy may be examined at the place or places where notices to employees are normally posted, and by other appropriate means.

            A description of how employees have been informed shall be contained in the certification. The information to employees shall also inform them of their right to petition the Secretary for a hearing.

  C. The Secretary is authorized to grant a variance from any standard or portion thereof whenever he determines, or the Secretary of Health and Human Services certifies, that such variance is necessary to permit an employer to participate in an experiment approved by him or the Secretary of Health and Human Services designed to demonstrate or validate new and improved techniques to safeguard the health or safety of workers.

7. Any standard promulgated under this subsection shall prescribe the use of labels or other appropriate forms of warning as are necessary to insure that employees are apprised of all hazards to which they are exposed, relevant symptoms and appropriate emergency treatment, and proper conditions and precautions of safe use or exposure. Where appropriate, such standard shall also prescribe suitable protective equipment and control or technological procedures to be used in connection with such hazards and shall provide for monitoring or measuring employee exposure at such locations and intervals, and in such manner as may be necessary for the protection of employees. In addition, where appropriate, any such standard shall prescribe the type and frequency of medical examinations or other tests which shall be made available, by the employer or at his cost, to employees exposed to such hazards in order to most effectively determine whether the health of such employees is adversely affected by such exposure. In the event such medical examinations are in the nature of research, as determined by the Secretary of Health and Human Services, such examinations may be furnished at the expense of the Secretary of Health and Human Services. The results of such examinations or tests shall be furnished only to the Secretary or the Secretary of Health and Human Services, and, at the request of the employee, to his physician. The Secretary, in consultation with the Secretary of Health and Human Services, may by

rule promulgated pursuant to Section 553 of title 5, United States Code, make appropriate modifications in the foregoing requirements relating to the use of labels or other forms of warning, monitoring or measuring, and medical examinations, as may be warranted by experience, information, or medical or technological developments acquired subsequent to the promulgation of the relevant standard.

8. Whenever a rule promulgated by the Secretary differs substantially from an existing national consensus standard, the Secretary shall, at the same time, publish in the Federal Register a statement of the reasons why the rule as adopted will better effectuate the purposes of this Act than the national consensus standard.

c.

1. The Secretary shall provide, without regard to the requirements of Chapter 5, title 5, Unites States Code, for an emergency temporary standard to take immediate effect upon publication in the Federal Register if he determines —

   A. That employees are exposed to grave danger from exposure to substances or agents determined to be toxic or physically harmful or from new hazards, and

   B. That such emergency standard is necessary to protect employees from such danger.

2. Such standard shall be effective until superseded by a standard promulgated in accordance with the procedures prescribed in paragraph (3) of this subsection.

3. Upon publication of such standard in the Federal Register the Secretary shall commence a proceeding in accordance with Section 6(b) of this Act, and the standard as published shall also serve as a proposed rule for the proceeding. The Secretary shall promulgate a standard under this paragraph no later than six months after publication of the emergency standard as provided in paragraph (2) of this subsection.

d. Any affected employer may apply to the Secretary for a rule or order for a variance from a standard promulgated under this section. Affected employees shall be given notice of each such application and an opportunity to participate in a hearing. The Secretary shall issue such rule or order if he determines on the record, after opportunity for an inspection where appropriate and a hearing, that the proponent of the variance has demonstrated by a preponderance of the evidence that the conditions, practices, means, methods, operations, or processes used or proposed to be used by an employer will provide employment and places of employment to his employees which are as safe and healthful as those which would prevail if he complied with the standard. The rule or order so issued shall prescribe the conditions the employer must maintain, and the practices, means, methods, operations, and processes which he must adopt and utilize to the extent they differ from the standard in question. Such a rule or order may be modified or revoked upon application by an employer, employees, or by the Secretary on his own motion, in the manner prescribed for its issuance under this subsection at any time after six months from its issuance.

e. Whenever the Secretary promulgates any standard, makes any rule, order, or decision, grants any exemption or extension of time, or compromises, mitigates, or settles any penalty assessed under this Act, he shall include a statement of the reasons for such action, which shall be published in the Federal Register.

f. Any person who may be adversely affected by a standard issued under this section may at any time prior to the sixtieth day after such standard is promulgated file a petition challenging the validity of such standard with the United States court of appeals for the circuit wherein such person resides or has his principal place of business, for a judicial review of such standard. A copy of the petition shall be forthwith transmitted by the clerk of the court to the Secretary. The filing of such petition shall not, unless otherwise ordered by the court, operate as a stay of the standard. The determinations of the Secretary shall be conclusive if supported by substantial evidence in the record considered as a whole.

g. In determining the priority for establishing standards under this section, the Secretary shall give due regard to the urgency of the need for mandatory safety and health standards for particular industries, trades, crafts, occupations, businesses, workplaces or work environments. The Secretary shall also give due regard to the recommendations of the Secretary of Health and Human Services regarding the need for mandatory standards in determining the priority for establishing such standards.

SEC. 7.   ADVISORY COMMITTEES; ADMINISTRATION

a.

1. There is hereby established a National Advisory Committee on Occupational Safety and Health consisting of twelve members appointed by the Secretary, four of whom are to be designated by the Secretary of Health and Human Services, without regard to the provisions of title 5, United States Code, governing appointments in the competitive service, and composed of representatives of management, labor, occupational safety and occupational health professions, and of the public. The Secretary shall designate one of the public members as Chairman. The members shall be selected upon the basis of their experience and competence in the field of occupational safety and health.

   29 USC 656

2. The Committee shall advise, consult with, and make recommendations to the Secretary and the Secretary of Health and Human Services on matters relating to the administration of the Act. The Committee shall hold no fewer than two meetings during each calendar year. All meetings of the Committee shall be open to the public and a transcript shall be kept and made available for public inspection.

3. The members of the Committee shall be compensated in accordance with the provisions of Section 3109 of title 5, United States Code.

4. The Secretary shall furnish to the Committee an executive secretary and such secretarial, clerical, and other services as are deemed necessary to the conduct of its business.

b. An advisory committee may be appointed by the Secretary to assist him in his standard-setting functions under Section 6 of this Act. Each such committee shall consist of not more than fifteen members and shall include as a member one or more designees of the Secretary of Health and Human Services, and shall include among its members an equal number of persons qualified by experience and affiliation to present the viewpoint of the employers involved, and of persons similarly qualified to present the viewpoint of the workers involved, as well as one or more representatives of health and safety agencies of the States. An advisory committee may also include such other persons as the Secretary may appoint who are qualified by knowledge and experience to make a useful contribution to the work of such committee, including one or more representatives of professional organizations of technicians or professionals specializing in occupational safety or health, and one or more representatives of nationally recognized standards producing organizations, but the number of persons so appointed to any such advisory committee shall not exceed the number appointed to such committee as representatives of Federal and State agencies. Persons appointed to advisory committees from private life shall be compensated in the same manner as consultants or experts under Section 3109 of title 5, United States Code. The Secretary shall pay to any State which is the employer of a member of such a committee who is a representative of the health or safety agency of that State, reimbursement sufficient to cover the actual cost to the State resulting from such representative's membership on such committee. Any meeting of such committee shall be open to the public and an accurate record shall be kept and made available to the public. No member of such committee (other than representatives of employers and employees) shall have an economic interest in any proposed rule.

c. In carrying out his responsibilities under this Act, the Secretary is authorized to —

1. Use, with the consent of any Federal agency, the services, facilities, and personnel of such agency, with or without reimbursement, and with the consent of any State or political subdivision thereof, accept and use the services, facilities, and personnel of any agency of such State or subdivision with reimbursement; and

2. Employ experts and consultants or organizations thereof as authorized by Section 3109 of title 5, United States Code, except that contracts for such employment may be renewed annually; compensate individuals so employed at rates not in excess of the rate specified at the time of service for grade GS-18 under Section 5332 of title 5, United States Code, including travel time, and allow them while away from their homes or regular places of business, travel expenses (including per diem in lieu of subsistence) as authorized by Section 5703 of title 5, United States

Code, for persons in the Government service employed intermittently, while so employed.

SEC. 8.   INSPECTIONS, INVESTIGATIONS, AND RECORDKEEPING

a. In order to carry out the purposes of this Act, the Secretary, upon presenting appropriate credentials to the owner, operator, or agent in charge, is authorized —

     29 USC 657

  1. To enter without delay and at reasonable times any factory, plant, establishment, construction site, or other area, workplace or environment where work is performed by an employee of an employer; and
  2. To inspect and investigate during regular working hours and at other reasonable times, and within reasonable limits and in a reasonable manner, any such place of employment and all pertinent conditions, structures, machines, apparatus, devices, equipment, and materials therein, and to question privately any such employer, owner, operator, agent or employee.

b. In making his inspections and investigations under this Act the Secretary may require the attendance and testimony of witnesses and the production of evidence under oath. Witnesses shall be paid the same fees and mileage that are paid witnesses in the courts of the United States. In case of a contumacy, failure, or refusal of any person to obey such an order, any district court of the United States or the United States courts of any territory or possession, within the jurisdiction of which such person is found, or resides or transacts business, upon the application by the Secretary, shall have jurisdiction to issue to such person an order requiring such person to appear to produce evidence if, as, and when so ordered, and to give testimony relating to the matter under investigation or in question, and any failure to obey such order of the court may be punished by said court as a contempt thereof.

c.

  1. Each employer shall make, keep and preserve, and make available to the Secretary or the Secretary of Health and Human Services, such records regarding his activities relating to this Act as the Secretary, in cooperation with the Secretary of Health and Human Services, may prescribe by regulation as necessary or appropriate for the enforcement of this Act or for developing information regarding the causes and prevention of occupational accidents and illnesses. In order to carry out the provisions of this paragraph such regulations may include provisions requiring employers to conduct periodic inspections. The Secretary shall also issue regulations requiring that employers, through posting of notices or other appropriate means, keep their employees informed of their protections and obligations under this Act, including the provisions of applicable standards.
  2. The Secretary, in cooperation with the Secretary of Health and Human Services, shall prescribe regulations requiring employers to maintain

accurate records of, and to make periodic reports on, work-related deaths, injuries and illnesses other than minor injuries requiring only first aid treatment and which do not involve medical treatment, loss of consciousness, restriction of work or motion, or transfer to another job.

3. The Secretary, in cooperation with the Secretary of Health and Human Services, shall issue regulations requiring employers to maintain accurate records of employee exposures to potentially toxic materials or harmful physical agents which are required to be monitored or measured under Section 6. Such regulations shall provide employees or their representatives with an opportunity to observe such monitoring or measuring, and to have access to the records thereof. Such regulations shall also make appropriate provision for each employee or former employee to have access to such records as will indicate his own exposure to toxic materials or harmful physical agents. Each employer shall promptly notify any employee who has been or is being exposed to toxic materials or harmful physical agents in concentrations or at levels which exceed those prescribed by an applicable occupational safety and health standard promulgated under Section 6, and shall inform any employee who is being thus exposed of the corrective action being taken.

d. Any information obtained by the Secretary, the Secretary of Health and Human Services, or a State agency under this Act shall be obtained with a minimum burden upon employers, especially those operating small businesses. Unnecessary duplication of efforts in obtaining information shall be reduced to the maximum extent feasible.

e. Subject to regulations issued by the Secretary, a representative of the employer and a representative authorized by his employees shall be given an opportunity to accompany the Secretary or his authorized representative during the physical inspection of any workplace under subsection (a) for the purpose of aiding such inspection. Where there is no authorized employee representative, the Secretary or his authorized representative shall consult with a reasonable number of employees concerning matters of health and safety in the workplace.

f.

1. Any employees or representative of employees who believe that a violation of a safety or health standard exists that threatens physical harm, or that an imminent danger exists, may request an inspection by giving notice to the Secretary or his authorized representative of such violation or danger. Any such notice shall be reduced to writing, shall set forth with reasonable particularity the grounds for the notice, and shall be signed by the employees or representative of employees, and a copy shall be provided the employer or his agent no later than at the time of inspection, except that, upon the request of the person giving such notice, his name and the names of individual employees referred to therein shall not appear in such copy or on any record published, released, or made available pursuant to subsection (g) of this section.

If upon receipt of such notification the Secretary determines there are reasonable grounds to believe that such violation or danger exists, he shall make a special inspection in accordance with the provisions of this section as soon as practicable, to determine if such violation or danger exists. If the Secretary determines there are no reasonable grounds to believe that a violation or danger exists he shall notify the employees or representative of the employees in writing of such determination.

2. Prior to or during any inspection of a workplace, any employees or representative of employees employed in such workplace may notify the Secretary or any representative of the Secretary responsible for conducting the inspection, in writing, of any violation of this Act which they have reason to believe exists in such workplace. The Secretary shall, by regulation, establish procedures for informal review of any refusal by a representative of the Secretary to issue a citation with respect to any such alleged violation and shall furnish the employees or representative of employees requesting such review a written statement of the reasons for the Secretary's final disposition of the case.

g.

1. The Secretary and Secretary of Health and Human Services are authorized to compile, analyze, and publish, either in summary or detailed form, all reports or information obtained under this section.

2. The Secretary and the Secretary of Health and Human Services shall each prescribe such rules and regulations as he may deem necessary to carry out their responsibilities under this Act, including rules and regulations dealing with the inspection of an employer's establishment.

h. The Secretary shall not use the results of enforcement activities, such as the number of citations issued or penalties assessed, to evaluate employees directly involved in enforcement activities under this Act or to impose quotas or goals with regard to the results of such activities.

Pub. L. 105-198 added subsection (h).

SEC. 9.   CITATIONS

a. If, upon inspection or investigation, the Secretary or his authorized representative believes that an employer has violated a requirement of Section 5 of this Act, of any standard, rule or order promulgated pursuant to Section 6 of this Act, or of any regulations prescribed pursuant to this Act, he shall with reasonable promptness issue a citation to the employer. Each citation shall be in writing and shall describe with particularity the nature of the violation, including a reference to the provision of the Act, standard, rule, regulation, or order alleged to have been violated. In addition, the citation shall fix a reasonable time for the abatement of the violation. The Secretary may prescribe procedures for the issuance of a notice in lieu of a citation with respect to de minimis violations which have no direct or immediate relationship to safety or health.

29 USC 658

b. Each citation issued under this section, or a copy or copies thereof, shall be prominently posted, as prescribed in regulations issued by the Secretary, at or near each place a violation referred to in the citation occurred.

c. No citation may be issued under this section after the expiration of six months following the occurrence of any violation.

SEC. 10.   PROCEDURE FOR ENFORCEMENT

a. If, after an inspection or investigation, the Secretary issues a citation under Section 9(a), he shall, within a reasonable time after the termination of such inspection or investigation, notify the employer by certified mail of the penalty, if any, proposed to be assessed under Section 17 and that the employer has fifteen working days within which to notify the Secretary that he wishes to contest the citation or proposed assessment of penalty. If, within fifteen working days from the receipt of the notice issued by the Secretary the employer fails to notify the Secretary that he intends to contest the citation or proposed assessment of penalty, and no notice is filed by any employee or representative of employees under subsection (c) within such time, the citation and the assessment, as proposed, shall be deemed a final order of the Commission and not subject to review by any court or agency.

29 USC 659

b. If the Secretary has reason to believe that an employer has failed to correct a violation for which a citation has been issued within the period permitted for its correction (which period shall not begin to run until the entry of a final order by the Commission in the case of any review proceedings under this section initiated by the employer in good faith and not solely for delay or avoidance of penalties), the Secretary shall notify the employer by certified mail of such failure and of the penalty proposed to be assessed under Section 17 by reason of such failure, and that the employer has fifteen working days within which to notify the Secretary that he wishes to contest the Secretary's notification or the proposed assessment of penalty. If, within fifteen working days from the receipt of notification issued by the Secretary, the employer fails to notify the Secretary that he intends to contest the notification or proposed assessment of penalty, the notification and assessment, as proposed, shall be deemed a final order of the Commission and not subject to review by any court or agency.

c. If an employer notifies the Secretary that he intends to contest a citation issued under Section 9(a) or notification issued under subsection (a) or (b) of this section, or if, within fifteen working days of the issuance of a citation under Section 9(a), any employee or representative of employees files a notice with the Secretary alleging that the period of time fixed in the citation for the abatement of the violation is unreasonable, the Secretary shall immediately advise the Commission of such notification, and the Commission shall afford an opportunity for a hearing (in accordance with Section 554 of title 5, United States Code, but without regard to subsection (a)(3) of such section). The Commission shall thereafter issue an order, based on findings of fact, affirming, modifying, or vacating the Secretary's citation or proposed penalty, or directing other appropriate relief, and such order shall become final thirty days after its issuance. Upon a showing by an employer of a good faith effort to comply with the abatement requirements of a citation, and that abatement has not been completed because of factors beyond his reasonable control, the Secretary, after an opportunity for a hearing as provided in this subsection, shall issue an order affirming or modifying the abatement requirements in such citation. The rules of procedure prescribed by the Commission shall provide affected employees or representatives of affected employees an opportunity to participate as parties to hearings under this subsection.

SEC. 11. JUDICIAL REVIEW

a. Any person adversely affected or aggrieved by an order of the Commission issued under subsection (c) of Section 10 may obtain a review of such order in any United States court of appeals for the circuit in which the violation is alleged to have occurred or where the employer has its principal office, or in the Court of Appeals for the District of Columbia Circuit, by filing in such court within sixty days following the issuance of such order a written petition praying that the order be modified or set aside. A copy of such petition shall be forthwith transmitted by the clerk of the court to the Commission and to the other parties, and thereupon the Commission shall file in the court the record in the proceeding as provided in Section 2112 of title 28, United States Code. Upon such filing, the court shall have jurisdiction of the proceeding and of the question determined therein, and shall have power to grant such temporary relief or restraining order as it deems just and proper, and to make and enter upon the pleadings, testimony, and proceedings set forth in such record a decree affirming, modifying, or setting aside in whole or in part, the order of the Commission and enforcing the same to the extent that such order is affirmed or modified. The commencement of proceedings under this subsection shall not, unless ordered by the court, operate as a stay of the order of the Commission. No objection that has not been urged before the Commission shall be considered by the court, unless the failure or neglect to urge such objection shall be excused because of extraordinary circumstances. The findings of the Commission with respect to questions of fact, if supported by substantial evidence on the record considered as a whole, shall be conclusive. If any party shall apply to the court for leave to adduce additional evidence and shall show to the satisfaction of the court that such additional evidence is material and that there were reasonable grounds for the failure to adduce such evidence in the hearing before the Commission, the court may order such additional evidence to be taken before the Commission and to be made a part of the record. The Commission may modify its findings as to the facts, or make new findings, by reason of additional evidence so taken and filed, and it shall file such modified or new findings, which findings with respect to questions of fact, if supported by substantial evidence on the record considered as a whole, shall be conclusive, and its recommendations, if any, for the modification or setting aside of its original order. Upon the filing of the record with it, the jurisdiction of the court shall be exclusive and its judgment and decree shall be final, except that the same shall be subject to review by the Supreme Court of the United States, as provided in Section 1254 of title 28, United States Code.

> 29 USC 660

b. The Secretary may also obtain review or enforcement of any final order of the Commission by filing a petition for such relief in the United States court of appeals for the circuit in which the alleged violation occurred or in which the employer has its principal office, and the provisions of subsection (a) shall govern such proceedings to the extent applicable. If no petition for review, as provided in subsection (a), is filed within sixty days after service of the Commission's order, the Commission's findings of fact and order shall be conclusive in connection with any petition for enforcement which is filed by the Secretary after the expiration of such sixty-day period. In any such case, as well as in the case of a noncontested citation or notification by the Secretary which has become a final order of the Commission under subsection (a) or (b) of Section 10, the clerk of the court, unless otherwise ordered by the court, shall forthwith enter a decree enforcing the order and shall transmit a copy of such decree to the Secretary and the employer named in the petition. In any contempt proceeding brought to enforce a decree of a court of appeals entered pursuant to this subsection or subsection (a), the court of appeals may assess the penalties provided in Section 17, in addition to invoking any other available remedies.

> Pub. L. 98-620

c.

1. No person shall discharge or in any manner discriminate against any employee because such employee has filed any complaint or instituted or caused to be instituted any proceeding under or related to this Act or has testified or is about to testify in any such proceeding or because of the exercise by such employee on behalf of himself or others of any right afforded by this Act.

2. Any employee who believes that he has been discharged or otherwise discriminated against by any person in violation of this subsection may, within thirty days after such violation occurs, file a complaint with the Secretary alleging such discrimination. Upon receipt of such complaint, the Secretary shall cause such investigation to be made as he deems appropriate. If upon such investigation, the Secretary determines that the provisions of this subsection have been violated, he shall bring an action in any appropriate United States district court against such person. In any such action the United States district courts shall have jurisdiction, for cause shown to restrain violations of paragraph (1) of this subsection and order all appropriate relief including rehiring or reinstatement of the employee to his former position with back pay.

3. Within 90 days of the receipt of a complaint filed under this subsection the Secretary shall notify the complainant of his determination under paragraph 2 of this subsection.

SEC. 12.   THE OCCUPATIONAL SAFETY AND HEALTH REVIEW COMMISSION

a. The Occupational Safety and Health Review Commission is hereby established. The Commission shall be composed of three members who shall be appointed by the President, by and with the advice and consent of the Senate, from among persons who by reason of training, education, or experience are qualified to carry out the functions of the Commission under this Act. The President shall designate one of the members of the Commission to serve as Chairman.

29 USC 661

b. The terms of members of the Commission shall be six years except that
1. The members of the Commission first taking office shall serve, as designated by the President at the time of appointment, one for a term of two years, one for a term of four years, and one for a term of six years, and
2. A vacancy caused by the death, resignation, or removal of a member prior to the expiration of the term for which he was appointed shall be filled only for the remainder of such unexpired term.
   A member of the Commission may be removed by the President for inefficiency, neglect of duty, or malfeasance in office.
c. (Text omitted.)
See notes on omitted text.
d. The principal office of the Commission shall be in the District of Columbia. Whenever the Commission deems that the convenience of the public or of the parties may be promoted, or delay or expense may be minimized, it may hold hearings or conduct other proceedings at any other place.
e. The Chairman shall be responsible on behalf of the Commission for the administrative operations of the Commission and shall appoint such administrative law judges and other employees as he deems necessary to assist in the performance of the Commission's functions and to fix their compensation in accordance with the provisions of Chapter 51 and subchapter III of Chapter 53 of title 5, United States Code, relating to classification and General Schedule pay rates: *Provided,* That assignment, removal and compensation of administrative law judges shall be in accordance with Sections 3105, 3344, 5372, and 7521 of title 5, United States Code.

Pub. L. 95-251

f. For the purpose of carrying out its functions under this Act, two members of the Commission shall constitute a quorum and official action can be taken only on the affirmative vote of at least two members.
g. Every official act of the Commission shall be entered of record, and its hearings and records shall be open to the public. The Commission is

authorized to make such rules as are necessary for the orderly transaction of its proceedings. Unless the Commission has adopted a different rule, its proceedings shall be in accordance with the Federal Rules of Civil Procedure.

h. The Commission may order testimony to be taken by deposition in any proceedings pending before it at any state of such proceeding. Any person may be compelled to appear and depose, and to produce books, papers, or documents, in the same manner as witnesses may be compelled to appear and testify and produce like documentary evidence before the Commission. Witnesses whose depositions are taken under this subsection, and the persons taking such depositions, shall be entitled to the same fees as are paid for like services in the courts of the United States.

i. For the purpose of any proceeding before the Commission, the provisions of Section 11 of the National Labor Relations Act (29 U.S.C. 161) are hereby made applicable to the jurisdiction and powers of the Commission.

j. An administrative law judge appointed by the Commission shall hear, and make a determination upon, any proceeding instituted before the Commission and any motion in connection therewith, assigned to such administrative law judge by the Chairman of the Commission, and shall make a report of any such determination which constitutes his final disposition of the proceedings. The report of the administrative law judge shall become the final order of the Commission within thirty days after such report by the administrative law judge, unless within such period any Commission member has directed that such report shall be reviewed by the Commission.

k. Except as otherwise provided in this Act, the administrative law judges shall be subject to the laws governing employees in the classified civil service, except that appointments shall be made without regard to Section 5108 of title 5, United States Code. Each administrative law judge shall receive compensation at a rate not less than that prescribed for GS-16 under Section 5332 of title 5, United States Code.

SEC. 13. PROCEDURES TO COUNTERACT IMMINENT DANGERS

a. The United States district courts shall have jurisdiction, upon petition of the Secretary, to restrain any conditions or practices in any place of employment which are such that a danger exists which could reasonably be expected to cause death or serious physical harm immediately or before the imminence of such danger can be eliminated through the enforcement procedures otherwise provided by this Act. Any order issued under this section may require such steps to be taken as may be necessary to avoid, correct, or remove such imminent danger and prohibit the employment or presence of any individual in locations or under conditions where such imminent danger exists, except individuals whose presence is necessary to avoid, correct, or remove such imminent danger or to maintain the capacity

of a continuous process operation to resume normal operations without a complete cessation of operations, or where a cessation of operations is necessary, to permit such to be accomplished in a safe and orderly manner.
   29 USC 662

b. Upon the filing of any such petition the district court shall have jurisdiction to grant such injunctive relief or temporary restraining order pending the outcome of an enforcement proceeding pursuant to this Act. The proceeding shall be as provided by Rule 65 of the Federal Rules, Civil Procedure, except that no temporary restraining order issued without notice shall be effective for a period longer than five days.

c. Whenever and as soon as an inspector concludes that conditions or practices described in subsection (a) exist in any place of employment, he shall inform the affected employees and employers of the danger and that he is recommending to the Secretary that relief be sought.

d. If the Secretary arbitrarily or capriciously fails to seek relief under this section, any employee who may be injured by reason of such failure, or the representative of such employees, might bring an action against the Secretary in the United States district court for the district in which the imminent danger is alleged to exist or the employer has its principal office, or for the District of Columbia, for a writ of mandamus to compel the Secretary to seek such an order and for such further relief as may be appropriate.

SEC. 14.   REPRESENTATION IN CIVIL LITIGATION

Except as provided in Section 518(a) of title 28, United States Code, relating to litigation before the Supreme Court, the Solicitor of Labor may appear for and represent the Secretary in any civil litigation brought under this Act but all such litigation shall be subject to the direction and control of the Attorney General.
   29 USC 663

SEC. 15.   CONFIDENTIALITY OF TRADE SECRETS

All information reported to or otherwise obtained by the Secretary or his representative in connection with any inspection or proceeding under this Act which contains or which might reveal a trade secret referred to in Section 1905 of title 18 of the United States Code shall be considered confidential for the purpose of that section, except that such information may be disclosed to other officers or employees concerned with carrying out this Act or when relevant in any proceeding under this Act. In any such proceeding the Secretary, the Commission, or the court shall issue such orders as may be appropriate to protect the confidentiality of trade secrets.
   29 USC 664

16.   VARIATIONS, TOLERANCES, AND EXEMPTIONS

The Secretary, on the record, after notice and opportunity for a hearing may provide such reasonable limitations and may make such rules and regulations allowing reasonable variations, tolerances, and exemptions to and from any or all provisions of this Act as he may find necessary and proper to avoid serious impairment of the national defense. Such action shall not be in effect for more than six months without notification to affected employees and an opportunity being afforded for a hearing.

29 USC 665

SEC. 17. PENALTIES

a. Any employer who willfully or repeatedly violates the requirements of Section 5 of this Act, any standard, rule, or order promulgated pursuant to Section 6 of this Act, or regulations prescribed pursuant to this Act, may be assessed a civil penalty of not more than $70,000 for each violation, but not less than $5,000 for each willful violation.

   29 USC 666

   Pub. L. 101-508 increased the civil penalties in subsections (a)–(d) & (i). *See Historical notes.*

b. Any employer who has received a citation for a serious violation of the requirements of Section 5 of this Act, of any standard, rule, or order promulgated pursuant to Section 6 of this Act, or of any regulations prescribed pursuant to this Act, shall be assessed a civil penalty of up to $7,000 for each such violation.

c. Any employer who has received a citation for a violation of the requirements of Section 5 of this Act, of any standard, rule, or order promulgated pursuant to Section 6 of this Act, or of regulations prescribed pursuant to this Act, and such violation is specifically determined not to be of a serious nature, may be assessed a civil penalty of up to $7,000 for each violation.

d. Any employer who fails to correct a violation for which a citation has been issued under Section 9(a) within the period permitted for its correction (which period shall not begin to run until the date of the final order of the Commission in the case of any review proceeding under Section 10 initiated by the employer in good faith and not solely for delay or avoidance of penalties), may be assessed a civil penalty of not more than $7,000 for each day during which such failure or violation continues.

e. Any employer who willfully violates any standard, rule, or order promulgated pursuant to Section 6 of this Act, or of any regulations prescribed pursuant to this Act, and that violation caused death to any employee, shall, upon conviction, be punished by a fine of not more than $10,000 or by imprisonment for not more than six months, or by both; except that if the conviction is for a violation committed after a first conviction of such person, punishment shall be by a fine of not more than $20,000 or by imprisonment for not more than one year, or by both.

   Pub. L. 98-473 Maximum criminal fines are increased by the Sentencing Reform Act of 1984, 18 USC § 3551 et seq. *See Historical notes.*

f. Any person who gives advance notice of any inspection to be conducted under this Act, without authority from the Secretary or his designees, shall, upon conviction, be punished by a fine of not more than $1,000 or by imprisonment for not more than six months, or by both.

   See historical notes.

g. Whoever knowingly makes any false statement, representation, or certification in any application, record, report, plan, or other document filed or required to be maintained pursuant to this Act shall, upon conviction, be punished by a fine of not more than $10,000, or by imprisonment for not more than six months, or by both.

h.

1. Section 1114 of title 18, United States Code, is hereby amended by striking out "designated by the Secretary of Health and Human Services to conduct investigations, or inspections under the Federal Food, Drug, and Cosmetic Act" and inserting in lieu thereof "or of the Department of Labor assigned to perform investigative, inspection, or law enforcement functions."

2. Notwithstanding the provisions of Sections 1111 and 1114 of title 18, United States Code, whoever, in violation of the provisions of Section 1114 of such title, kills a person while engaged in or on account of the performance of investigative, inspection, or law enforcement functions added to such Section 1114 by paragraph (1) of this subsection, and who would otherwise be subject to the penalty provisions of such Section 1111, shall be punished by imprisonment for any term of years or for life.

i. Any employer who violates any of the posting requirements, as prescribed under the provisions of this Act, shall be assessed a civil penalty of up to $7,000 for each violation.

j. The Commission shall have authority to assess all civil penalties provided in this section, giving due consideration to the appropriateness of the penalty with respect to the size of the business of the employer being charged, the gravity of the violation, the good faith of the employer, and the history of previous violations.

k. For purposes of this section, a serious violation shall be deemed to exist in a place of employment if there is a substantial probability that death or serious physical harm could result from a condition which exists, or from one or more practices, means, methods, operations, or processes which have been adopted or are in use, in such place of employment unless the employer did not, and could not with the exercise of reasonable diligence, know of the presence of the violation.

l. Civil penalties owed under this Act shall be paid to the Secretary for deposit into the Treasury of the United States and shall accrue to the United States and may be recovered in a civil action in the name of the United States brought in the United States district court for the district where the violation is alleged to have occurred or where the employer has its principal office.

SEC. 18.   STATE JURISDICTION AND STATE PLANS

a. Nothing in this Act shall prevent any State agency or court from asserting jurisdiction under State law over any occupational safety or health issue with respect to which no standard is in effect under Section 6.

   29 USC 667

b. Any State which, at any time, desires to assume responsibility for development and enforcement therein of occupational safety and health standards relating to any occupational safety or health issue with respect to which a Federal standard has been promulgated under Section 6 shall submit a State plan for the development of such standards and their enforcement.

c. The Secretary shall approve the plan submitted by a State under subsection (b), or any modification thereof, if such plan in his judgement —

   1. Designates a State agency or agencies as the agency or agencies responsible for administering the plan throughout the State,

   2. Provides for the development and enforcement of safety and health standards relating to one or more safety or health issues, which standards (and the enforcement of which standards) are or will be at least as effective in providing safe and healthful employment and places of employment as the standards promulgated under Section 6 which relate to the same issues, and which standards, when applicable to products which are distributed or used in interstate commerce, are required by compelling local conditions and do not unduly burden interstate commerce,

   3. Provides for a right of entry and inspection of all workplaces subject to the Act which is at least as effective as that provided in Section 8, and includes a prohibition on advance notice of inspections,

   4. Contains satisfactory assurances that such agency or agencies have or will have the legal authority and qualified personnel necessary for the enforcement of such standards,

   5. Gives satisfactory assurances that such State will devote adequate funds to the administration and enforcement of such standards,

   6. Contains satisfactory assurances that such State will, to the extent permitted by its law, establish and maintain an effective and comprehensive occupational safety and health program applicable to all employees of public agencies of the State and its political subdivisions, which program is as effective as the standards contained in an approved plan,

   7. Requires employers in the State to make reports to the Secretary in the same manner and to the same extent as if the plan were not in effect, and

   8. Provides that the State agency will make such reports to the Secretary in such form and containing such information, as the Secretary shall from time to time require.

d. If the Secretary rejects a plan submitted under subsection (b), he shall afford the State submitting the plan due notice and opportunity for a hearing before so doing.

e. After the Secretary approves a State plan submitted under subsection (b), he may, but shall not be required to, exercise his authority under Sections 8, 9, 10, 13, and 17 with respect to comparable standards promulgated under Section 6, for the period specified in the next sentence. The Secretary may exercise the authority referred to above until he determines, on the basis of actual operations under the State plan, that the criteria set forth in subsection (c) are being applied, but he shall not make such determination for at least three years after the plan's approval under subsection (c). Upon making the determination referred to in the preceding sentence, the provisions of Sections 5(a)(2), 8 (except for the purpose of carrying out subsection (f) of this section), 9, 10, 13, and 17, and standards promulgated under Section 6 of this Act, shall not apply with respect to any occupational safety or health issues covered under the plan, but the Secretary may retain jurisdiction under the above provisions in any proceeding commenced under Section 9 or 10 before the date of determination.

f. The Secretary shall, on the basis of reports submitted by the State agency and his own inspections make a continuing evaluation of the manner in which each State having a plan approved under this section is carrying out such plan. Whenever the Secretary finds, after affording due notice and opportunity for a hearing, that in the administration of the State plan there is a failure to comply substantially with any provision of the State plan (or any assurance contained therein), he shall notify the State agency of his withdrawal of approval of such plan and upon receipt of such notice such plan shall cease to be in effect, but the State may retain jurisdiction in any case commenced before the withdrawal of the plan in order to enforce standards under the plan whenever the issues involved do not relate to the reasons for the withdrawal of the plan.

g. The State may obtain a review of a decision of the Secretary withdrawing approval of or rejecting its plan by the United States court of appeals for the circuit in which the State is located by filing in such court within thirty days following receipt of notice of such decision a petition to modify or set aside in whole or in part the action of the Secretary. A copy of such petition shall forthwith be served upon the Secretary, and thereupon the Secretary shall certify and file in the court the record upon which the decision complained of was issued as provided in Section 2112 of title 28, United States Code. Unless the court finds that the Secretary's decision in rejecting a proposed State plan or withdrawing his approval of such a plan is not supported by substantial evidence the court shall affirm the Secretary's decision. The judgment of the court shall be subject to review by the Supreme Court of the United States upon certiorari or certification as provided in Section 1254 of title 28, United States Code.

h. The Secretary may enter into an agreement with a State under which the State will be permitted to continue to enforce one or more occupational health and safety standards in effect in such State until final action is taken by the Secretary with respect to a plan submitted by a State under subsection (b) of this section, or two years from the date of enactment of this Act, whichever is earlier.

SEC. 19.   FEDERAL AGENCY SAFETY PROGRAMS AND RESPONSIBILITIES

a. It shall be the responsibility of the head of each Federal agency (not including the United States Postal Service) to establish and maintain an effective and comprehensive occupational safety and health program which is consistent with the standards promulgated under Section 6. The head of each agency shall (after consultation with representatives of the employees thereof) —
   29 USC 668
   1. Provide safe and healthful places and conditions of employment, consistent with the standards set under Section 6;
        Pub. L. 50-241
   2. Acquire, maintain, and require the use of safety equipment, personal protective equipment, and devices reasonably necessary to protect employees;
   3. Keep adequate records of all occupational accidents and illnesses for proper evaluation and necessary corrective action;
   4. Consult with the Secretary with regard to the adequacy as to form and content of records kept pursuant to subsection (a)(3) of this section; and
   5. Make an annual report to the Secretary with respect to occupational accidents and injuries and the agency's program under this section. Such report shall include any report submitted under Section 7902(e)(2) of title 5, United States Code.
b. The Secretary shall report to the President a summary or digest of reports submitted to him under subsection (a)(5) of this section, together with his evaluations of and recommendations derived from such reports.
        Pub. L. 97-375
c. Section 7902(c)(1) of title 5, United States Code, is amended by inserting after "agencies" the following: "and of labor organizations representing employees."
d. The Secretary shall have access to records and reports kept and filed by Federal agencies pursuant to subsections (a)(3) and (5) of this section unless those records and reports are specifically required by Executive order to be kept secret in the interest of the national defense or foreign policy, in which case the Secretary shall have access to such information as will not jeopardize national defense or foreign policy.

SEC. 20.   RESEARCH AND RELATED ACTIVITIES

a.
   1. The Secretary of Health and Human Services, after consultation with the Secretary and with other appropriate Federal departments or

agencies, shall conduct (directly or by grants or contracts) research, experiments, and demonstrations relating to occupational safety and health, including studies of psychological factors involved, and relating to innovative methods, techniques, and approaches for dealing with occupational safety and health problems.

29 USC 669

2. The Secretary of Health and Human Services shall from time to time consult with the Secretary in order to develop specific plans for such research, demonstrations, and experiments as are necessary to produce criteria, including criteria identifying toxic substances, enabling the Secretary to meet his responsibility for the formulation of safety and health standards under this Act; and the Secretary of Health and Human Services, on the basis of such research, demonstrations, and experiments and any other information available to him, shall develop and publish at least annually such criteria as will effectuate the purposes of this Act.

3. The Secretary of Health and Human Services, on the basis of such research, demonstrations, and experiments, and any other information available to him, shall develop criteria dealing with toxic materials and harmful physical agents and substances which will describe exposure levels that are safe for various periods of employment, including but not limited to the exposure levels at which no employee will suffer impaired health or functional capacities or diminished life expectancy as a result of his work experience.

4. The Secretary of Health and Human Services shall also conduct special research, experiments, and demonstrations relating to occupational safety and health as are necessary to explore new problems, including those created by new technology in occupational safety and health, which may require ameliorative action beyond that which is otherwise provided for in the operating provisions of this Act. The Secretary of Health and Human Services shall also conduct research into the motivational and behavioral factors relating to the field of occupational safety and health.

5. The Secretary of Health and Human Services, in order to comply with his responsibilities under paragraph (2), and in order to develop needed information regarding potentially toxic substances or harmful physical agents, may prescribe regulations requiring employers to measure, record, and make reports on the exposure of employees to substances or physical agents which the Secretary of Health and Human Services reasonably believes may endanger the health or safety of employees. The Secretary of Health and Human Services also is authorized to establish such programs of medical examinations and tests as may be necessary for determining the incidence of occupational illnesses and the susceptibility of employees to such illnesses. Nothing in this or any other provision of this Act shall be deemed to authorize or require medical examination, immunization, or treatment for those who object thereto

on religious grounds, except where such is necessary for the protection of the health or safety of others. Upon the request of any employer who is required to measure and record exposure of employees to substances or physical agents as provided under this subsection, the Secretary of Health and Human Services shall furnish full financial or other assistance to such employer for the purpose of defraying any additional expense incurred by him in carrying out the measuring and recording as provided in this subsection.

6. The Secretary of Health and Human Services shall publish within six months of enactment of this Act and thereafter as needed but at least annually a list of all known toxic substances by generic family or other useful grouping, and the concentrations at which such toxicity is known to occur. He shall determine following a written request by any employer or authorized representative of employees, specifying with reasonable particularity the grounds on which the request is made, whether any substance normally found in the place of employment has potentially toxic effects in such concentrations as used or found; and shall submit such determination both to employers and affected employees as soon as possible. If the Secretary of Health and Human Services determines that any substance is potentially toxic at the concentrations in which it is used or found in a place of employment, and such substance is not covered by an occupational safety or health standard promulgated under Section 6, the Secretary of Health and Human Services shall immediately submit such determination to the Secretary, together with all pertinent criteria.

7. Within two years of enactment of the Act, and annually thereafter the Secretary of Health and Human Services shall conduct and publish industry wide studies of the effect of chronic or low-level exposure to industrial materials, processes, and stresses on the potential for illness, disease, or loss of functional capacity in aging adults.

b. The Secretary of Health and Human Services is authorized to make inspections and question employers and employees as provided in Section 8 of this Act in order to carry out his functions and responsibilities under this section.

c. The Secretary is authorized to enter into contracts, agreements, or other arrangements with appropriate public agencies or private organizations for the purpose of conducting studies relating to his responsibilities under this Act. In carrying out his responsibilities under this subsection, the Secretary shall cooperate with the Secretary of Health and Human Services in order to avoid any duplication of efforts under this section.

d. Information obtained by the Secretary and the Secretary of Health and Human Services under this section shall be disseminated by the Secretary to employers and employees and organizations thereof.

e. The functions of the Secretary of Health and Human Services under this Act shall, to the extent feasible, be delegated to the Director of the National Institute for Occupational Safety and Health established by Section 22 of this Act.

EXPANDED RESEARCH ON WORKER SAFETY AND HEALTH

The Secretary of Health and Human Services (referred to in this section as the "Secretary"), acting through the Director of the National Institute of Occupational Safety and Health, shall enhance and expand research as deemed appropriate on the health and safety of workers who are at risk for bioterrorist threats or attacks in the workplace, including research on the health effects of measures taken to treat or protect such workers for diseases or disorders resulting from a bioterrorist threat or attack. Nothing in this section may be construed as establishing new regulatory authority for the Secretary or the Director to issue or modify any occupational safety and health rule or regulation.

29 USC 669a

Pub. L. 107-188, Title I, § 153 added this text.

SEC. 21. TRAINING AND EMPLOYEE EDUCATION

a. The Secretary of Health and Human Services, after consultation with the Secretary and with other appropriate Federal departments and agencies, shall conduct, directly or by grants or contracts —

   29 USC 670

   1. Education programs to provide an adequate supply of qualified personnel to carry out the purposes of this Act, and
   2. Informational programs on the importance of and proper use of adequate safety and health equipment.

b. The Secretary is also authorized to conduct, directly or by grants or contracts, short-term training of personnel engaged in work related to his responsibilities under this Act.

c. The Secretary, in consultation with the Secretary of Health and Human Services, shall -—

   1. Provide for the establishment and supervision of programs for the education and training of employers and employees in the recognition, avoidance, and prevention of unsafe or unhealthful working conditions in employments covered by this Act, and
   2. Consult with and advise employers and employees, and organizations representing employers and employees as to effective means of preventing occupational injuries and illnesses.

   Pub. L. 105-97, §2 added subsection (d). *See Historical notes.*

d.
   1. The Secretary shall establish and support cooperative agreements with the States under which employers subject to this Act may consult with State personnel with respect to —

      A. The application of occupational safety and health requirements under this Act or under State plans approved under Section 18; and
      B. Voluntary efforts that employers may undertake to establish and maintain safe and healthful employment and places of employment. Such agreements may provide, as a condition of receiving funds

under such agreements, for contributions by States towards meeting the costs of such agreements.

2. Pursuant to such agreements the State shall provide on-site consultation at the employer's worksite to employers who request such assistance. The State may also provide other education and training programs for employers and employees in the State. The State shall ensure that on-site consultations conducted pursuant to such agreements include provision for the participation by employees.

3. Activities under this subsection shall be conducted independently of any enforcement activity. If an employer fails to take immediate action to eliminate employee exposure to an imminent danger identified in a consultation or fails to correct a serious hazard so identified within a reasonable time, a report shall be made to the appropriate enforcement authority for such action as is appropriate.

4. The Secretary shall, by regulation after notice and opportunity for comment, establish rules under which an employer —

   A. Which requests and undergoes an on-site consultative visit provided under this subsection;

   B. Which corrects the hazards that have been identified during the visit within the time frames established by the State and agrees to request a subsequent consultative visit if major changes in working conditions or work processes occur which introduce new hazards in the workplace; and

   C. Which is implementing procedures for regularly identifying and preventing hazards regulated under this Act and maintains appropriate involvement of, and training for, management and non-management employees in achieving safe and healthful working conditions, may be exempt from an inspection (except an inspection requested under Section 8(f) or an inspection to determine the cause of a workplace accident which resulted in the death of one or more employees or hospitalization for three or more employees) for a period of one year from the closing of the consultative visit.

5. A State shall provide worksite consultations under paragraph (2) at the request of an employer. Priority in scheduling such consultations shall be assigned to requests from small businesses which are in higher hazard industries or have the most hazardous conditions at issue in the request.

SEC. 22.   NATIONAL INSTITUTE FOR OCCUPATIONAL SAFETY AND HEALTH

a. It is the purpose of this section to establish a National Institute for Occupational Safety and Health in the Department of Health and Human Services in order to carry out the policy set forth in Section 2 of this Act and to perform the functions of the Secretary of Health and Human Services under Sections 20 and 21 of this Act.

 29 USC 671

b. There is hereby established in the Department of Health and Human Services a National Institute for Occupational Safety and Health. The Institute shall be headed by a Director who shall be appointed by the Secretary of Health and Human Services, and who shall serve for a term of six years unless previously removed by the Secretary of Health and Human Services.

c. The Institute is authorized to —

 1. Develop and establish recommended occupational safety and health standards; and

 2. Perform all functions of the Secretary of Health and Human Services under Sections 20 and 21 of this Act.

d. Upon his own initiative, or upon the request of the Secretary of Health and Human Services, the Director is authorized (1) to conduct such research and experimental programs as he determines are necessary for the development of criteria for new and improved occupational safety and health standards, and (2) after consideration of the results of such research and experimental programs make recommendations concerning new or improved occupational safety and health standards. Any occupational safety and health standard recommended pursuant to this section shall immediately be forwarded to the Secretary of Labor, and to the Secretary of Health and Human Services.

e. In addition to any authority vested in the Institute by other provisions of this section, the Director, in carrying out the functions of the Institute, is authorized to —

 1. Prescribe such regulations as he deems necessary governing the manner in which its functions shall be carried out;

 2. Receive money and other property donated, bequeathed, or devised, without condition or restriction other than that it be used for the purposes of the Institute and to use, sell, or otherwise dispose of such property for the purpose of carrying out its functions;

 3. Receive (and use, sell, or otherwise dispose of, in accordance with paragraph (2)), money and other property donated, bequeathed, or devised to the Institute with a condition or restriction, including a condition that the Institute use other funds of the Institute for the purposes of the gift;

 4. In accordance with the civil service laws, appoint and fix the compensation of such personnel as may be necessary to carry out the provisions of this section;

 5. Obtain the services of experts and consultants in accordance with the provisions of Section 3109 of title 5, United States Code;

 6. Accept and utilize the services of voluntary and noncompensated personnel and reimburse them for travel expenses, including per diem, as authorized by Section 5703 of title 5, United States Code;

 7. Enter into contracts, grants or other arrangements, or modifications thereof to carry out the provisions of this section, and such contracts or

modifications thereof may be entered into without performance or other bonds, and without regard to Section 3709 of the Revised Statutes, as amended (41 U.S.C. 5), or any other provision of law relating to competitive bidding;

8. Make advance, progress, and other payments which the Director deems necessary under this title without regard to the provisions of Section 3324 (a) and (b) of Title 31; and

9. Make other necessary expenditures.
      Pub. L. 97-258

f. The Director shall submit to the Secretary of Health and Human Services, to the President, and to the Congress an annual report of the operations of the Institute under this Act, which shall include a detailed statement of all private and public funds received and expended by it, and such recommendations as he deems appropriate.

g. Lead-Based Paint Activities.
      Pub. L. 102-550 added subsection (g).

1. Training Grant Program.

    A. The Institute, in conjunction with the Administrator of the Environmental Protection Agency, may make grants for the training and education of workers and supervisors who are or may be directly engaged in lead-based paint activities.

    B. Grants referred to in subparagraph (A) shall be awarded to nonprofit organizations (including colleges and universities, joint labor-management trust funds, States, and nonprofit government employee organizations) —

        i. Which are engaged in the training and education of workers and supervisors who are or who may be directly engaged in lead-based paint activities (as defined in Title IV of the Toxic Substances Control Act),

        ii. Which have demonstrated experience in implementing and operating health and safety training and education programs, and

        iii. With a demonstrated ability to reach, and involve in lead-based paint training programs, target populations of individuals who are or will be engaged in lead-based paint activities. Grants under this subsection shall be awarded only to those organizations that fund at least 30 percent of their lead-based paint activities training programs from non-Federal sources, excluding in-kind contributions. Grants may also be made to local governments to carry out such training and education for their employees.

    C. There are authorized to be appropriated, a minimum, $10,000,000 to the Institute for each of the fiscal years 1994 through 1997 to make grants under this paragraph.

2. Evaluation of Programs. The Institute shall conduct periodic and comprehensive assessments of the efficacy of the worker and supervisor training programs developed and offered by those receiving grants under this section. The Director shall prepare reports on the results of

these assessments addressed to the Administrator of the Environmental Protection Agency to include recommendations as may be appropriate for the revision of these programs. The sum of $500,000 is authorized to be appropriated to the Institute for each of the fiscal years 1994 through 1997 to carry out this paragraph.

WORKERS' FAMILY PROTECTION

a. Short title

This section may be cited as the "Workers' Family Protection Act."

29 USC 671a

b. Findings and purpose

1. Findings

Congress finds that—

Pub. L. 102-522, Title II, §209 added this text.

A. Hazardous chemicals and substances that can threaten the health and safety of workers are being transported out of industries on workers' clothing and persons;

B. These chemicals and substances have the potential to pose an additional threat to the health and welfare of workers and their families;

C. Additional information is needed concerning issues related to employee transported contaminant releases; and

D. Additional regulations may be needed to prevent future releases of this type.

2. Purpose

It is the purpose of this section to—

A. Increase understanding and awareness concerning the extent and possible health impacts of the problems and incidents described in paragraph (1);

B. Prevent or mitigate future incidents of home contamination that could adversely affect the health and safety of workers and their families;

C. Clarify regulatory authority for preventing and responding to such incidents; and

D. Assist workers in redressing and responding to such incidents when they occur.

c. Evaluation of employee transported contaminant releases

1. Study

A. In general

Not later than 18 months after October 26, 1992, the Director of the National Institute for Occupational Safety and Health (hereafter in this section referred to as the "Director"), in cooperation with the Secretary of Labor, the Administrator of the Environmental Protection Agency, the Administrator of the Agency for Toxic Substances and Disease Registry, and the heads of other Federal Government agencies as determined to be appropriate by the

Director, shall conduct a study to evaluate the potential for, the prevalence of, and the issues related to the contamination of workers' homes with hazardous chemicals and substances, including infectious agents, transported from the workplaces of such workers.

B. Matters to be evaluated

In conducting the study and evaluation under subparagraph (A), the Director shall—

   i.   Conduct a review of past incidents of home contamination through the utilization of literature and of records concerning past investigations and enforcement actions undertaken by—

       I.   The National Institute for Occupational Safety and Health;

      II.   The Secretary of Labor to enforce the Occupational Safety and Health Act of 1970 (29 U.S.C. 651 et seq.);

    III.   States to enforce occupational safety and health standards in accordance with Section 18 of such Act (29 U.S.C. 667); and

   IV.   Other government agencies (including the Department of Energy and the Environmental Protection Agency), as the Director may determine to be appropriate;

  ii.   Evaluate current statutory, regulatory, and voluntary industrial hygiene or other measures used by small, medium and large employers to prevent or remediate home contamination;

 iii.   Compile a summary of the existing research and case histories conducted on incidents of employee transported contaminant releases, including—

       I.   The effectiveness of workplace housekeeping practices and personal protective equipment in preventing such incidents;

      II.   The health effects, if any, of the resulting exposure on workers and their families;

    III.   The effectiveness of normal house cleaning and laundry procedures for removing hazardous materials and agents from workers' homes and personal clothing;

   IV.   Indoor air quality, as the research concerning such pertains to the fate of chemicals transported from a workplace into the home environment; and

    V.   Methods for differentiating exposure health effects and relative risks associated with specific agents from other sources of exposure inside and outside the home;

  iv.   Identify the role of Federal and State agencies in responding to incidents of home contamination;

   v.   Prepare and submit to the Task Force established under paragraph (2) and to the appropriate committees of Congress, a report concerning the results of the matters studied or evaluated under clauses (i) through (iv); and

    vi. Study home contamination incidents and issues and worker and family protection policies and practices related to the special circumstances of firefighters and prepare and submit to the appropriate committees of Congress a report concerning the findings with respect to such study.

2. Development of investigative strategy

   A. Task Force

    Not later than 12 months after October 26, 1992, the Director shall establish a working group, to be known as the "Workers' Family Protection Task Force." The Task Force shall—

      i. Be composed of not more than 15 individuals to be appointed by the Director from among individuals who are representative of workers, industry, scientists, industrial hygienists, the National Research Council, and government agencies, except that not more than one such individual shall be from each appropriate government agency and the number of individuals appointed to represent industry and workers shall be equal in number;

     ii. Review the report submitted under paragraph (1)(B)(v);

    iii. Determine, with respect to such report, the additional data needs, if any, and the need for additional evaluation of the scientific issues related to and the feasibility of developing such additional data; and

    iv. If additional data are determined by the Task Force to be needed, develop a recommended investigative strategy for use in obtaining such information.

   B. Investigative strategy

      i. Content

        The investigative strategy developed under subparagraph (A)(iv) shall identify data gaps that can and cannot be filled, assumptions and uncertainties associated with various components of such strategy, a timetable for the implementation of such strategy, and methodologies used to gather any required data.

     ii. Peer review

        The Director shall publish the proposed investigative strategy under subparagraph (A)(iv) for public comment and utilize other methods, including technical conferences or seminars, for the purpose of obtaining comments concerning the proposed strategy.

    iii. Final strategy

        After the peer review and public comment is conducted under clause (ii), the Director, in consultation with the heads of other government agencies, shall propose a final strategy for investigating issues related to home contamination that shall be implemented by the National Institute for Occupational Safety and

Health and other Federal agencies for the period of time necessary to enable such agencies to obtain the information identified under subparagraph (A)(iii).

  C. Construction

Nothing in this section shall be construed as precluding any government agency from investigating issues related to home contamination using existing procedures until such time as a final strategy is developed or from taking actions in addition to those proposed in the strategy after its completion.

3. Implementation of investigative strategy

Upon completion of the investigative strategy under subparagraph (B)(iii), each Federal agency or department shall fulfill the role assigned to it by the strategy.

d. Regulations

1. In general

Not later than four years after October 26, 1992, and periodically thereafter, the Secretary of Labor, based on the information developed under subsection (c) of this section and on other information available to the Secretary, shall—

  A. Determine if additional education about, emphasis on, or enforcement of existing regulations or standards is needed and will be sufficient, or if additional regulations or standards are needed with regard to employee transported releases of hazardous materials; and

  B. Prepare and submit to the appropriate committees of Congress a report concerning the result of such determination.

2. Additional regulations or standards If the Secretary of Labor determines that additional regulations or standards are needed under paragraph (1), the Secretary shall promulgate, pursuant to the Secretary's authority under the Occupational Safety and Health Act of 1970 (29 U.S.C. 651 et seq.), such regulations or standards as determined to be appropriate not later than three years after such determination.

e. Authorization of appropriations There are authorized to be appropriated from sums otherwise authorized to be appropriated, for each fiscal year such sums as may be necessary to carry out this section.

SEC. 23. GRANTS TO THE STATES

a. The Secretary is authorized, during the fiscal year ending June 30, 1971, and the two succeeding fiscal years, to make grants to the States which have designated a State agency under Section 18 to assist them —

29 USC 672

1. In identifying their needs and responsibilities in the area of occupational safety and health,

2. In developing State plans under Section 18, or

3. In developing plans for —

    A. Establishing systems for the collection of information concerning the nature and frequency of occupational injuries and diseases;

    B. Increasing the expertise and enforcement capabilities of their personnel engaged in occupational safety and health programs; or

    C. Otherwise improving the administration and enforcement of State occupational safety and health laws, including standards thereunder, consistent with the objectives of this Act.

b. The Secretary is authorized, during the fiscal year ending June 30, 1971, and the two succeeding fiscal years, to make grants to the States for experimental and demonstration projects consistent with the objectives set forth in subsection (a) of this section.

c. The Governor of the State shall designate the appropriate State agency for receipt of any grant made by the Secretary under this section.

d. Any State agency designated by the Governor of the State desiring a grant under this section shall submit an application therefor to the Secretary.

e. The Secretary shall review the application, and shall, after consultation with the Secretary of Health and Human Services, approve or reject such application.

f. The Federal share for each State grant under subsection (a) or (b) of this section may not exceed 90 per centum of the total cost of the application. In the event the Federal share for all States under either such subsection is not the same, the differences among the States shall be established on the basis of objective criteria.

g. The Secretary is authorized to make grants to the States to assist them in administering and enforcing programs for occupational safety and health contained in State plans approved by the Secretary pursuant to Section 18 of this Act. The Federal share for each State grant under this subsection may not exceed 50 per centum of the total cost to the State of such a program. The last sentence of subsection (f) shall be applicable in determining the Federal share under this subsection.

h. Prior to June 30, 1973, the Secretary shall, after consultation with the Secretary of Health and Human Services, transmit a report to the President and to the Congress, describing the experience under the grant programs authorized by this section and making any recommendations he may deem appropriate.

SEC. 24.   STATISTICS

a. In order to further the purposes of this Act, the Secretary, in consultation with the Secretary of Health and Human Services, shall develop and maintain an effective program of collection, compilation, and analysis of occupational safety and health statistics. Such program may cover all employments whether or not subject to any other provisions of this Act but shall not cover employments excluded by Section 4 of the Act. The Secretary shall compile accurate statistics on work injuries and illnesses which shall include all disabling, serious, or significant injuries and illnesses, whether or not involving loss of time from work, other than minor injuries requiring only first aid treatment and which do not involve medical treatment, loss of consciousness, restriction of work or motion, or transfer to another job.

b. To carry out his duties under subsection (a) of this section, the Secretary may —

1. Promote, encourage, or directly engage in programs of studies, information and communication concerning occupational safety and health statistics;

2. Make grants to States or political subdivisions thereof in order to assist them in developing and administering programs dealing with occupational safety and health statistics; and

3. Arrange, through grants or contracts, for the conduct of such research and investigations as give promise of furthering the objectives of this section.

c. The Federal share for each grant under subsection (b) of this section may be up to 50 per centum of the State's total cost.

d. The Secretary may, with the consent of any State or political subdivision thereof, accept and use the services, facilities, and employees of the agencies of such State or political subdivision, with or without reimbursement, in order to assist him in carrying out his functions under this section.

e. On the basis of the records made and kept pursuant to section 8(c) of this Act, employers shall file such reports with the Secretary as he shall prescribe by regulation, as necessary to carry out his functions under this Act.

f. Agreements between the Department of Labor and States pertaining to the collection of occupational safety and health statistics already in effect on the effective date of this Act shall remain in effect until superseded by grants or contracts made under this Act.

SEC. 25.   AUDITS

a. Each recipient of a grant under this Act shall keep such records as the Secretary or the Secretary of Health and Human Services shall prescribe, including records which fully disclose the amount and disposition by such recipient of the proceeds of such grant, the total cost of the project or undertaking in connection with which such grant is made or used, and the amount of that portion of the cost of the project or undertaking supplied by other sources, and such other records as will facilitate an effective audit.
29 USC 674

b. The Secretary or the Secretary of Health and Human Services, and the Comptroller General of the United States, or any of their duly authorized representatives, shall have access for the purpose of audit and examination to any books, documents, papers, and records of the recipients of any grant under this Act that are pertinent to any such grant.

SEC. 26.   ANNUAL REPORT

Within one hundred and twenty days following the convening of each regular session of each Congress, the Secretary and the Secretary of Health and Human Services shall each prepare and submit to the President for transmittal to the Congress a report upon the subject matter of this Act, the progress toward achievement of the purpose of this Act, the needs and requirements in the field of occupational safety and health, and any other relevant information. Such reports shall include information regarding occupational safety and health standards, and criteria for such standards, developed during the preceding year; evaluation of standards and criteria previously developed under this Act, defining areas of emphasis for new criteria and standards; an evaluation of the degree of observance of applicable occupational safety and health standards, and a summary of inspection and enforcement activity undertaken; analysis and evaluation of research activities for which results have been obtained under governmental and nongovernmental sponsorship; an analysis of major occupational diseases; evaluation of available control and measurement technology for hazards for which standards or criteria have been developed during the preceding year; description of cooperative efforts undertaken between Government agencies and other interested parties in the implementation of this Act during the preceding year; a progress report on the development of an adequate supply of trained manpower in the field of occupational safety and health, including estimates of future needs and the efforts being made by Government and others to meet those needs; listing of all toxic substances in industrial usage for which labeling requirements, criteria, or standards have not yet been established; and such recommendations for additional legislation as are deemed necessary to protect the safety and health of the worker and improve the administration of this Act.

29 USC 675 Pub. L. 104-66 §3003 terminated provision relating to transmittal of report to Congress.

SEC. 27.   NATIONAL COMMISSION ON STATE WORKMEN'S COMPENSATION LAWS

(Text omitted.)
29 USC 676

SEC. 28.   ECONOMIC ASSISTANCE TO SMALL BUSINESSES

(Text omitted.)
See notes on omitted text.

SEC. 29.   ADDITIONAL ASSISTANT SECRETARY OF LABOR

(Text omitted.)
See notes on omitted text.

SEC. 30.   ADDITIONAL POSITIONS

(Text omitted.)
See notes on omitted text.

SEC. 31.   EMERGENCY LOCATOR BEACONS

(Text omitted.)
See notes on omitted text.

SEC. 32.   SEPARABILITY

If any provision of this Act, or the application of such provision to any person or circumstance, shall be held invalid, the remainder of this Act, or the application of such provision to persons or circumstances other than those as to which it is held invalid, shall not be affected thereby.

29 USC 677

SEC. 33.   APPROPRIATIONS

There are authorized to be appropriated to carry out this Act for each fiscal year such sums as the Congress shall deem necessary.

29 USC 678

SEC. 34.   EFFECTIVE DATE

This Act shall take effect one hundred and twenty days after the date of its enactment.
Approved December 29, 1970.
As amended through January 1, 2004.

HISTORICAL NOTES

This reprint generally retains the section numbers originally created by Congress in the Occupational Safety and Health (OSH) Act of 1970, Pub. L. 91-596, 84 Stat 1590. This document includes some editorial changes, such as changing the format to make it easier to read, correcting typographical errors, and updating some of the margin notes. Because Congress enacted amendments to the Act since 1970, this version differs from the original version of the OSH Act. It also differs slightly from the version published in the United States Code at 29 U.S.C. 661 *et seq.* For example, this reprint refers to the statute as the "Act" rather than the "chapter."

This reprint reflects the provisions of the OSH Act that are in effect as of January 1, 2004. Citations to Public Laws which made important amendments to the OSH Act since 1970 are set forth in the margins and explanatory notes are included below.

NOTE: Some provisions of the OSH Act may be affected by the enactment of, or amendments to, other statutes. Section 17(h)(1), 29 U.S.C. 666, is an example. The original provision amended Section 1114 of title 18 of the United States Code to include employees of "the Department of Labor assigned to perform investigative, inspection, or law enforcement functions" within the list of persons protected by the provisions to allow prosecution of persons who have killed or attempted to kill an officer or employee of the U.S. government while performing official duties. This reprint sets forth the text of Section 17(h) as enacted in 1970. However, since 1970,

Congress has enacted multiple amendments to 18 U.S.C. 1114. The current version does not specifically include the Department of Labor in a list; rather it states that "Whoever kills or attempts to kill any officer or employee of the United States or of any agency in any branch of the United States Government (including any member of the uniformed services) while such officer or employee is engaged in or on account of the performance of official duties, or any person assisting such an officer or employee in the performance of such duties or on account of that assistance shall be punished…" as provided by the statute. Readers are reminded that the official version of statutes can be found in the current volumes of the United States Code, and more extensive historical notes can be found in the current volumes of the United States Code Annotated.

AMENDMENTS

On January 2, 1974, Section 2(c) of Pub. L. 93-237 replaced the phrase "7(b)(6)" in Section 28(d) of the OSH Act with "7(b)(5)." 87 Stat. 1023. Note: The text of Section 28 (Economic Assistance to Small Business) amended Sections 7(b) and Section 4(c)(1) of the Small Business Act. Because these amendments are no longer current, the text of Section 28 is omitted in this reprint. For the current version, see 15 U.S.C. 636.

In 1977, the U.S. entered into the Panama Canal Treaty of 1977, Sept. 7, 1977, U.S.-Panama, T.I.A.S. 10030, 33 U.S.T. 39. In 1979, Congress enacted implementing legislation. Panama Canal Act of 1979, Pub. L. 96-70, 93 Stat. 452 (1979). Although no corresponding amendment to the OSH Act was enacted, the Canal Zone ceased to exist in 1979. The U.S. continued to manage, operate and facilitate the transit of ships through the Canal under the authority of the Panama Canal Treaty until December 31, 1999, at which time authority over the Canal was transferred to the Republic of Panama.

On March 27, 1978, Pub. L. 95-251, 92 Stat. 183, replaced the term "hearing examiner(s)" with "administrative law judge(s)" in all federal laws, including Sections 12(e), 12(j), and 12(k) of the OSH Act, 29 U.S.C. 661.

On October 13, 1978, Pub. L. 95-454, 92 Stat. 1111, 1221, which redesignated section numbers concerning personnel matters and compensation, resulted in the substitution of Section 5372 of Title 5 for Section 5362 in Section 12(e) of the OSH Act, 29 U.S.C. 661.

On October 17, 1979, Pub. L. 96-88, Title V, Section 509(b), 93 Stat. 668, 695, redesignated references to the Department of Health, Education, and Welfare to the Department of Health and Human Services and redesignated references to the Secretary of Health, Education, and Welfare to the Secretary of Health and Human Services.

On September 13, 1982, Pub. L. 97-258, §4(b), 96 Stat. 877, 1067, effectively substituted "Section 3324(a) and (b) of Title 31" for "Section 3648 of the Revised Statutes, as amended (31 U.S.C. 529)" in Section 22 (e)(8), 29 U.S.C. 671, relating to NIOSH procurement authority.

On December 21, 1982, Pub. L. 97-375, 96 Stat. 1819, deleted the sentence in Section 19(b) of the Act, 29 U.S.C. 668, that directed the President of the

United≈States to transmit annual reports of the activities of federal agencies to the House of Representatives and the Senate.

On October 12, 1984, Pub. L. 98-473, Chapter II, 98 Stat. 1837, 1987, (commonly referred to as the "Sentencing Reform Act of 1984") instituted a classification system for criminal offenses punishable under the United States Code. Under this system, an offense with imprisonment terms of "six months or less but more than thirty days, "such as that found in 29 U.S.C. 666(e) for a willful violation of the OSH Act, is classified as a criminal "Class B misdemeanor." 18 U.S.C. 3559(a)(7).

The criminal code increases the monetary penalties for criminal misdemeanors beyond what is provided for in the OSH Act: a fine for a Class B misdemeanor resulting in death, for example, is not more than $250,000 for an individual, and is not more than $500,000 for an organization. 18 U.S.C. 3571(b)(4), (c)(4). The criminal code also provides for authorized terms of probation for both individuals and organizations. 18 U.S.C. 3551, 3561. The term of imprisonment for individuals is the same as that authorized by the OSH Act. 18 U.S.C. 3581(b)(7).

On November 8, 1984, Pub. L. 98-620, 98 Stat. 3335, deleted the last sentence in Section 11(a) of the Act, 29 U.S.C. 660, that required petitions filed under the subsection to be heard expeditiously.

On November 5, 1990, Pub. L. 101-508, 104 Stat. 1388, amended Section 17 of the Act, 29 U.S.C. 666, by increasing the penalties in Section 17(a) from $10,000 for each violation to "$70,000 for each violation, but not less than $5,000 for each willful violation," and increased the limitation on penalties in Sections (b), (c), (d), and (i) from $1,000 to $7,000.

On October 26, 1992, Pub. L. 102-522, 106 Stat. 3410, 3420, added to Title 29, Section 671a "Workers' Family Protection" to grant authority to the Director of NIOSH to evaluate, investigate and if necessary, for the Secretary of Labor to regulate employee transported releases of hazardous material that result from contamination on the employee's clothing or person and may adversely affect the health and safety of workers and their families. Note: Section 671a was enacted as Section 209 of the Fire Administration Authorization Act of 1992, but it is reprinted here because it is codified within the chapter that comprises the OSH Act.

On October 28, 1992, the Housing and Community Development Act of 1992, Pub. L. 102-550, 106 Stat. 3672, 3924, amended Section 22 of the Act, 29 U.S.C. 671, by adding subsection (g), which requires NIOSH to institute a training grant program for lead-based paint activities.

On July 5, 1994, Section 7(b) of Pub. L. 103-272, 108 Stat. 745, repealed Section 31 of the OSH Act, "Emergency Locator Beacons." Section 1(e) of the same Public Law, however, enacted a modified version of Section 31 of the OSH Act. This provision, titled "Emergency Locator Transmitters," is codified at 49 U.S.C. 44712.

On December 21, 1995, Section 3003 of Pub. L. 104-66, 109 Stat. 707, as amended, effective May 15, 2000, terminated the provisions relating to the transmittal to Congress of reports under Section 26 of the OSH Act. 29 U.S.C. 675.

On July 16, 1998, Pub. L. 105-197, 112 Stat. 638, amended Section 21 of the Act, 29 U.S.C. 670, by adding subsection (d), which required the Secretary to establish a compliance assistance program by which employers can consult with state personnel regarding the application of and compliance with OSHA standards.

On July 16, 1998, Pub. L. 105-198, 112 Stat. 640, amended Section 8 of the Act, 29 U.S.C. 657, by adding subsection (h), which forbids the Secretary to use the results of enforcement activities to evaluate the employees involved in such enforcement or to impose quotas or goals.

On September 29, 1998, Pub. L. 105-241, 112 Stat. 1572, amended Sections 3(5) and 19(a) of the Act, 29 U.S.C. 652 and 668, to include the United States Postal Service as an "employer" subject to OSHA enforcement.

On June 12, 2002, Pub. L. 107-188, Title I, Section 153, 116 Stat. 631, Congress enacted 29 U.S.C. 669a, to expand research on the "health and safety of workers who are at risk for bioterrorist threats or attacks in the workplace."

Jurisdictional Note

Although no corresponding amendments to the OSH Act have been made, OSHA no longer exercises jurisdiction over the entity formerly known as the Trust Territory of the Pacific Islands. The Trust Territory, which consisted of the Former.

Japanese Mandated Islands, was established in 1947 by the Security Council of the United Nations, and administered by the United States. *Trusteeship Agreement for the Former Japanese Mandated Islands,* April 2–July 18, 1947, 61 Stat. 3301, T.I.A.S. 1665, 8 U.N.T.S. 189.

From 1947 to 1994, the people of these islands exercised the right of self-determination conveyed by the Trusteeship four times, resulting in the division of the Trust Territory into four separate entities. Three entities: the Republic of Palau, the Federated States of Micronesia, and the Republic of the Marshall Islands, became "Freely Associated States," to which U.S. Federal Law does not apply. Since the OSH Act is a generally applicable law that applies to Guam, it applies to the Commonwealth of Northern Mariana Islands, which elected to become a "Flag Territory" of the United States. *See Covenant to Establish a Commonwealth of the Northern Mariana Islands in Political Union with the United States of America,* Article V, Section 502(a) as contained in Pub. L. 94-24, 90 Stat. 263 (March 24, 1976)[citations to amendments omitted]; 48 U.S.C. 1801 and note (1976); *see also Saipan Stevedore Co., Inc. v. Director, Office of Workers'Compensation Programs,* 133 F.3d 717, 722 (9th Cir. 1998)(Longshore and Harbor Workers' Compensation Act applies to the Commonwealth of Northern Mariana Islands pursuant to Section 502(a) of the Covenant because the Act has general application to the states and to Guam). For up-to-date information on the legal status of these freely associated states and territories, contact the Office of Insular Affairs of the Department of the Interior. (Web address: http://www.doi.gov/oia/)

Omitted Text. Reasons for textual deletions vary. Some deletions may result from amendments to the OSH Act; others to subsequent amendments to other statutes which the original provisions of the OSH Act may have amended in 1970. In some instances, the original provision of the OSH Act was date-limited and is no longer operative.

The text of Section 12(c), 29 U.S.C. 661, is omitted. Subsection (c) amended Sections 5314 and 5315 of Title 5, United States Code, to add the positions of Chairman and members of the Occupational Safety and Health Review Commission.

The text of Section 27, 29 U.S.C. 676, is omitted. Section 27 listed Congressional findings on workers' compensation and established the National Commission on State Workmen's Compensation Laws, which ceased to exist ninety days after the submission of its final report, which was due no later than July 31, 1972.

The text of Section 28 (Economic Assistance to Small Business) amended Sections 7(b) and Section 4(c)(1) of the Small Business Act to allow for small business loans in order to comply with applicable standards. Because these amendments are no longer current, the text is omitted here. For the current version see 15 U.S.C. 636.

The text of Section 29, (Additional Assistant Secretary of Labor), created an Assistant Secretary for Occupational Safety and Health, and Section 30 (Additional Positions) created additional positions within the Department of Labor and the Occupational Safety and Health Review Commission in order to carry out the provisions of the OSH Act. The text of these sections is omitted here because it no longer reflects the current statutory provisions for staffing and pay. For current provisions, see 29 U.S.C. 553 and 5 U.S.C. 5108 (c).

Section 31 of the original OSH Act amended 49 U.S.C. 1421 by inserting a section entitled "Emergency Locator Beacons." The text of that section is omitted in this reprint because Pub. L. 103-272, 108 Stat.745, (July 5, 1994), repealed the text of Section 31 and enacted a modified version of the provision, entitled "Emergency Locator Transmitters," which is codified at 49 U.S.C. 44712.

Notes on other legislation affecting the administration of the Occupational Safety and Health Act. Sometimes legislation does not directly amend the OSH Act, but does place requirements on the Secretary of Labor either to act or to refrain from acting under the authority of the OSH Act. Included below are some examples of such legislation. Please note that this is not intended to be a comprehensive list.

Standards Promulgation

For example, legislation may require the Secretary to promulgate specific standards pursuant to authority under Section 6 of the OSH Act, 29 U.S.C. 655. Some examples include the following:

Hazardous Waste Operations. Pub. L. 99-499, Title I, Section 126(a)-(f), 100 Stat. 1613 (1986), as amended by Pub. L. 100-202, Section 101(f), Title II, Section 201, 101 Stat. 1329 (1987), required the Secretary of Labor to promulgate standards concerning hazardous waste operations.

Chemical Process Safety Management. Pub. L. 101-549, Title III, Section 304, 104 Stat. 2399 (1990), required the Secretary of Labor, in coordination with the Administrator of the Environmental Protection Agency, to promulgate a chemical process safety standard.

Hazardous Materials. Pub. L. 101-615, Section 29, 104 Stat. 3244 (1990), required the Secretary of Labor, in consultation with the Secretaries of Transportation and Treasury, to issue specific standards concerning the handling of hazardous materials.

Bloodborne Pathogens Standard. Pub. L. 102-170, Title I, Section 100, 105 Stat. 1107 (1991), required the Secretary of Labor to promulgate a final Bloodborne Pathogens standard.

Lead Standard. The Housing and Community Development Act of 1992, Pub. L. 102-550, Title X, Sections 1031 and 1032, 106 Stat. 3672 (1992), required the Secretary of Labor to issue an interim final lead standard.

Extension of Coverage

Sometimes a statute may make some OSH Act provisions applicable to certain entities that are not subject to those provisions by the terms of the OSH Act. For example, the Congressional Accountability Act of 1995, Pub. L. 104-1, 109 Stat. 3, (1995), extended certain OSH Act coverage, such as the duty to comply with Section 5 of the OSH Act, to the Legislative Branch. Among other provisions, this legislation authorizes the General Counsel of the Office of Compliance within the Legislative Branch to exercise the authority granted to the Secretary of Labor in the OSH Act to inspect places of employment and issue a citation or notice to correct the violation found. This statute does not make all the provisions of the OSH Act applicable to the Legislative Branch. Another example is the Medicare Prescription Drug, Improvement, and Modernization Act of 2003, Title IX, Section 947, Pub. L. 108-173, 117 Stat. 2066 (2003), which requires public hospitals not otherwise subject to the OSH Act to comply with OSHA's Bloodborne Pathogens standard, 29 CFR 1910.1030. This statute provides for the imposition and collection of civil money penalties by the Department of Health and Human Services in the event that a hospital fails to comply with OSHA's Bloodborne Pathogens standard.

Program Changes Enacted through Appropriations Legislation

Sometimes an appropriations statute may allow or restrict certain substantive actions by OSHA or the Secretary of Labor. For example, sometimes an appropriations statute may restrict the use of money appropriated to run the Occupational Safety and Health Administration or the Department of Labor. One example of such a restriction, that has been included in OSHA's appropriation for many years, limits the applicability of OSHA requirements with respect to farming operations that employ ten or fewer workers and do not maintain a temporary labor camp. Another example is a restriction that limits OSHA's authority to conduct certain enforcement activity with respect to employers of ten or fewer employees in low hazard industries. See Consolidated Appropriations Act, 2004, Pub. L. 108-199, Div. E ¿ Labor, Health and Human Services, and Education, and Related Agencies Appropriations, 2004, Title I ¿ Department of Labor, 118 Stat. 3 (2004). Sometimes an appropriations statute may allow OSHA to retain some money collected to use for occupational safety and health training or grants. For example, the Consolidated Appropriations Act, 2004, Div. E, Title I, cited above, allows OSHA to retain up to $750,000 of training institute course tuition fees per fiscal year for such uses. For the statutory text of currently applicable appropriations provisions, consult the OSHA appropriations statute for the fiscal year in question.

OSH Act of 1970- Table of Contents

Appendix B: Selected State Laws

ALABAMA

{66.01} LABOR RELATIONS LAWS

Collective Bargaining Rights of Firefighters
  Code of Alabama, Sections 11-43-143 and 11-43-144.
  Right to Work Statue
  Code of Alabama, Section 25-7-30, et seq.
  Code of Alabama, Section 25-7-32.
  Code of Alabama, Section 25-7-34.

{66.02} STRIKES, PICKETING, AND BOYCOTT LAWS

Conspiracy to Interfere with Business
  Code of Alabama, Section 13A-11-122.
  Garner v. Teamsters Union, 346 U.S. 485 (1953).
  Interference with Employment Relationship
  Code of Alabama, Section 27-7-9.

{66.03} MEDIATION AND ARBITRATION LAWS

Code of Alabama, Section 25-7-50.

{66.04} REGULATION OF UNION ACTIVITIES

Code of Alabama, Sections 25-7-1, et seq.

{66.05} REGULATION OF EMPLOYMENT PRACTICES

Jury Duty:
  Code of Alabama, Section 12-16-8.
  Blacklisting:
  Code of Alabama, Section 13A-11-123.
  Resident Workmen Requirements:
  Code of Alabama, Section 39-3-2.

{66.06} Wage and Hour Laws

Child Labor:
Code of Alabama, Section 25-8-5.
Code of Alabama, Sections 25-8-4 and 25-8-2, Sections 25-8-2 and 25-8-11.
Code of Alabama, Sections 25-8-13 and 25-8-14.
Voting
Code of Alabama, Sections 17-23-10 and 17-23-11.
Wage Claims
Code of Alabama, Section 25-3-2.

{66.07} Safety and Health Laws

Code of Alabama, Section 25-1-1.

{66.08} Unemployment Compensation Laws

Code of Alabama, Section 25-4-78.
Code of Alabama, Section 25-4-78.

{66.09} Workers' Compensation Laws

Code of Alabama, Sections 25-5-1, et seq.
Code of Alabama, Section 25-5-51.

{66.10} Employment-at-will Developments

"Independent Consideration" Exception.
Scott v. Lane, 409 S.2d 791 (Ala. 1982).
Peters v. Alabama Power Co., No. 82-248 (Ala. S. Ct. 1931).
Intentional Infliction of Emotional Distress Exception:
Rice v. United Ins. Co. of America, Case No. 83-84 (Ala. S. Ct., 1984).

ALASKA

{67.01} Labor Relations Laws

Public Employment Relations Act.
Section 23.40.070, et seq.
Alaska Statutes, Section 23.40.080.
Alaska Statutes, Section 23.40.70 through 23.40.220.
Teachers Collective Bargaining Rights.
Section 14.20.550, et seq.
Alaska Statutes, Section 14.20.550 through 14.20.610.
Nonright-to-Work Police.
Section 14(b) of the Labor Management Relations Act.

{67.02} Strikes, Picketing, and Boycott Laws

Riots.
Alaska Statutes, Section 11.45.020.
Unlawful Assembly.
Alaska Statutes, Section 11.45.020.

{67.03} Mediation and Arbitration Laws

Alaska Statutes, Section 09.43.010.
Alaska Statutes, Section 09.43.010.

{67.04} Regulation of Union Activities

Alaska Statutes, Section 23.40.20.
Alaska Public Acts, S.B. 123, Section 1 (L.1959).
Alaska Public Acts, S.B. 123, Section 1 (L.1959).

{67.05} Regulation of Employment Practices

Anti-discrimination Laws.
Alaska Statutes, Section 18.80.220.
Polygraph Restrictions.
Alaska Statutes, Section 23.10.37.
False Representations to Procure Employees.
Alaska Statutes, Section 23.10.015.
Equal Pay.
Alaska Statutes, Section 18.80.220.

{67.06} Wage and Hour Laws

Child Labor.
Alaska Statutes, Section 23.10.340.
Alaska Statutes, Section 23.10.350.
Alaska Statutes, Section 23.10.332.
Hourly Rate of Pay.
Alaska Statutes, Section 23.10.065.
Payment of Wages Upon Termination.
Alaska Statutes, Section 23.05.140.
Voting Time.
Alaska Statutes, Section 15.56.100.
Garnishment.
Alaska Statutes, Section 47.23.070 (b).

{67.07} Safety and Health Laws

General Provisions.
Alaska Statutes, Section 18.60.075.

Toxic Substances-Right to know.
Alaska Statutes, Section 18.60.066.
Alaska Statutes, Section 18.60.068.
Alaska Statutes, Section 18.60.067.

{67.08} UNEMPLOYMENT COMPENSATION LAWS

Alaska statutes, Section 23.20.350.

{67.09} WORKERS COMPENSATION LAWS

Alaska Statutes, Section 23.30.005, et seq.
Alaska Statutes, Section 23.30.005, et seq.
Alaska Statutes, Section 23.30.040.

{67.10} EMPLOYMENT-AT-WILL DEVELOPMENTS

Covenant of Good Faith and Dealing Exception.
Mitford v. lasala, 666 p.2d 1000 (Alaska, 1983).
"Permanent Employment" Exception.
Eales v. Tanana valley medical surgical group, Inc., 663 p.2d 958 (Alaska,1983).

ARIZONA

New Law: Minimum Wage
AZ ST § 23-363 Arizona Revised Statutes Annotated Title 23. Labor

{68.01} LABOR RELATIONS LAWS

Collective Bargaining Rights of Agricultural Employees.
Arizona Revised Statutes, Section 23-1381, et seq.
Arizona Revised Statutes, Section 23-1385.
Arizona Revised Statutes, Section 23-1385 and 23-1389.
Right- to-Work Law.
Arizona Revised Statutes, Section 23-1301, et seq.
"Yellow-Dog" Contracts.
Arizona Statutes, Section 23-1342.

{68.02} STRIKES, PICKETING, AND BOYCOTT LAWS

Anti-injunction Statute.
Arizona Revised Statutes, Section 23-1393.
Unlawful Assembly.
Arizona Statutes, Section 13-2902.
Secondary Boycotts.
Arizona Statutes, Section 23-1322.

{68.03} MEDIATION AND ARBITRATION LAWS

Arizona revised Statutes, Section 12-1517 (although such agreements are recognized by the federal labor policy).

{68.04} REGULATION OF UNION ACTIVITIES

Arizona Revised Statutes, Section 44-1453.
  Arizona Revised Statutes, Section16-471.

{68.05} REGULATION OF EMPLOYMENT PRACTICES

Anti-discrimination Laws.
  Arizona Statutes, Section 41-1463.
  Jury Duty.
  Arizona Revised Statutes, Section 21-236.
  Backlisting.
  Arizona Constitution, Article 18, Section 8.
  Employment Under False Pretenses.
  Arizona Revised Statutes, Section 23-201 and 23-202.
  Protection of Employees Political and Voting Freedom.
  Arizona Revised Statutes, Section 16-1012.
  Employee Right of Access to Consumer Reports.
  Arizona Revised Statutes, Section 44-1693.
  National Guard Member Protection.
  Arizona Revised Statutes, Section 26-167 and 26-168.
  Equal Pay.
  Arizona Revised Statutes, Section 23-340 and 23-341.

{68.06} WAGE AND HOUR LAWS

Child Labor.
  Arizona Revised Statutes, Section 23-231 and 23-233.
  Payment of Wages.
  Arizona Revised Statutes, Section 23-351.
  Payment Upon Termination.
  Arizona Revised Statutes, Section 23-353.
  Voting Time.
  Arizona Revised Statutes, Section 16-897.

{68.07} SAFETY AND HEALTH LAWS

Arizona Revised Statutes, Section 23-403 and 23-404.

{68.08} UNEMPLOYMENT COMPENSATION LAWS

Arizona Revised Statutes, Section 23-601, et seq.

See generally Arizona Revised Statutes, Section 23-601, et seq.
See generally Arizona Revised Statutes, Section 23-771 and 23-776.

{68.09} Workers Compensation Laws

Arizona Revised Statutes, Section 23-901, et seq.
Arizona Revised Statutes, Section 23-902.
See, for example, Arizona Revised Statutes, Section 23-1044 through 24-1046.

{68.10} Employment-at-will Developments

Public Policy Exception.
Vermillon u. AAA Pro Moving and storage, Case No. CA-CIV 5297 (Ariz. Ct. of App.,1985).
Implied Contract Exception
Wagenseller u. Scottsdale Memorial Hosp., Case No. 17646-PR (Ariz.S.ct., 1985).

ARKANSAS

{69.01} Labor Relations Laws

Right-to-Work Law.
Arkansas Statutes, Section 81-202.
Collective Bargaining Policy.
Arkansas Statutes, Section 81-201.
See Arkansas Attorney General Opinion No. 77-99.

{69.02} Strike, Picketing, and Boycott Laws

Interference with Lawful Employment.
Arkansas Statutes, Section 81-206.
Interference with Railroad Trains During Picketing.
Arkansas Statutes, Section 81-214.

{69.03} Mediation and Arbitration Laws

Arkansas Statutes, Section 81-107.

{69.04} Regulation of Union Activities

Arkansas Statutes, Section 71-201.

{69.05} Regulation of Employment Practices

Anti-discrimination Laws.
Arkansas Statutes, Section 6-1506 and 81-405

Interference with Employment.
Arkansas Statutes, Section 81-210.
Blacklisting.
Arkansas Statutes, Section 81-211.
Wrongful Discharge.
Arkansas Statutes, Section 81-310.
Jury Service.
Arkansas Statutes, Section 39-103.
Discrimination Against Political and Voting Activates.
Arkansas Statutes, Section 3-1105(0).
Protection of Public Employees.
Arkansas Public Acts, no.46, Section 1 (L.1961).
Arkansas Public Acts, no.406, Section 2 (L.1973).
Medical Examination Payments.
Arkansas Statutes, Section 81-212.
Equal Pay.
Arkansas Statutes, Section 81-624.

{69.06} WAGE AND HOUR LAWS

Child Labor.
Arkansas Statutes, Section 81-701.
Arkansas Statutes, Section 81-702 and 81-703.
Arkansas Statutes, Section 81-708 through 81-711.
Payment of Wages Upon Termination.
Arkansas Statutes, Section 81-308.
Access to Medical Reports.
Arkansas Statutes, Section 81-212.
Voting Time.
Arkansas Statutes, Section 3-1602.
Medical Insurance Continuance.
Arkansas Public Laws, Acts 8115:854(L.1985).

{69.07} SAFETY AND HEALTH LAWS

Arkansas Statutes, Section 81-108.

{69.08} UNEMPLOYMENT COMPENSATION LAWS

Arkansas Statutes, Section 81.1101, et saq.
    See for example: Arkansas Statutes, Section 81-1105, et seq.

{69.09} WORKERS COMPENSATION LAWS

Arkansas Statutes, Section 81-1301, et seq.

{69.10} EMPLOYMENT-AT-WILL DEVELOPMENTS

Public Policy Exception.
Lucas u. brown and root, 736 f.2d 1202(ca-8,1984).
Intentional Infliction of Emotional Distress Exception.
M.b.m.co., Inc. u. counce, 268 ark. 269, 596 s. w.2d 681(1980).

CALIFORNIA

New Law: § 1182.12. **Minimum Wage**; scheduled **Increases**; adjusted **Minimum Wage**; temporary suspension of **Increases**.

{70.01} LABOR RELATIONS LAWS

Collective Bargaining Rights of Public Employees.
California Government code, Section 3502.
California Government code, Section 3502.5.
California Government code, Section 3505.
Collective Bargaining Rights of Agricultural Employees.
See California Labor Code Section 1152, et seq.
California Labor Code Section 1152-1154.
California Labor Code Section 1156, et seq.
California Labor Code Section 1160.
Higher Education Employees Bargaining Rights.
See California Government Code, Section 3560, et seq.
Public School Employees Bargaining Rights.
California Government Code, Section 3540.
See a discussion of the California law regulating the collective bargaining rights
of public employees at {70.01}
Firefighters Bargaining Rights.
California Code, Section 1960, et seq.
Nonright-to-Work Police.
Section 14(b) of the Labor Management Relations Act.
"Yellow-Dog" Contracts.
California Code, Section 920, et seq.

{70.02} STRIKES, PICKETING, AND BOYCOTT LAWS

Striker Replacements and Strikebreakers.
California Labor Code Section 973-974.
California Labor Code Section 1134.
California Labor Code Section 1112-1113.
California Penal Code Section 12590(a)(1).
Jurisdictional Strikes.
California Labor Code Section 1115-1116.

Unlawful Assembly.
California Penal Code Section 407.
Anti-injunction Statutes.
See California civil procedure Code Section 527, et seq.

{70.03} Mediation and Arbitration Laws

Code Section 1280, et seq.

{70.04} Regulation of Union Activities

California business and professions Code, Section 9972.
California business and professions Code, Section 9988.
California Labor Code Section 1010, et seq.
California Labor Code Section 1017.

{70.05} Regulation of Employment Practices

California Government Code, Section 12940, et seq.
California Government Code, Section 12941, et seq.
California Government Code, Section 12940(I).
California Government Code, Section 12943 and 12945.
Protection of Political Freedom.
California Labor Code, Section 1101, et seq.
Registration of Employment Applications.
California Labor Code Section 430, et seq.
Jury Duty.
California Labor Code Section 230.
Sterilization.
California Government Code, Section 12945.5.
Investigative Consumer Reports.
California civil Code, Section 1786.
Arrest Record.
California Labor Code Section 432.7.
Access to Personnel Records.
California Labor Code, Section 1198.5.
Confidentiality of Medical Information.
California civil Code, Section 56.20.
Employment Under False Pretense.
California Labor Code, Section 970.
Polygraph Restrictions.
California Labor Code, Section 432.2.
California Penal Code Section 637.
Protection of Military Personnel.
California Code, Section 394.

California military and veterans Code, Section 394.
Blacklisting, Photographing, and Fingerprinting.
California Labor Code, Section 1051.
Whistle-Blowing Statute.
California Government Code, Section 10545.
Cancer Recovery.
California Government Code, Section 12926.
Alcoholic Rehabilitation.
California Labor Code, Section 1025, et seq.
Medical Examination Payments.
California Labor Code, Section 222.5.
Equal Pay.
California Labor Code, Section 1197.

{70.06} WAGE AND HOUR LAWS

Child Labor.
California Labor Code, Section 1290.
California Labor Code, Section 1308.
Hours of Work.
California Labor Code, Section 552, et seq.
Payment of Wages.
California Labor Code, Section 204-210.
Payment Upon Termination.
California Labor Code, Section 201-203.
Garnishment.
California Labor Code, Section 2929.
Medical Insurance Conversion.
California Health and Safety Code, Section 1373.6.
Voting Time.
California Elections Code, Section 14350.
Anti-reprisal Statute.
California Labor Code, Section 98.6.

{70.07} SAFETY AND HEALTH LAWS

General Provisions.
California Labor Code, Section 6400, et seq.
California Labor Code, Section 6399.7.
Toxic Substances-Right to Know.
California Labor Code, Section 6399, et seq.

{70.08} UNEMPLOYMENT COMPENSATION LAWS

California Unemployment Ins. Code, Section 1, et seq.
California Unemployment Ins. Code, Section 2601, et seq.

{70.09} WORKERS COMPENSATION LAWS

California Labor Code, Section 3201, et seq.
  California Labor Code, Section 132a.

{70.10} EMPLOYMENT-AT-WILL DEVELOPMENTS

Implied Contract Exception.
  Walker v. northern san Diego county hosp. dist.,135 cal. App. 3d 896, 185 Cal.
Rptr. 617 (1982).
  Covenant of Good Faith and Fair Dealing Exception.
  Pugh v. see's candies, Inc., 116 Cal. app. 3d 311, 171 Cal. Rptr. 917 (1981), see also:
cancellier v. federated dept. stores, 672 f. 2d1312 (CA-9, 1982).
    "Independent Consideration" Exception.
    Alvarez v. dart Industries, ins., 55 Cal. App.3d 91, 127 Cal. Rptr. 222(1976).
    Public Policy Exception.
    Tameny v. Atlantic Richfield Co., 27 Cal. 3d 167,610 p.2d 1330, 164 Cal. Rptr.
    839(1980); Petermann v. International Brotherhood of Teamsters, 174 Cal. App. 2d
    184, 344, p.2d 25 (1959); Crossen v. foremost McKesson. Inc., 537 F. Supp.
1067(ND Cal., 1982).

COLORADO

{71.01} LABOR RELATIONS LAWS

Collective Bargaining Laws.
  Colorado Revised Statutes, Section 8-13-101, et seq.
  Colorado Revised Statutes, Section 80-3-106, et seq.
  Nonright-to-Work Policy.
  Section 14(b) of the Labor Management Relations Act.
  "Yellow-Dog" Contracts.
  Colorado Revised Statutes, Section 8-3-108.

{71.02} STRIKES, PICKETING, AND BOYCOTT LAWS

Prohibition of Injunctions to Restrain Strikes.
  Colorado Revised Statutes, Section 8-3-118.
  Interference with Employment.
  Colorado Revised Statutes, Section 8-2-101, et seq.
  Unlawful Assembly.
  Colorado Revised Statutes, Section 18-9-108.
  Secondary Boycotts.
  Colorado Revised Statutes, Section 8-3-108(g).
  Colorado Revised Statutes, Section 8-2-112.
  Striker Replacements.
  Colorado Revised Statutes, Section 12-24-109.
  Colorado Revised Statutes, Section 8-2-104, et seq.

Strikebreakers.
Colorado Revised Statutes, Section 8-2-104.

{71.03} MEDIATION AND ARBITRATION LAWS

Colorado Revised Statutes, Section 8-3-12, et seq.
Colorado Revised Statutes, Section 8-3-113.

{71.04} REGULATION OF UNION ACTIVITIES

Colorado Revised Statutes, Section 7-70-101, et seq.

{71.05} REGULATION OF EMPLOYMENT PRACTICES

Anti-discrimination Laws.
Colorado Revised Statutes, Section 24-34-402.
Colorado Revised Statutes, Section 8-2-116.
Employment Under False Pretenses.
Colorado Revised Statutes, Section 8-2-104, et seq.
Protection of Political Freedom.
Colorado Revised Statutes, Section 1-13-719.
Military Leaves of Absence.
Colorado Revised Statutes, Section 28-3-609, et seq.
Jury Duty.
Colorado Revised Statutes, Section 13-71-118.
Blacklisting.
Colorado Revised Statutes, Section 8-2-111.
Medical Examination Payments.
Colorado Revised Statutes, Section 8-2-118.
Equal Pay.
Colorado Revised Statutes, Section 8-5-101, et seq.

{71.06} WAGE AND HOUR LAWS

Child Labor.
Colorado Revised Statutes, Section 8-12-101, et seq.
Colorado Revised Statutes, Section 8-12-110.
Colorado Revised Statutes, Section 8-12-111 through 8-12-113.
Payment of Wages.
Colorado Revised Statutes, Section 8-4-105 and Section 8-4-106.
Payment Upon Termination.
Colorado Revised Statutes, Section 8-4-104.
Voting Time.
Colorado Revised Statutes, Section 31-10-603.
Garnishments.
Colorado Revised Statutes, Section 5-5-106, et seq.

{71.07} SAFETY AND HEALTH LAWS

Colorado Revised Statutes, Section 8-11-101, et seq.
   Colorado Revised Statutes, Section 8-11-108.

{71.08} UNEMPLOYMENT COMPENSATION LAWS

Colorado Revised Statutes, Section 8-70-103, et seq.
   Colorado Revised Statutes, Section 8-70-101, et seq.

{71.09} WORKERS COMPENSATION LAWS

Colorado Revised Statutes, Section 8-40-101, et seq.

{71.10} EMPLOYMENT-AT-WILL DEVELOPMENTS

See Lampe v. Presbyterian medical center, 41 Colo. App. 465, 590 P.2d 513(1978);
Rawson V. Sears, Roebuck and co., 530 F. Supp. 776 (D. Colo. 1982).
   Brooks v. Trans World Airlines, Inc., 574 F. Supp.805 (D. Colo. 1983).

CONNECTICUT

{72.01} LABOR RELATIONS LAWS

Connecticut Labor Relations Act.
   Connecticut General Statutes, Section 31-101, et seq.
   Connecticut General Statutes, Section 31-101.
   State Employees Bargaining Rights.
   Connecticut General Statutes, Section 5-270, et seq.
   Connecticut General Statutes, Section 5-272.
   Connecticut General Statutes, Section 5-271.
   Municipal Employees Bargaining Rights.
   Connecticut General Statutes, Section 7-467, et seq.
   Teachers Bargaining Rights.
   Connecticut General Statutes, Section 10-153.
   Nonright-to-Work policy
   Section 14(b) of the Labor Management Relations Act.
   "Yellow-Dog" Contracts.
   Connecticut General Statutes, Section 31-90.

{72.02} STRIKES, PICKETING, AND BOYCOTT LAWS

Limitation of Anti-Strike Injunctions.
   Connecticut General Statutes, Section 31-113.
   Unlawful Assembly.
   Connecticut General Statutes, Section 53a-177.

Striker Replacements.
Connecticut General Statutes, Section 31-121.
Strikebreakers.
Connecticut General Statutes, Section 31-121, et seq.
Use of Municipal Police Officers During Strike.
Connecticut Public Acts, No. 77 (L.1981).

{72.03} MEDIATION AND ARBITRATION LAWS

Connecticut General Statutes, Section 52-408, et seq.

{72.04} REGULATION OF UNION ACTIVITIES

Connecticut General Statutes, Section 31-77.

{72.05} REGULATION OF EMPLOYMENT PRACTICES

Anti-discrimination Laws.
Connecticut General Statutes, Section 46a-51, et seq.
Inquiries Regarding Arrest Record.
Connecticut General Statutes, Section 31-51(I).
Employment of Illegal Aliens.
Connecticut General Statutes, Section 31-51(k).
Polygraphs Prohibited.
Connecticut General Statutes, Section 31-51(g).
Electronic Surveillance Forbidden.
Connecticut General Statutes, Section 31-48 (b).
Protection of Political Freedom.
Connecticut General Statutes, Section 9-365.
Jury Duty.
Connecticut General Statutes, Section 51-247(a).
Witness Duty.
Connecticut General Statutes, Section 54-85(b).
Military Leaves of Absence.
Connecticut General Statutes, Section 27-33, et seq.
Access to Personnel Records.
Connecticut General Statutes, Section 31-128a, et seq.
See Connecticut General Statutes, Section 31-128a, et seq.
Whistle-Blowing Statute.
Connecticut Public Acts, No.289 (L.1982).
Blacklisting.
Connecticut General Statutes, Section 31-51.
Plant Closures.
Connecticut Public Acts, No.451 (L.1983).
Equal Pay.
Connecticut General Statutes, Section 31-75.

{72.06} Wage and Hour Laws

Child Labor.
Connecticut General Statutes, Section 10-189 and 10-193.
Hours of Work.
Connecticut General Statutes, Section 31-21.
Payment of Wages.
Connecticut General Statutes, Section 31-71a, et seq.
Payment Upon Termination.
Connecticut General Statutes, Section 31-71c.
Garnishments.
Connecticut Public Laws, No.83-581 (L.1983).
Medical Insurance Conversion
Connecticut General Statutes, Section 38-262(d).

{72.07} Safety and Health Laws

General Provisions.
Connecticut General Statutes, Section 31-370.
Toxic Substances-Right to know.
Connecticut General Statutes, Section 31-40j, et seq.

{72.08} Unemployment Compensation Laws

Connecticut General Statutes, Section 31-222, et seq.

{72.09} Workers Compensation Laws

Connecticut General Statutes, Section 31-275, et seq.
Connecticut General Statutes, Section 31-284.

{72.10} Employment at-will Developments

Violation of Public Policy.
Sheet v. Teddy's frosted foods, Inc., 179 Conn. 472 A.2d 385 (1980).
Covenant of Good Faith and Fair Dealing.
Magnan v. Anaconda Industries, Inc., 37 Conn. Super. 38 (1980).
"Independent Consideration" Exception.
Fisher v. Jackson, 142 Conn. 734,118 A.2d 316 (1955).

DELAWARE

{73.01} Labor Relations Laws

Public Employees Bargaining Rights.
Delaware Code, Sections 19-1301.
Delaware Code, Sections 19-1305 through 19-1308.

School Employees Bargaining Rights.
Delaware Code, Sections 14-4001, et seq.
Delaware Code, Sections 14-4003.
Nonright-to-work policy.
Section 14(b) of the Labor Management Relations Act.

{73.02} STRIKES, PICKETING, AND BOYCOTT LAWS

Unlawful Assembly.
Delaware Code, Sections 11-1302, et seq.
Strikebreakers.
Delaware Code, Sections 19-704.
Delaware Code, Sections 19-703.

{73.03} MEDIATION AND ARBITRATION LAWS

Delaware Public Acts, S.B.No.425 (L.1972).

{73.04} REGULATION OF UNION ACTIVITIES

Delaware Code, Sections 6-3331.
Delaware Code, Sections 6-3305.

{73.05} REGULATION OF EMPLOYMENT PRACTICES

Anti-discrimination Laws.
Delaware Code, Sections 19-711, et seq.
Polygraph Restrictions.
Delaware Code, Sections 19-705.
Protection of Political Freedom.
Delaware Code, Sections 15-5302.
National Guard Members.
Delaware Code, Sections 20-905.
Whistle-Blowing Statute.
Delaware Code, Sections 29-5115.
Access to Personnel Records.
Delaware Public Acts, Chapter 473(L.1984).

{73.06} WAGE AND HOUR LAWS

Delaware Code, Sections 19-512.
Delaware Code, Sections 19-542.
Delaware Code, Sections 19-541.
Payment of Wages.
Delaware Code, Sections 19-1102.

Payment on Termination.
Delaware Code, Sections 19-1103.
Garnishments.
Delaware Code, Sections 1-3509.

{73.07} SAFETY AND HEALTH LAWS

General Provisions.
Delaware Code, Sections 19-106.
Toxic Substances-Right to Know.
Delaware Public Laws, S.B. 436 (L.1984).

{73.08} UNEMPLOYMENT COMPENSATION LAWS

Delaware Code, Sections 19-3301, et seq.

{73.09} WORKERS COMPENSATION LAWS

Delaware Code, Sections 19-2101, et seq.
Delaware Code, Sections 19-2301, et seq.

{73.10} EMPLOYMENT-AT-WILL DEVELOPMENTS

Heideck v. Kent General Hospital, Inc., 446 A.2d 1095 (Del. 1982).

DISTRICT OF COLUMBIA

{74.01} LABOR RELATIONS LAWS

Public Employees Bargaining Rights
D.C. Code, Section 1-618.1, et seq.
D.C. Code, Section 1-618.6.
D.C. Code, Section 1-618.4.
D.C. Code, Section 1-618.5.

{74.02} STRIKES, PICKETING, AND BOYCOTT LAWS

Unlawful Assembly
D.C. Code, Section 22-1107.
Threats of Violence
D.C. Code, Section 22-507.

{74.03} MEDIATION AND ARBITRATION

D.C. Code, Section 16-4301, et seq.

{74.05} Regulation of Employment Practices

Anti-Discrimination Laws.
D.C. Code, Section 1-2512, et seq.
D.C. Code, Section 1-2502(17), 1-2512.
Access to Personnel Records.
D.C. Code, Section 3105.
Polygraph Restrictions.
D.C. Code, Section 36-801, et seq.

{74.06} Wage and Hour Laws

Child Labor.
D.C. Code, Section 36-501.
D.C. Code, Section 36-502.
D.C. Code, Section 36-507, et seq.
Payment of Wages.
D.C. Code, Section 36-102.
Payment Upon Termination.
D.C. Code, Section 36-103.

{74.07} Safety and Health Laws

D.C. Code, Section 36-228.

{74.08} Unemployment Compensation

D.C. Code, Section 46-101, et seq.
D.C. Code, Section 46-110.

{74.09} Workers Compensation Laws

The Longshoremen and Harbor Workers Compensation Act is discussed in Chapter 62.
D.C. Code, Section36-301, et seq.

{74.10} Employment-at-Will Developments

Prouty v. National R.R. Passenger Corp., 572 F.Supp.200 (D. D.C. 1982).
Little v. Evening star Newspaper Co., 120 F.2d 36 (D.C. Cir. 1941).
Kitzmiller v. Washington Post, 115 LRRM 3015 (D.D.C. 1984).

FLORIDA

{75.01} Labor Relations Acts

Employees Sights of Self-Organization.
Florida Statutes, Section 447.03.

Public Employees Bargaining Rights.
Florida Statutes, Section 447.209, et seq.
Florida Statutes, Section 447.501.
See generally Florida Statutes, Section 447.201, et seq.
Right-to-Work Statute.
Florida Revised Constitution Section 6, Art. 1.

{75.02} STRIKES, PICKETING, AND BOYCOTT LAWS

Regulation of Strike Activity.
Florida Statutes, Section 447.09(11) through (13).
Unlawful Assembly
Florida Statutes, Section 870.01, et seq.
Striker Replacements.
Florida Statutes, Section 449.07.

{75.03} MEDIATION AND ARBITRATION LAWS

Florida Statutes, Section 453.01, et seq.
Florida Statutes, Section 682.02.

{75.04} REGULATION OF UNION ACTIVITIES

Florida Statutes, Section 447.01.
Florida Statutes, Section 447.09.
Florida Statutes, Section 506.06.

{75.05} REGULATION OF EMPLOYMENT PRACTICES

Anti-Discrimination Laws.
Florida Statutes, Section 760.01, et seq.
Florida Statutes, Section 448.075.
Jury Duty.
Florida Statutes, Section 40.271.
Employment of Illegal Aliens.
Florida Statutes, Section 448.09.
Protection of Political Freedom.
Florida Statutes, Section 104.081.
Protection of National Guard Members.
Florida Statutes, Section 250.48.
Blacklisting.
Florida Statutes, Section 448.045.
Equal pay.
Florida statutes, Section 448.07.

{75.06} Wage and Hour Laws

Child Labor.
  Florida Statutes, Section 450.021.
  Florida Statutes, Section 450.061.
  Payment of Wages.
  Florida Statutes, Section 532.01.
  Medical Insurance Conversion.
  Florida Statutes, Section 627.6675.

{75.07} Safety and Health Laws

Florida Statutes, Section 440.56.
  Toxic Substances-Right to Know.
  Florida Public Laws, Chapters 84-223(L. 1984).

{75.08} Unemployment Compensation Laws

Florida Statutes, Section 443.011, et seq.

{75.09} Workers Compensation Laws

Florida Statutes, Section 440.01, et seq.
  Florida Statutes, Section 440.205.

{75.10} Employment-at-Will Developments

See, for example: Muller v. Stromberg Carlson Corp., 427 So.2d 266(2d Dist. Ct. Fla. App.1983).
  Public Police Exception.
  Smith v. Piezo Technology, 427 So.2d 182 (Fla. 1983).
  "Independent Consideration" Exception.
  Chatelier v. Robertson, 118 So.2d 241(2d Dist. Ct. Fla. App. 1960).

GEORGIA

{76.01} Firefighters Bargaining Rights

Georgia Public Acts, H.B. 569 (L.1971).
  Right-to-Work Statute.
  Section 34-6-23 of the Georgia code.

{76.02} Strikes, Picketing, and Boycott Laws

Anti-picketing Statute.
  Section 34-6-2 of the Georgia code.

Unlawful Assembly.
Georgia Code Annotated, Section 16-11-30, et seq.
Interference with Employment Right.
Georgia Code Annotated, Section 34-6-4.
Mass Picketing Prohibited.
Georgia Code Annotated, Section 34-6-5.
Prohibition Against Public Employee Strikes.
Georgia Code Annotated, Section 45-19-1, et seq.

{76.03} MEDIATION AND ARBITRATION LAWS

Georgia Code Annotated, Section 9-9-30, et seq.
 Georgia Code Annotated, Section 34-2-6.

{76.04} REGULATION OF UNION ACTIVITIES

Georgia Code Annotated, Section 10-1-451.
 Georgia Code Annotated, Section 34-6-8.

{76.05} REGULATION OF EMPLOYMENT PRACTICES

Anti-discrimination Laws (Public Sector).
 Georgia Code Annotated, Section 45-19-29.
 Georgia Code Annotated, Section 34-1-2.
 Georgia Code Annotated, Section 34-6A-4.
 Unlawful Enticement of Employees.
 Georgia Code Prohibited, Section 60-9904, et seq.
 Forged Letters of Reference Restrictions.
 Georgia Code Annotated, Section 34-10-14.
 Lie Detector Restrictions.
 Georgia Code Annotated, Section 43-36-14.
 Military Leave (Public Employees).
 Georgia Code Annotated, Section 38-2-279.
 Equal Pay.
 Georgia code Annotated, Section 45-19-29.

{76.06} WAGE AND HOUR LAWS

Child Labor.
 See, Georgia Child Labor Regulations, Section 300-7-1, et seq.
 Garnishments.
 Georgia Code forbids, Section 18-4-7.
 Terms of Employment.
 Georgia Code Annotated, Section 34-7-1.
 Voting Time.
 Georgia Code Annotated, Section 21-1-404.

Payment of Wages.
Georgia Code Annotated, Section 34-7-2.

{76.07} SAFETY AND HEALTH LAWS

Georgia Code Annotated, Section 34-2-10.

{76.08} UNEMPLOYMENT COMPENSATION LAWS

Georgia Code Annotated, Section 34-8-1, et seq.

{76.09} WORKER COMPENSATION LAWS

Georgia Code Annotated, Section 34-9-1, et seq.

{76.10} EMPLOYMENT-AT-WILL DEVELOPMENTS

See, for example: Troy v. Interincisal, Inc., 320 S.E.2d 872(Ga. Ct. of App., 1984).
   Nelson v. M and M Products Co., 168 Ga. App. 280, 308 S.E.2d 607 (Ga. Ct. of App., 1983).
   Cox v. Brazo, 303 S.E.2d 71 (Ga. Ct. of App., 1983).
   Beavers v. Johnson, 145 S.E.2d 776 (Ga. Ct. of App., 1965).
   Smith v. Rich's, Inc., 104 Ga.App. 883, 123 S.E.2.d 316(Ga. Ct. of App., 1961).

HAWAII

{77.01} LABOR RELATIONS LAWS

Hawaii Employment Relations Act.
   Hawaii Revised Statutes, Section 377-1, et seq.
   Public Employee's Bargaining Rights
   Hawaii Revised Statutes, Section 89-3.
   Hawaii Revised Statutes, Section 89-7 and 89-8.
   Hawaii Revised Statutes, Section 89-6.
   Hawaii Revised Statutes, Section 89-12.
   Nonright-to-Work Policy
   Section 14(b) of the Labor Management Relations Act.

{77.02} STRIKER, PICKETING, AND BOYCOTT LAWS

Unlawful Assembly.
   Hawaii Revised Statutes, Section 711-1104.
   Picketing of residence or Dwelling.
   Hawaii Revised Statutes, Section 379-A-1.
   Striker Replacements and Strikebreakers.
   Hawaii Revised Statutes, Section 379-3.

Hawaii Revised Statutes, Section 379-2.
Anti-Injunction Laws.
Hawaii Revised Statutes, Section 380-1, et seq.
Interference with Ingress or Egress.
Hawaii Revised Statutes, Section 711-1105.
Restrictions in Stevedore Strikes.
Hawaii Revised Statutes, Section 382-1, et seq.

{77.03} MEDIATION AND ARBITRATION LAWS

Hawaii Public Acts, No. 146 (L.1949).
Hawaii Public Acts, No. 146, Section 4163(L.1949).

{77.04} REGULATION OF UNION ACTIVITIES

Hawaii Revised Statutes, Section 482-4.
Hawaii Revised Statutes, Section 337-14.
Hawaii Revised Statutes, Section 377-10.

{77.05} REGULATION OF EMPLOYMENT PRACTICES

Anti-Discrimination.
Hawaii Revised Statutes, Section 378-1, et seq.
Unlawful Enticement.
Hawaii Public Acts, Chapter 70 (L.1911).
Jury Pay.
Hawaii Revised Statutes, Section 612-25. See also: Sections 95-26 and
79-14.
Polygraph Restrictions.
Hawaii Revised Statutes, Section 378-21.
Witness Appearances.
Hawaii Public Acts, No. 621 (L.1978).
Criminal and Arrest Records (State Employees).
Hawaii Revised Statutes, Section 378-2.
Military Leave.
Hawaii Revised Statutes, Section 79-23.
Hawaii Revised Statutes, Section 121-43.
Equal Pay.
Hawaii Revised Statutes, Section 387-4.

{77.06} WAGE AND HOUR LAWS

Child Labor.
Hawaii Revised Statutes, Section 390-1, et seq.
Voting Time.
Hawaii Revised Statutes, Section 11-95.

Payment of Wages.
Hawaii Revised Statutes, Section 388-2.
Payment Upon Termination.
Hawaii Revised Statutes, Section 388-3(a).
Hawaii Revised Statutes, Section 388-3(b).
Garnishments.
Hawaii Revised Statutes, Section 378-32(1).

{77.07} Safety and Health Laws

General Provisions.
Hawaii Revised Statutes, Section 396-6(a) and (c).
Hawaii Revised Statutes, Section 396-8(e) (1).
Toxic Substances-Right to Know.
Hawaii Revised Statutes, Section 396-7.

{77.08} Unemployment Compensation Laws

Hawaii Revised Statutes, Section 383-1, et seq.

{77.09} Worker Compensation Laws

Hawaii Revised Statutes, Section 386-10, et seq.
Hawaii Revised Statutes, Section 386-1, et seq.
Hawaii Revised Statutes, Section 378-32(2).

{77.10} Employment-at-will Developments

Lim v. Motor Supply Co., 45 Hawaii 111, 364 P.2d 38 (1961).
Public Policy Exception.
Parnar v. Americana Hotels, Inc., 652P.2d 625 (Hawaii, 1982).
Promissory Estoppel Exception.
Ravelo v. County of Hawaii, 66 Hawaii 197, 658 P.2d 883 (1983).

IDAHO

{78.01} Labor Relations Laws

Agricultural Employees Bargaining Rights.
Idaho Code, Section 22-4101, et seq.
Teachers Bargaining Rights.
Idaho Code, Section 33-1271.
Idaho Code, Section 33-1274.
Municipal Employees' and Firefighters' Bargaining Rights.
Idaho Code, Section 44-1801, et seq.
Idaho Code, Section 50-901.

Right-to-Work Statute.
Idaho Code, Section 44-2001, et seq.
"Yellow-Dog."
Idaho Code, Section 44-901.

{78.02} STRIKES, PICKETING, AND BOYCOTT LAWS

Anti-injunction Laws.
Idaho Code, Section 44-701, et seq.
Unlawful Assembly.
Idaho Code, Section 18-6402.
Strikebreakers.
Idaho Code, Section 18-712.

{78.03} MEDIATION AND ARBITRATION LAWS

Idaho Code, Section 44-106.
Idaho Code, Section 7-901, et seq.

{78.04} REGULATION OF UNION ACTIVITIES

Idaho Code, Section 44-601, et seq.

{78.05} REGULATION OF EMPLOYMENT PRACTICES

Anti-Discrimination Laws.
Idaho Code, Section 67-5909, et seq.
Freedom of Political Activities.
Idaho Code, Section 18-2319.
Jury or Witness Duty.
Idaho Code, Section 2-218.
Employment Under False Pretense.
Idaho Code, Section 18-3101.
National Guard Duty.
Idaho Code, Section 46-224.
Polygraph Restrictions.
Idaho Code, Section 44-903.
Equal Pay.
Idaho Code, Section 44-1702.

{78.06} WAGE AND HOUR LAWS

Child Labor.
Idaho Code, Section 44-1301, et seq.
Idaho Code, Section 44-1301.
Idaho Code, Section 44-1302.

Idaho Code, Section 44-1301, et seq.
Payment of Wages.
Idaho Code, Section 45-610.
Payment Upon Termination.
Idaho Code, Section 45-606.
Garnishments.
Idaho Code, Section 28-35-106.

{78.07} SAFETY AND HEALTH LAWS

Idaho Code, Section 44-104.
Idaho Code, Section 72-1101.

{78.08} UNEMPLOYMENT COMPENSATION

Idaho Code, Section 72-1361, et seq.

{78.09} WORKERS COMPENSATION LAWS

Idaho Code, Section 72-101, et seq.

{78.10} EMPLOYMENT-AT-WILL DEVELOPMENTS

Implied Contract Exception.
MacNeil v. Minidoka memorial Hospital, 701 P. 2d 208 (Idaho S. Ct., 1985).
Fraud.
Verway v. Blinkcoe packing Co., Case No. 15189 (Idaho Ct. of App., 1985).

ILLINOIS

New Law (HB 3554/ PA 99-0762). Amends Illinois Wage and Collection Act.

{79.01} LABOR RELATIONS LAWS

Public Employees Bargaining Rights.
Illinois Executive Order No. 6 of 1973.
Bargaining Rights of Teachers.
Illinois Public Acts, No. 1014 (L.1984).
Nonright-to-Work Policy
Section 14(b) of the labor management relations act
"Yellow-Dog" Contracts.
Illinois Revised Statutes, Ch. 48, Section 2b.

{79.02} STRIKES, PICKETING, AND BOYCOTT LAWS

Interference with Employment
Illinois Revised Statutes, Chapter 38, Section 12.6

Unlawful Assemble.
Illinois Revised Statutes, Chapter 38, Section 25.1.
Striker Replacements.
Illinois Revised Statutes, Chapter 48, Section 2d.
Strikebreakers.
Illinois Revised Statutes, Chapter 48, Section 2f.
Anti-Injunction Statute.
Illinois Revised Statutes, Chapter 48, Section 2a.
Picketing of Residence or Dwelling.
Illinois Revised Statutes, Chapter 38, Section 21.1-1.
Inciting Strikes.
Illinois Revised Statutes, Chapter 38, Section 201.11.
Restriction of Railroad Picketing
Illinois Revised Statutes, Chapter 114, Section 101, et seq.

{79.03} MEDIATION AND ARBITRATION LAWS

Illinois Revised Statutes, Chapter 10, Section 101, et seq.
Illinois Revised Statutes, Chapter 10, Section 20, et seq.
{79.04} Regulation of Union Activities.
Illinois Revised Statutes, Chapter 38, Section 242.
Illinois Public Acts, S.B. 192 (L.1961).

{79.05} REGULATION OF EMPLOYMENT PRACTICES

Anti-Discrimination Laws.
Illinois Revised Statutes, Chapter 68, Section 1-102, et seq.
Military Personnel Leave.
Illinois Revised Statutes, Chapter.126 ½ Section 31, et seq.
Arrest Records.
Illinois Revised Statutes, Chapter 48, Section 2-103.
Jury and Witness Duty.
Illinois Revised Statutes, Chapter 78, Section 4.1.
Whistle-Blowing Statute (Public Employees).
Illinois Public Acts, No.82-734 (L.1981).
Polygraph restrictions.
Illinois Revised Statutes, Chapter111, Section 2415.1.
Access to Personnel Records.
Illinois Revised Statutes, Chapter 48. Section 2001.
Illinois Revised Statutes, Chapter 48, Section 2001, et seq.
Medical Examination Payments.
Illinois Revised Statutes, Chapter 48, Section 172d.
Equal Pay.
Illinois Revised Statutes, Chapter 48, Section 4(a).

{79.06} Wage and Hour Laws

Child Labor.
Illinois Revised statutes, Chapter 48, Section 31, et seq.
Payment of wages.
Illinois Revised Statutes, Chapter 48, Section 39m.
Payment on Termination.
Illinois Revised Statutes, Chapter 48, Section 39m.
Garnishments.
Illinois Revised Statutes, Chapter 110, Section 12-818.

{79.07} Safety and Health Laws

General Provisions.
Illinois Revised Statutes, Chapter 48, Section 137.3.
Toxic Substances-Right to Know.
Illinois Revised Statutes, Chapter 48, Section 1401, et seq.

{79.08} Unemployment Compensation Laws

Illinois Revised Statutes, Chapter 48, Section 300, et seq.
Illinois Revised Statutes, Chapter 48, Section 401, et seq.

{79.09} Workers Compensation Laws

Illinois Revised Statutes, Chapter 48, Section 138, et seq.
Illinois Revised Statutes, Chapter 48, Section 138h.

{79.10} Employment-at-Will Developments

Public Policy Exception.
Kelsay v. Motorola, Inc., 74 Ill.2d 172,384 N.E.2d 353(1978).
Palmateer v. International Harvester, 85 Ill. App. 2d 124, 421 N.E.2d 876 (1981).
"Independent Consideration" Exception.
Martin v. Federated Life Insurance Co., 109 Ill. App.3d 596, 440 N.E.2d 998(1982).
Intentional Infliction of Emotional Distress Exception.
Harris v. First Federal Savings and loan Assn. of Chicago, 473 N.E.2d 457(Ill. Ct. of App., 1984).

INDIANA

New Law - HB 1183 **Employee** Paid Sick Leave

{80.01} Labor Relations Laws

Teachers' Bargaining Rights.
Indiana Statutes, Section 20-7.5-1-1.

Indiana Statutes, Section 20-7.5-1-7.
Indiana Statutes, Section 20-7.5-1-10.
Indiana Statutes, Section 20-7.5-1-14.
Right to Organize.
Indiana Public Acts, senate Bill No. 251 (1957).
Nonright-to-Work Policy.
Section 14(b) of the Labor Management Relations Act.
"Yellow-Dog."
Indiana Statutes, Section 35-15-3-1.

{80.02} STRIKES, PICKETING, AND BOYCOTT LAWS

Anti-Injunction Statute.
Indiana Statutes, Section 22-6-1, et seq.
Striker Replacements.
Indiana Statutes, Section 25-16-1-12.
Unlawful Interference with Employment.
Indiana Statutes, Section 35-15-4-2.

{80.03} MEDIATION AND ARBITRATION LAWS

Indiana Statutes, Section 22-1-1-8.
Indiana Statutes, Section 34-4-1-1.

{80.04} REGULATION OF UNION ACTIVITIES

Indiana Statutes, Section 23-116

{80.05} REGULATION OF EMPLOYMENT PRACTICES

Anti-Discrimination Laws.
Indiana Statutes, Section 22-9-1-2, et seq.
Freedom of Political Activities.
Indiana Statutes, Section 3-4-7-3.
Service Letter.
Indiana Statutes, Section 22-6-3-1.
Whistle-Blowing Statute.
Indiana Statutes, Section 4-15-10-4.
Military Personnel Leaves.
Indiana Statutes, Section 10-5-9-2.
Blacklisting.
Indiana Statutes, Section 22-5-3-2.
Jury Service.
Indiana Statutes, Section 35-44-3-10.
Equal Pay.
Indiana Statutes, Section 22-2-2-4.

{80.06} Wage and Hour Laws

Child Labor.
  Indiana Statutes, Section 20-8-1-4-1, et seq.
  Indiana Statutes, Section 20-8.1-4-21.
  Indiana Statutes, Section 20-8.1-4-27.
  Voting Time.
  Indiana Statutes, Section 3-1-21-7.
  Payment of Wages.
  Indiana Statutes, Section 22-2-4-1.
  Payment Upon Termination.
  Indiana Statutes, Section 22-2-5-1.
  Garnishments.
  Indiana Statutes, Section 24-4.5-5-106.

{80.07} Safety and Health Laws

Indiana Code annotated, Section 22-8-1.1-1.
  Indiana Code annotated, Section 22-8-1.1-4.

{80.08} Unemployment Compensation Laws

Indiana Code Annotated, Section 22-2-14-1, et seq.
  Indiana Code Annotated, Section 22-5-14-3.

{80.09} Workers Compensation Laws

Indiana Code Annotated, Section 22-3-2-1 et seq.
  Indiana Code Annotated, Section 22-3-2-1, et seq.
  Indiana Code Annotated, Section 22-3-7-1, et seq.

{80.10} Employment-at-will Developments

Public Policy Exception.
  Frampton v. Central Indiana Gas Co., 297 N, E.2d 425 (Ind.1973).
  Perry v. Hartz Mountain Corp., F. Supp. 1387 (S.D. Ind. 1982).
  Promissory Estoppel Exception.
  Eby v. York Division, Borg Warner, 455 N.E.2d 623 (Ind. App. 1983); Pepsi-cola
General Bottlers, Inc. v. Woods, 440 N.E.2d 969 (Ind. App. 1982).

LOWA

{81.01} Labor Relations Laws

Public Employees Bargaining Rights.
  Code of Lowa, Section 20.8.

Code of Lowa, Section 20.7.
Code of Lowa, Section 20.10.
Code of Lowa, Section 20.15.
Code of Lowa, Section 20.12.
Right-to-Work-Statute.
Code of Lowa, Section 731.1.

{81.02} Strikes, Picketing and Boycott Laws

Unlawful Assembly.
Code of Lowa, Section 723.2.
Secondary Boycotts.
Code of Lowa, Section 732.1.
Jurisdictional Disputes.
Chapter 732.3 of the Lowa Public Acts.
Strikebreakers.
Code of Lowa, Section 732.6.

{81.03} Mediation and Arbitration Laws

Code of Lowa, Section 679.1. et seq.
Code of Lowa, Section 90.1.

{81.04} Regulation of Union Activity

Code of Lowa, Section 548.10.

{81.05} Regulation of Employment Practices

Anti-Discrimination Statutes.
Code of Lowa, Section 601A.6.
Military Leaves of Absence.
Code of Lowa, Section 29A.43.
Drunk Driving Rehabilitation.
Code of Lowa, Section 321.283(8).
Blacklisting.
Code of Lowa, Section 730.2.
Whistle-Blowing Statute (Public Employees).
Code of Lowa, Section 19A.19.
Polygraph Restrictions.
Code of Lowa, Section 730.4(2).
Comparable Work Law (Public Employees).
Code of Lowa, Section 79.18.

{81.06} Wage and Hour Laws

Child Labor.
Lowa Public Acts, Section 2.1, H. B. 1251{1970}.

Lowa Public Acts, Section 4, H. B. 1251{1970}.
Lowa Public Acts, Section 5, H. B. 1251{1970}.
Voting Time.
Code of Iowa, Chapter 49 Section 109.
Payment of Wages.
Code of Iowa, Chapter 91A Section 3(1).
Payment upon Termination.
Code of Iowa, Section 91A.4.
Garnishments.
Code of Iowa, Chapter 642 Section 21.

{81.07} SAFETY AND HEALTH LAWS

General Provisions
   Code of Iowa, Section 88.4.
   Toxic substances - Right to Know
   Code of Iowa, Section 455D.1.

{81.08} UNEMPLOYMENT COMPENSATION LAWS

Code of Iowa, Chapter 96 Section 1, et seq.

{81.09} WORKERS COMPENSATION LAWS

Code of Iowa, Section 85.1, et seq.

{81.10} EMPLOYMENT-AT-WILL DEVELOPMENTS

Allen v. Highway Equipment Co., 239 N.W.2d 135 (Iowa S. Ct., 1976).
   Abrisz v. Pulley Freight Lines, Inc., 270 N.W.2d 454 (Iowa S. Ct., 1978).
   Covenant of Good Faith and Fair Dealing Excepting.
   High v. Sperry Crop., 581 F.Supp. 1246 (S.D. Iowa, 1984).
   "Independent Consideration" Exception
   Collins v. Parsons College, 203 N. W2d 594 (Iowa, 1973).

KANSAS

{82.01} LABOR RELATIONS LAWS

Kansas LMRA.
   Section 44-801, et seq. of the Kansas statutes.
   Agricultural Employees Bargaining Rights.
   Kansas statutes Annotated, Section 44-818, et seq.
   Teachers' Bargaining Rights.
   Kansas statutes Annotated, Section 72-5411 et seq.
   Kansas statutes Annotated, Section 72-5414.

Kansas statutes Annotated, Section 72-5430.
Public Employees' Bargaining Rights.
Kansas statutes Annotated, Section 75-4321et seq.
Right-to-Work Statute.
Kansas statutes Annotated, Section 44-831.

{82.02} STRIKES, PICKETING, AND BOYCOTT LAWS

Anti-Injunction Laws.
Kansas statutes Annotated, Section 60-904, et seq.
Unlawful Assembly
Kansas statutes Annotated, Section 21-1001.
Interference with Railroads
Kansas statutes Annotated, Section 21-1901.
Kansas statutes Annotated, Section 21-1901, et seq.
Strikebreakers
Kansas statutes Annotated, Section 21-1616, et seq.
Secondary Boycotts and Jurisdictional Disputes
Kansas statutes Annotated, Section 44.809(a).

{82.03} MEDIATION AND ARBITRATION LAWS

Kansas statutes Annotated, Section 5-201, et seq.
Kansas statutes Annotated, Section 44-603.

{82.04} REGULATION OF UNION ACTIVITIES

Kansas statutes Annotated, Section 81-105 et seq.
Kansas statutes Annotated, Section 44-809(6).

{82.05} REGULATION OF EMPLOYMENT PRACTICES

Anti-Discrimination Laws.
Kansas statutes Annotated, Section 44-1001, et seq.
Protection of Political Freedom
Kansas statutes Annotated, Section 25-418.
Service Letter
Kansas statutes Annotated, Section 44-808(3).
Hiring of Illegal Aliens.
Kansas statutes Annotated, Section 21-4409.
Whistle-Blowing Statute (State Employees)
Kansas public laws, H.B. 2621 (L.1984).
Blacklisting
Kansas statutes Annotated, Section 44-118.
Equal Pay
Kansas statutes Annotated, Section 44-1210(b).

{82.06} Wage and Hour Laws

Child Labor
  Kansas statutes Annotated, Section 38-614.
  Voting Time
  Kansas statutes Annotated, Section 25-418.
  Payment of Wages
  Kansas statutes Annotated, Section 44-314.
  Payment Upon Termination
  Kansas statutes Annotated, Section 44-315 (a).
  Garnishments
  Kansas statutes Annotated, Section 60-2311(a).
  Medical Insurance Conversion
  Kansas statutes Annotated, Section 40-2209.

{82.07} Safety and Health Laws

Kansas statutes Annotated, Section 44-636.

{82.08} Unemployment Compensation Laws

Kansas statutes Annotated, Section 44-701, et seq.

{82.10} Employment-at-Will Developments

Public Policy Exception
  Murphy v. City of Topeka-Shawnee County Dept., 630 P.2d 186 (Kan., 1981).
  Promissory Estoppel Exception
  Lorson v. Falcon Coach, Inc., 522 P.2d 449 (Kan 1974).
  Implied Contract Exception
  Owens v. City of derby, 586 F.Supp. 37 (D. Kan 1984).
  Rouse v. People's National Gas Co., 116 LRRM 2875 (D. Kan., 1984).

KENTUCKY

{83.01} Labor Relations Laws

Employees' Right of Self-Organization
  Kentucky revised statutes, Section 345.010, et seq.
  Firefighters and Police Officers
  Kentucky public acts, H.B.217 (1.1972).
  Kentucky revised statutes, Section 340.050.
  Nonright-to-Work Police
  Section 14(b) of the Labor Management Relations Act.

{83.02} Strikes, Picketing, and Boycott Laws

Unlawful Assembly
Kentucky revised statutes, Section 437.010.
Striker Replacements
Kentucky revised statutes, Section 340.050.
Interference with Transportation
Kentucky revised statutes, Section 433.370.

{83.03} Mediation and Arbitration Laws

Kentucky revised statutes, Section 417.010.
Kentucky revised statutes, Section 336.140.

{83.04} Regulation of Union Activities

Kentucky revised statutes, Section 336.170.
Kentucky revised statutes, Section 365.120
Kentucky public acts, H. B. 362 (1962).

{83.05} Regulation of Employment Practices

Anti-Discrimination Laws
Kentucky revised statutes, Section 344.040.
Kentucky revised statutes, Section 207.130.
Kentucky revised statutes, Section 344.030.
Jury Duty
Kentucky public acts, H. B. 23-x (L.1976).
Unlawful Enticement
Kentucky revised statutes, Section 433.310.
Protection of Political Activities
Kentucky revised statutes, Section 121.310.
Employment of Convicted Persons
Kentucky public acts, H. B. 100 (1978): see also Kentucky revised statutes,
Section 335B.2(1).
National Guard Members
Kentucky revised statutes, Section 38.460.
Equal Pay
Kentucky revised statutes, Section 337.423.

{83.06} Wage and Hour Laws

Child Labor
Kentucky revised statutes, Section 339.210, et seq.
Kentucky revised statutes, Section 339.230.

Voting Time
Kentucky revised statutes, Section 118.035.
Payment of Wages
Kentucky revised statutes, Section 337.020.
Payment Upon Terminating
Kentucky revised statutes, Section 337.055.
Garnishments
Kentucky revised statutes, Section 427.140.
Medical Insurance Conversion
Kentucky revised statutes, Section 304.18-110.

{83.07} Safety and Health Laws

Kentucky revised statutes, Section 338.031.

{83.08} Unemployment Compensation Laws

Kentucky revised statutes, Section 341.350, et seq.

{83.09} Workers Compensation Laws

Kentucky revised statutes, Section 342.630:342.650.

{83.10} Employment-at-Will Developments

Public Policy Exception
Firestone Textile Co. Division v. Meadows, 666 S.W.2d &30 (Ky., 1983).
Implied Contract Exception
Shah v. American Synthetic Rubber Crop., 655 S.W.2d 489 (Ky., 1983).
Presumption of Term Exception
Moore v. Young Women's Christian Ass'n, Case No. 84-CA-1508-MR (Ky., Ct of App., 1985).

LOUISIANA

{84.01} Labor Relations Laws

General Right to Organize
Louisiana Revised of the Section 23:822
Public Transit Employees Bargaining Rights
Louisiana public acts No. 127, Section 4 (1964).
Louisiana public acts No. 127, Section 5 (1964).
Right-to-Work Statute
Louisiana Revised Statutes, Section 23:983.
"Yellow-Dog" Contracts
Louisiana Revised Statutes, Section 23:823.

{84.02} Strikes, Picketing, and Boycott Laws

Anti-Injunction Laws
Louisiana Revised Statutes, Section 23:841.
Strikebreakers
Louisiana Revised Statutes, Section 23:898.
Louisiana Revised Statutes, Section 23:901.
Obstruction of Commerce or Passageways
Louisiana Revised Statutes, Section 14:100.
Picketing of Courts
Louisiana Revised Statutes, Section 14:401.

{84.03} Mediation and Arbitration Laws

Louisiana Revised Statutes, Section 23:6.

{84.04} Regulation of Union Activities

Louisiana Revised Statutes, Section 51:211, et seq.

{84.05} Regulation of Employment Practices

Anti-Discrimination Laws.
Louisiana Revised Statutes, Section 23:1006.
Louisiana Revised Statutes, Section 23:973.
Louisiana Revised Statutes, Section 46:2254(1).
Hiring of Illegal Aliens
Louisiana Revised Statutes, Section 23:992.
Whistle-Blowing Statutes (Environmental Conditions)
Louisiana Revised Statutes, Section 30:1074.1.
Reemployment Right of Veterans
Louisiana Revised Statutes, Section 29:28.
Protection of Political Activities
Louisiana Revised Statutes, Section 23:962.
Jury Duty
Louisiana Revised Statutes, Section 23:965.
Prior Criminal Convictions
Louisiana Revised Statutes, Section 37:2950.
Access to Medical Records
Louisiana Revised Statutes, Section 23:1125.
Medical Examination Payments
Louisiana Revised Statutes, Section 23:897.

{84.06} Wage and Hour Laws

Child Labor
Louisiana Revised Statutes, Section 23:151, et seq.

Louisiana Revised Statutes, Section 23:161.
Payment of Wages
Louisiana Revised Statutes, Section 23:633.
Payment Upon Termination
Louisiana Revised Statutes, Section 23:631, et seq.
Garnishments
Louisiana Revised Statutes, Section 23:731(c)

{84.07} Safety and Health Laws

General Provisions
Louisiana Revised Statutes, Section 23:8.
Toxic Substances-Right to Know
Louisiana Revised Statutes, Section 23:1126.

{84.08} Unemployment Compensation Laws

Louisiana Revised Statutes, Section 23:1600, et seq.

{84.09} Workers Compensation Laws

Louisiana Revised Statutes, Section 23:1021, et seq.

{84.10} Employment-at-Will Developments

Gil v. metal service Crop., 412 So.2d 706 (La. Ct. of App., 1982).
Williams v. Delta Haven, Inc., 416 So.2d 637 (La. Ct. of App., 1928).

MAINE

New Law §664. Minimum wage; overtime rate

{85.01} Labor Relations Laws

State Employees Bargaining Rights
Main Revised Statutes Annotated, Tile 26, Section 979.
Main Revised Statutes Annotated, Tile 26, Section 979-E and F.
Main Revised Statutes Annotated, Tile 26, Section 979-K.
Public Employees Bargaining Rights
Main Revised Statutes Annotated, Tile 26, Section 963, et seq.
Main Revised Statutes Annotated, Tile 26, Section 964.
University Employees Bargaining Rights
Main Revised Statutes Annotated, Tile 26, Section 10.21, et seq.
Bargaining Rights to Judicial Employees
Maine public acts, Chapter 702 (L.1984).
General Right to Organize Statute

Main Revised Statutes Annotated, Tile 26, Section 911.
Nonright-to-Work Policy
Section 14(b) of the Labor Management Relations Act.

{85.02} STRIKES, PICKETING, AND BOYCOTT LAWS

Anti-Injunction Laws
Maine public acts, Chapter 620 (L.1972).
Unlawful Assembly
Main Revised Statutes Annotated, Tile 17, Section 3352.
Interference with Railroads
Main Revised Statutes Annotated, Tile 17, Section 3605.
Strikebreakers
Main Revised Statutes Annotated, Tile 26, Section 851.
Striker Replacement
Main Revised Statutes Annotated, Tile 26, Section 921.
Mass Picketing
Main Revised Statutes Annotated, Tile 17, Section 3606.
Cancellation of Health Insurance During Strike
Main Revised Statutes Annotated, Tile 24-A, Section 2894.
Main Revised Statutes Annotated, Tile 26, Section 634.
Interference with Public Utilities Employment
Main Revised Statutes Annotated, Tile 17, Section 3601.

{85.03} MEDIATION AND ARBITRATION LAWS

Main Revised Statutes Annotated, Tile 14, Section 1151, et seq.
Main Revised Statutes Annotated, Tile 26, Section 891.

{85.04} REGULATION OF UNION ACTIVITIES

Main Revised Statutes Annotated, Tile 16, Section 1341.

{85.05} REGULATION OF EMPLOYMENT PRACTICES

Anti-Discrimination Laws
Main Revised Statutes Annotated, Tile 5, Section 4572-A.
Blacklisting
Main Revised Statutes Annotated, Tile 17, Section 401.
Polygraph Restrictions
Main Revised Statutes Annotated, Tile 32, Section 7166.
National Guard Members
Main Revised Statutes Annotated, Tile 26, Section 811.
Military Leaves of Absence
Main Revised Statutes Annotated, Tile 26, Section 811.
Hiring of Illegal Aliens

Main Revised Statutes Annotated, Tile 26, Section 871.
Plant Closures
Main Revised Statutes Annotated, Tile 26, Section 625 B (6).
Main Revised Statutes Annotated, Tile 26, Section 625 B (2).
Disclosure of Consumer Reports
Main Revised Statutes Annotated, Tile 10, Section 1320.
Access to Employment Records
Main Revised Statutes Annotated, Tile 26, Section 631.
Whistle-Blowing Statute
Main Revised Statutes Annotated, Tile 26, Section 831, et seq.
Service Letter
Main Revised Statutes Annotated, Tile 26, Section 630.
Comparable Pay
Main Revised Statutes Annotated, Tile 26, Section 628.
Medical Examination Payments
Main Revised Statutes Annotated, Tile 26, Section 592.

{85.06} WAGE AND HOUR LAWS

Child Labor
Main Revised Statutes Annotated, Tile 26, Section 711, et seq.
Payment of Wages
Main Revised Statutes Annotated, Tile 26, Section 621.

{85.07} SAFETY AND HEALTH LAWS

General Provisions
Main Revised Statutes Annotated, Tile 26, Section 561, et seq.
Toxic Substances- Right to Know.
Main Revised Statutes Annotated, Tile 26, Section 1701, et seq.

{85.08} UNEMPLOYMENT COMPENSATION LAWS

Main Revised Statutes Annotated, Tile 26, Section 1192.

{85.09} WORKERS COMPENSATION LAWS

Main Revised Statutes Annotated, Tile 39, Section 1, et seq.
Merrill v. Western Union Tele. Co., 2 A.847 (Maine, 1886).
MacDonald v. Eastern Fine Paper Inc., 485 A.2d 228 (Maine, 1984).
Larrabee v. Penobscot Frozen Foods, Inc., 486 A.2d 97 (Maine, 1984).

MARYLAND

{86.01} LABOR RELATIONS LAWS

General Right to Organize
Annotated code of Maryland, art. 100, Section 63.

Public School Employees' Bargaining Rights.
Annotated code of Maryland, art. 77, Section 160A, et seq.
Nonright-to-Work Police
Section 14(b) of the labor management relations act
"Yellow-Dog" Contracts
Annotated code of Maryland, art. 100, Section 64.

{86.02} STRIKES, PICKETING, AND BOYCOTT LAWS

Anti-Injunction Laws
Annotated code of Maryland, art. 100, Section 70 and 71.
Strikebreakers
Annotated code of Maryland, art. 100, Section 51A.

{86.03} MEDIATION AND ARBITRATION LAWS

Annotated code of Maryland, art. 64A, Section 52, et seq.
Annotated code of Maryland, art. 723 (L.1978).

{86.04} REGULATION OF UNION ACTIVITIES

Annotated code of Maryland, art. 27, Section 187.

{86.05} REGULATION OF EMPLOYMENT PRACTICES

Anti-Discrimination Laws.
Annotated code of Maryland, art. 49A, Section 16.
Polygraph Restrictions
Annotated code of Maryland, art. 100, Section 95.
Discrimination Against Volunteer Public Service Forbidden
Annotated code of Maryland, art. 100, Section 109.
Reemployment Rights of Military Personnel
Annotated code of Maryland, art. 65, Section 32A.
Whistle-Blowing Statute (Public Employees)
Annotated code of Maryland, art. 64, Section 12(G).
Arrest Records
Annotated code of Maryland, art. 27, Section 740(A).
Medical Records
Annotated code of Maryland, art. 100, Section 95A
Jury Duty
Maryland courts and judicial proceedings code annotated, Section 8-105.
Comparable Pay
Annotated code of Maryland, art. 100, Section 55A.

{89.06} WAGE AND HOUR LAWS

Child Labor
Annotated code of Maryland, art. 100, Section 23(a)-(6).

Voting Time
Annotated code of Maryland, art. 33, Section 24-26.
Payment of Wages
Annotated code of Maryland, art. 100, Section 94.
Payment Upon Termination
Annotated code of Maryland, art. 100, Section 94 E.
Garnishments
Annotated code of Maryland, art. 15, Section 606.
Medical Insurance Conversion
Annotated code of Maryland, art. 95A, Section 5A.

{86.07} SAFETY AND HEALTH LAWS

Annotated code of Maryland, art. 89, Section 32A.

{86.08} UNEMPLOYMENT COMPENSATION LAWS

Annotated code of Maryland, art. 95A, Section 1, et seq.

{86.09} WORKERS COMPENSATION LAWS

Annotated code of Maryland, art. 101, Section 36, et seq.

{86.10} EMPLOYMENT-AT-WILL DEVELOPMENTS

Public Policy Exception
Adler v. American Standard Crop., 583 F.Supp. 572 (D.Md., 1982); Adler v. American standard Corp., 432 A.2d 464 (Md. Ct. of App., 1981).
Intentional Infliction of Emotional Distress Exception
Harris v. Jones, 380 A.2d 611 (Md. Ct. of App., 1977).
Implied Contract Exception
Staggs v. Blue Cross of Maryland, Inc., Case No. 538 (Md. Ct. of Sp. App., 1985).

MASSACHUSETTS

{87.01} LABOR RELATIONS LAWS

Massachusetts Labor Relations Law
Massachusetts General laws, Chapter 150A, Section 3.
Massachusetts General laws, Chapter 150A, Section 1, et seq.
Housing Employees Bargaining Rights.
Massachusetts General laws, Chapter 121B, Section 29.
Public Employees Bargaining Rights.
Massachusetts General laws, Chapter 150E, Section 2.
Massachusetts General laws, Chapter 150E, Section 10.
Massachusetts General laws, Chapter 150E, Section 1, et seq.

State Employee's Grievance Rights
Massachusetts General laws, Chapter 30, Section 53.
Prohibition Against Pay-Offs
Massachusetts General laws, Chapter 149 Section 20D.
Collective Bargaining Successor Clauses
Massachusetts General laws, Chapter 149, Section 179C.
Nonright-to-Work Policy
Section 14(b) of the labor management relations act.
"Yellow-Dog" Contracts
Massachusetts General laws, Chapter 149, Section 20A.

{87.02} Strikes, Picketing, and Boycott Laws

Anti-Injunction Act
Massachusetts General laws, Chapter 214, Section 6.
Unlawful Assembly
Massachusetts General laws, Chapter 269 Section 1.
Unlawful Interference with Employment
Massachusetts General laws, Chapter 149, Section 19 and 18.
Picketing of Courts
Massachusetts General laws, Chapter 268 Section 13a.
Declaration of Emergency During Transit Strikes.
Massachusetts General laws, Chapter 544, Section 19A.
Strikebreakers
Massachusetts General laws, Chapter 150D, Section 1, et seq.
Massachusetts General laws, Chapter 802, Section 22A.
Striker Replacements
Massachusetts General laws, Chapter 149 Section 22.
Use of Police Officers and Firefighters During Strike
Massachusetts General laws, Chapter 149, Section 23B.
Massachusetts General laws, Chapter 48, Section 88.

{87.03} Mediation and Conciliation Laws

Massachusetts General laws, Chapter150, Section 1-10.
Massachusetts General laws, Chapter 150B, Section 1-7.
Massachusetts public Acts, Chapter 154, (L-1979).
Massachusetts General laws, Chapter 161A, Section 19.

{87.04} Regulation of Union Activities

Massachusetts General laws, Chapter 612, Section 1-5.
Massachusetts General laws, Chapter 110, Section 7-11 and Chapter 266, Section 71A.
Massachusetts General laws, Chapter 151D, Section 1, et seq.
Massachusetts General laws, Chapter 149, Section 150B.

{87.05} Regulation of Employment Practices

Anti-Discrimination Laws

Massachusetts General laws, Chapter 151B, Section 4.

Massachusetts General laws, Chapter149. Section 24A.

Massachusetts General laws, Chapter 149 Section 24K.

Freedom of Political Activities

Massachusetts General laws, Chapter 54, Section 33.

Jury Duty

Massachusetts General laws, Chapter 234A, Section 61.

Military Leaves of Absence

Massachusetts General laws, Chapter 149, Section 52A.

Employment Under False Pretense.

Massachusetts General laws, Chapter 149, Section 21.

Polygraph Restrictions

Massachusetts General laws, Chapter 149, Section 19B.

Medical Examination Reports

Massachusetts General laws, Chapter 149, Section 19A.

Arrest Records

Massachusetts General laws, Chapter 276, Section 100A.

Hiring of Illegal Aliens

Massachusetts General laws, Chapter 149, Section 19C.

Disclosure of Consumer Reports

Massachusetts General laws, Chapter 93, Section 56.

Political Influence Relating to Public Utilities Employees

Massachusetts General laws, Chapter 271 Section 40.

Plant Closures

Massachusetts public laws, H.6120 (1984).

Equal Pay

Massachusetts General laws, Chapter 149, Section 105A.

{87.06} Wage and Hour Laws

Child Labor

Massachusetts General laws, Chapter 149, Section 56, et seq.

Voting Time

Massachusetts General laws, Chapter 149, Section 178.

Payment of Wages

Massachusetts General laws, Chapter 149, Section 148.

Payment Upon Termination

Massachusetts General laws, Chapter 149, Section 148.

Medical Insurance Continuance

Massachusetts General laws, Chapter 175, Section 110G.

{87.07} SAFETY AND HEALTH LAWS

General Provisions
   Massachusetts General laws, Chapter 149, Section 6-8.
   Toxic Substances- Right to Know
   Massachusetts General laws, Chapter 111F, Section 1, et seq.

{87.08} UNEMPLOYMENT COMPENSATION LAWS

Massachusetts General laws, Chapter 151A Section 1, et seq.
   Massachusetts General laws, Chapter 151A Section 24, et seq.

{87.09} WORKERS COMPENSATION LAWS

Massachusetts General laws, Chapter 152 Section 1, et seq.
   Massachusetts General laws, Chapter 152 Section 25A, et seq.

{87.10} EMPLOYMENT-AT-WILL DEVELOPMENT

Public Policy Exception
   McKinney v. National Dairy Council, 491 F.Supp. 1108 (D. Mass., 1980).
   Implied Contract Exception
   Garrity v. Valley View Nursing Home, Inc., 406 N.E.2d 423 (Mass. Ct. of App.,
1980).
   Covenant of Good Faith and Fair Dealing Exception
   Fortune v. National Cash Register Co., N.E.2d 1251 (Mass 1977).
   Intentional Infliction of Emotional Distress Exception
   Agis v. Howard Johnson Co., 355 N.E.2d 315 (Mass., 1976).

MICHIGAN

{88.01} LABOR RELATIONS LAWS

Public Employees Bargaining Rights
   Michigan Compiled laws, Section 423.209.
   Michigan Compiled laws, Section 423.201.
   Michigan Compiled laws, Section 423.201, et seq.
   Michigan LMRA (Bonnie-Tripp Act)
   Michigan Compiled laws, Annotated Section 423.8.
   Michigan Compiled laws, Annotated Section 423.3.
   Michigan Compiled laws, Annotated Section 423.1, et seq.
   Police Officers and Firefighters Labor Disputes.
   Michigan Compiled laws, Section 423.231, et seq.

Nonright-to-Work Policy
Section 14(b) of the labor management relations act

{88.02} Strikes, Picketing, and Boycott Laws

Michigan Compiled laws, Section 28-584.
  Michigan Compiled laws, Section 423.17.
  Sit-Down Strikes
  Michigan Compiled laws, Section 423.15
  Unlawful Picketing
  Michigan Compiled laws, Section 423.9F.
  Unlawful Assembly
  Michigan Compiled laws, Section 28-79.
  Interference with Transportation
  Michigan Compiled laws, Section 28-655.
  Strikebreakers and Replacements
  Michigan statutes, Annotated Section 17-456(1).

{88.03} Mediation and Conciliation Laws

Michigan Compiled laws, Section 423.9d
  Michigan Compiled laws, Section 423.231, et seq.
  Michigan public acts, No. 17 (1980), Section 1-16.

{88.04} Regulation of Union Activities

Michigan Compiled laws, Section 750.265a
  Michigan Compiled laws, Section 454.71, et seq.

{88.05} Regulation of Employment Practices

Anti- Discrimination Laws
  Michigan Compiled laws, Section 37.2202.
  Michigan Compiled laws, Section 37.1101, et seq.
  Freedom of Political Activities
  Michigan Compiled laws, Annotated Section 6.1931.
  Jury Duty
  Michigan Compiled laws, Section 600.1348.
  Polygraph Restrictions
  Michigan Compiled laws, Section 37.201, et seq.
  Whistle-Blowing Statute
  Michigan Compiled laws, Annotated Section 15.362.
  Reemployment Rights of Military Personnel
  Michigan Compiled laws, Annotated Section 32.271, et seq.
  Arrest Records
  Michigan Compiled laws, Section 37.2205a.

Access to Personnel Records
Michigan Compiled laws, Annotated Section 423.501, et seq.
Michigan Compiled laws, Annotated Section 4423.501, et seq.
Wage Disclosure
Michigan Compiled laws, Section 408.483.
Wage Evasion
Michigan Compiled laws, Section 408.396.
Equal Pay
Michigan Compiled laws, Section 408.397.

{88.06} WAGE AND HOUR LAWS

Child Labor
Michigan Compiled laws, Section 409.01 et seq.
Payment of Wages
Michigan Compiled laws, Section 408.472.
Payment Upon Termination
Michigan Compiled laws, Section 408.475.
Garnishment
Michigan Compiled laws, Section 600.4015.

{88.07} SAFETY AND HEALTH LAWS

General Provisions
Michigan Compiled laws, Section 408.1011.
Toxic Substances- Right to Know
Michigan Compiled laws, Section 408.1001, et seq.

{88.08} UNEMPLOYMENT COMPENSATION LAWS

Michigan Compiled laws, Section 421.1, et seq.

{88.09} WORKERS COMPENSATION LAWS

Michigan Compiled laws, Section 411.1, et seq.

{88.10} EMPLOYMENT-AT-WILL DEVELOPMENT

Public Policy Exception
Sventko v. Kroger Co., 245 N.W.2d 151(WD Mich., 1982).
Negligent Discharge Exception
Chamberlain v. Bissell, Inc., 547 F.Supp. 1067 (WD Mich., 1982).
Intentional Infliction of Emotional Distress Exception
See Novesel v. Sears, Roebuck & Co., 495 F.Supp. 344 (ED Mich., 1980).
Implied Contract Exception
See, for Example: Toussaint v. Blue Cross & Blue Shield of Michigan, 292 N.W.2d
880 (Mich. S. Ct., 1980).

MINNESOTA

{89.01} Labor Relations Laws

Minnesota Labor Relations Act
Minnesota Statutes, Section 179.10.
Minnesota Statutes, Section 179.01, et seq.
Public Employees Bargaining Rights
Minnesota Statutes, Section 179A.06.
Minnesota Statutes, Section 179A.01, et seq.
Nonright-to Work Policy
Section 14(b) of the labor management relations act
"Yellow-Dog" Contracts
Minnesota Statutes, Section 179.60.

{89.02} Strikes, Picketing, and Boycott Laws

Anti-Injunction Statute
Minnesota Statutes, Section 185.02.
Unlawful Assembly
Minnesota Statutes, Section 609.715.
Striker Replacements
Minnesota Statutes, Section 184.38(10).
False Advertisement and Representations in Hiring
Minnesota Statutes, Section 181.64.
Use of Police Office Limited During Strikes
Minnesota Statutes, Section 299c.03.
Use of Licensed Private Detectives During Strikes
Minnesota Statutes, Section 326.337.
Striker Employment Protection
Minnesota Statutes, Section 181.52.
Secondary Boycotts
Minnesota Statutes, Section 179.40, et seq.

{89.03} Mediation and Arbitration Laws

Minnesota Statutes, Section 572.08, et seq.
Minnesota Statutes, Section 179.61, et seq.

{89.04} Regulation of Union Activities

Minnesota Statutes, Section 179.11.

{89.05} Regulation of Employment Practices

Anti-Discrimination Laws
Minnesota Statutes, Section 363.01, et seq.

Protection of Political Freedom
Minnesota Statutes, Section 3.083.
Backlisting
Minnesota Statutes, Section 179.12.
Employment Under False Pretense
Minnesota Statutes, Section 181.64.
Polygraph Restrictions
Minnesota Statutes, Section 181.75.
National Guard Members
Minnesota Statutes, Section 192.34.
Equal Pay
Minnesota Statutes, Section 181.66-71.
Criminal and Arrest Records
Minnesota Statutes, Section 364.04.
Jure Duty
Minnesota public acts, chapter 286 (L.1977).
Mandatory Insurance Participation Restricted
Minnesota Statutes, Section 61A.091.
Pre-Employment Medical Exams
Minnesota Statutes, Section 363.02.
Maternity Leaves
Minnesota Statutes, Section 181.92.

{89.06} WAGE AND HOUR LAWS

Child Labor
Minnesota Statutes, Section 181A.05, et seq.
Voting Time
Minnesota Statutes, Section 204C.04.
Garnishment
Minnesota Statutes, Section 571.61
Medical Coverage Continuance
Minnesota Statutes, Section 62A.17.

{89.07} SAFETY AND HEALTH LAWS

General Provisions
Minnesota Statutes, Section 182.653.
Toxic Substances-Right to Know
Minnesota Statutes, Section 182.65, et seq.

{89.08} UNEMPLOYMENT COMPENSATION

Minnesota Statutes, Section 268.07-09.

{89.09} Workers Compensation Laws

Minnesota Statutes, Section 176.021, et seq.
  Minnesota Statutes, Section 176.66.

{89.10} Employment-at-will Developments

Promissory Estoppel Exception
  Grouse v. Group Health Plan, Inc., 306 N.W.2d 114 (Minn., 1981).
  Implied Contract Exception
  Pine River State Bank v. Mettille, 333 N.W.2d 155 (Minn., 1972).
  Independent Consideration Exception
  Bussard v. College of St. Thomas, Inc., 200 N.W.2d 155 (Minn., 1972).
  Intentional Infliction of Emotional Distress Exception
  Hubbard v. United Press International, Inc., 330 N.W.2d 428 (Minn., 1983).
  Covenant of Good Faith and Fair Dealing Exception
  Eklund v. Vincent Brass & Aluminum Co., 351 N.W.2d 371 (Minn., 1984).

MISSISSIPPI

{90.01} Labor Relations Laws

Union Telegrapher's Rights
  Mississippi code, Section 77-9-725, et seq.
  Right-to-Work Statute
  Mississippi Statutes, Section 71-1-47.
  "Yellow-Dog" Contracts
  Mississippi Statutes, Section 6984.5(1)(b).

{90.02} Strikes, Picketing, and Boycott Laws

Interference with Employment
  Mississippi Statutes, Section 97-1-1, et seq.
  Unlawful Assembly
  Mississippi Statutes, Section 219-25-67
  Interference with Business
  Mississippi Statutes, Section 97-23-83.
  Interference with Transportation
  Mississippi Statutes, Section 97-25-43.
  Restriction of Railroad Picketing
  Mississippi Statutes, Section 77-9-236.
  Use of Highway Patrol During Strikes
  Mississippi Statutes, Section 45-3-21.
  Use of Violence or Threats Forbidden
  Mississippi Statutes, Section 97-23-39.

{90.03} Mediation and Conciliation Laws

Mississippi Statutes, Section 11-15-1.

{90.04} Regulation of Union Activities

Mississippi Statutes, Section 97-21-53.
Mississippi Statutes, Section 71-1-49.
Mississippi public Acts, H.B.123 (L.1962).

{90.05} Regulation of Employment Practices

Anti-Discrimination Laws.
Mississippi Statutes, Section 25-9-103.
Jury Duty
Mississippi Statutes, Section 13-5-23.
Protection of Military Personnel
Mississippi Statutes, Section 33-1-19.
Unlawful Enticement
Mississippi Statutes, Section 97-23-29.
Protection of Political Activities
Mississippi Statutes, Section 23-3-29.

{90.06} Wage and Hour Laws

Child Labor
Mississippi Statutes, Section 71-1-1, et seq.
Payment of Wages
Mississippi Statutes, Section 71-1-35.

{90.07} Safety and Health Laws

Mississippi Statutes, Section 75-37-19.

{90.08} Unemployment Compensation

Mississippi Statutes, Section 71-5-1, et seq.
Mississippi Statutes, Section 71-5-511.

{90.09} Workers Compensation Laws

Mississippi Statutes, Section 71-3-1, et seq.

{90.10} Employment-at-will Developments

Implied Contract Exception
Conley v. Board of Trustees, 707 F.2d 175 (CA-5, 1983).
"Independent Consideration Exception"

McGlohn v. Gulf and S.I.R.R., 174 So. 250 (Miss., 1937); Sartin v. City of Columbus Utilities Commission, 421 F.Supp. 393 (N.D. Miss., 1976).

Intentional Tort Exception

Smith v. Atlas Off-shore Boat Service, 653 F.2d 1057 (CA-5, 1981); See Also: Moeller v. Fuselier, Ott & McKee, 115 LRRM 2600 (Miss., 1984).

MISSOURI

{91.01} Labor Relations Laws

Public Employees Bargaining Rights
Missouri revised statutes, Section 105.501, et seq.
Missouri revised statutes, Section 105.510.
Missouri revised statutes, Section 105.530.
Missouri revised statutes, Section 105.540.
Nonright-to-Work Policy
Section 14(b) of the labor management relations act

{91.02} Strikes, Picketing, and Boycott Laws

Interference with Employment
Missouri revised statutes, Section 559.460.
Unlawful Assembly
Missouri revised statutes, Section 562.150.
Importation of Private Detectives During Strikes
Missouri revised statutes, Section 562.200.
Restriction of Railroad Picketing
Missouri revised statutes, Section 560.315.
Illegal Seizure of Property
Missouri revised statutes, Section 560.435.

{91.03} Mediation and Arbitration Laws

Missouri revised statutes, Section 295.010, et seq.
Missouri revised statutes, Section 295.180.

{91.04} Regulation of Union Activities

Missouri revised statutes, Section 416.031.

{91.05} Regulation of Employment Practices

Anti-Discrimination Laws.
Missouri revised statutes, Section 296.010, et seq.
Protection of Political Freedom
Missouri revised statutes, Section 15.020(7).

Missouri revised statutes, Section 115.635(b).
Service Letter
Missouri revised statutes, Section 290.140.
Employment Rights of Military
Missouri revised statutes, Section 41.730.
Wage Reduction
Missouri revised statutes, Section 296.100.
Equal Pay
Missouri revised statutes, Section 290.400, et. seq.

{91.06} Wage and Hour Laws

Child Labor
Missouri revised statutes, Section 294.400, et. seq.
Voting Time
Missouri revised statutes, Section 115.639
Payment of Wages
Missouri revised statutes, Section 290.090.
Payment Upon Termination
Missouri revised statutes, Section 115.639.
Garnishments
Missouri revised statutes, Section 525.030.
Medical Coverage
Missouri revised statutes, Section 376.397.

{91.07} Safety and Health Laws

Missouri revised statutes, Section 291.101, et seq.
Missouri revised statutes, Section 291.130.

{91.08} Unemployment Compensation Laws.

Missouri revised statutes, Section 288.040.

{91.09} Workers Compensation Laws.

Missouri revised statutes, Section 287,780.

{91.10} Employment-at-will Developments

Public Policy Exception
Arie v. Intertherm, Inc., 644 S.W.2d 142 (Mo. App., 1983).
Intentional Infliction of Emotional Distress Exception
Bass v. Intertherm Co., 644 S.W.2d 765 (Mo. S. Ct., 1983).
Implied Contract Exception
Arie v. Intertherm, Inc., 648 S.W.2d 142 (Mo. App., 1983); Hinkeldey v. Cities Ins.
Co. Case No. 36426 (Mo. Ct. of App., 1985).

MONTANA

{92.01} Labor Relations Laws

Public Employees Bargaining Rights
Montana code Annotated, Section 39-31-201.
Nurses Bargaining Rights
Montana code Annotated, Section 39-32-101, et seq.
Nonright-to-Work Policy
Section 14(b) of the labor management relations act

{92.02} Strikes, Picketing, and Boycott Laws

Anti-Injunction Statutes
Montana code Annotated, Section 27-19-103.
Unlawful Assembly
Montana code Annotated, Section 45-8-103.
Strikebreakers
Montana code Annotated, Section 39-33-201, et seq.
Striker Replacements
Montana code Annotated, Section 45-8-106.
Sit-Down Strikes
Montana code Annotated, Section 45-6-203.
Importation of Private Detectives During Strikes
Montana code Annotated, Section 47-5-102 and 47-5-103.

{92.04} Regulation of Union Activities

Montana code Annotated, Section 39-33-101.

{92.05} Regulation of Employment Practices

Anti-Discrimination Laws
Montana code Annotated, Section 49-1-102, et seq.
Hiring of Illegal Aliens
Montana code Annotated, Section 39-2-305.
Polygraph Restrictions
Montana code Annotated, Section 39-2-304.
Blacklisting
Montana code Annotated, Section 39-2-802, et seq.
Service Letter
Montana code Annotated, Section 39-2-801.
Unlawful Enticement
Montana code Annotated, Section 39-2-303.
Comparable Pay
Montana code Annotated, Section 39-3-104.

{92.06} WAGE AND HOUR LAWS

Child Labor
Montana code Annotated, Section 41-2-101.
Payment of Wages
Montana code Annotated, Section 39-3-204.
Payment Upon Termination
Montana code Annotated, Section 39-3-205.
Garnishments
Montana code Annotated, Section 39-2-302.

{92.07} SAFETY AND HEALTH LAWS

Montana code Annotated, Section 50-70-113.

{92.08} UNEMPLOYMENT COMPENSATION LAWS

Montana code Annotated, Section 39-51-2103, et seq.
Montana code Annotated, Section 39-51-2103.

{92.09} WORKS COMPENSATION LAWS

Montana code Annotated, Section 39-71-701, et seq.

{92.10} EMPLOYMENT-AT-WILL DEVELOPMENTS

Montana code Annotated, Section 39-2-503.
Covenant of Good Faith and Fair Dealing Exception
Gates v. Life of Montana Insurance Co., 668 P.2d 213 (Mont. S. Ct., 1983).
Public Policy Exception
See Statement of legal principle in Keneally v. Orgain, 606 P2d 127 (Mont., 1980).

NEBRASKA

{93.01} LABOR RELATIONS LAWS

Teachers Bargaining Rights
Revised statutes of Nebraska, Section 79-1288.
Revised statutes of Nebraska, Section 79-1290.
Revised statutes of Nebraska, Section 79-1293.
Public Employees Bargaining Rights
Revised statutes of Nebraska, Section 48-801, et seq.
Revised statutes of Nebraska, Section 48-838.
Right-to-work-Statute
Revised statutes of Nebraska, Section 48-217.

{93.02} Strikes, Picketing, and Boycott Laws

Destruction of Property
Revised statutes of Nebraska, Section 25-580.
Unlawful Interference with Employment
Nebraska public acts, L.B. 38 (L.1977), Section 301.
Mass Picketing
Idib., Section 302.
Secondary Boycotts
Revised statutes of Nebraska, Section 48-901, et seq.

{92.03} Mediation and Conciliation Laws

Revised statutes of Nebraska, Section 25-2103.
Revised statutes of Nebraska, Section 43-801.

{92.04} Regulation of Union Activities

Revised statutes of Nebraska, Section 28-548.
Revised statutes of Nebraska, Section 4-106.
Nebraska public Acts, L.B. 672 (L. 1963).

{93.05} Regulation of Employment Practices

Anti-Discrimination Laws.
Revised statutes of Nebraska, Section 48-1001, et seq.
Protection of Political Freedom
Revised statutes of Nebraska, Section 32-1223.
Medical Examinations and Coverage Continuance
Revised statutes of Nebraska, Section 44-1633.
Revised statutes of Nebraska, Section 48-221.
Polygraph Restrictions
Nebraska public Acts, L.B. 485(L. 1980).
Military Leaves of Absence
Revised statutes of Nebraska, Section 55-161.
Jury Duty
Revised statutes of Nebraska, Section 25-1640.
Service Letter
Revised statutes of Nebraska, Section 48-211.
Equal Pay
Revised statutes of Nebraska, Section 48-1221.

{93.06} Wage and Hour Laws

Child Labor
Revised statutes of Nebraska, Section 48-304.
Revised statutes of Nebraska, Section 48-302,303.

Voting Time
Revised statutes of Nebraska, Section 32-1046.
Payment of Wages
Revised statutes of Nebraska, Section 48-1230.
Payment Upon Termination
Revised statutes of Nebraska, Section 48-1231.
Garnishments
Revised statutes of Nebraska, Section 25-1558(b).

{93.07} SAFETY AND HEALTH LAWS

Revised statutes of Nebraska, Section 48-401, et seq.
Revised statutes of Nebraska, Section 48-404.

{93.08} UNEMPLOYMENT COMPENSATION LAWS

Revised statutes of Nebraska, Section 24-601, et seq.

{93.09} WORKERS COMPENSATION LAWS

Revised statutes of Nebraska, Section 48-101, et seq.
Revised statutes of Nebraska, Section 48-101, et seq.

{93.10} EMPLOYMENT-AT-WILL DEVELOPMENTS

See, for example: Mau v. Omaha Nat'l Bank, 299 N.W.2d 147 (Neb., 1980).
Morris v. Lutheran Medical Center, 340 N.W.2d 388 (Neb., 1983); see also Corso v. Creighton University, 731 F.2d 529 (CA-8, 1984).

NEVADA

{94.01} LABOR RELATIONS LAWS

General Right to Organize.
Nevada Revised Statutes, Section 614.100.
Municipal Employees Bargaining Right
Nevada Revised Statutes, Section 288.140
Nevada Revised Statutes, Section 288.270.
Nevada Revised Statutes, Section 288.010, et seq.
Right-to-Work Statute
Nevada Revised Statutes, Section 613.230, et seq.
"Yellow-Dog" Contracts
Nevada Revised Statutes, Section 613.130.

{94.02} STRIKES, PICKETING, AND BOYCOTT LAWS

Interference with Employment
Nevada Revised Statutes, Section 613.100

Strike Notices
Nevada Revised Statutes, Section 611.290.
Nevada Revised Statutes, Section 614.120.

{94.03} MEDIATION AND CONCILIATION LAWS

Nevada Revised Statutes, Section 38.035, et seq.
  Nevada Revised Statutes, Section 614.020.

{94.04} REGULATION OF UNION ACTIVITIES

Nevada Revised Statutes, Section 205.205.

{94.05} REGULATION OF EMPLOYMENT PRACTICES

Anti-Discrimination Statutes
  Nevada Revised Statutes, Section 613.310, et seq.
  Polygraph Restrictions
  Nevada public Acts, chapter 676 (L.1981).
  Protection of Political Freedom
  Nevada Revised Statutes, Section 613.040.
  Employment Under False Pretense
  Nevada Revised Statutes, Section 613.010.
  Jury and Witness Duty
  Nevada public Acts, chapter 150 (L.1977).
  Nevada Revised Statutes, Section 50.070.
  Backlisting
  Nevada Revised Statutes, Section 613.210, et seq.
  Service Letter
  Nevada Revised Statutes, Section 613.240.
  Discharge of Volunteer Firefighters
  Nevada Public Acts, chapter 381(L.1983).
  Restrictions on Detectives and "Spotters"
  Nevada Revised Statutes, Section 613.160
  Equal Pay
  Nevada Revised Statutes, Section 608.017

{94.06} WAGE AND HOUR LAWS

Child Labor
  Nevada Revised Statutes, Section 609.220, et. seq.
  Voting Time
  Nevada Revised Statutes, Section 293.463.
  Payment of Wages.
  Nevada Revised Statutes, Section 608.060.

Payment Upon Termination
Nevada Revised Statutes, Section 6608.020 and 608.030.

{94.07} SAFETY AND HEALTH LAWS

General Provisions
Nevada Revised Statutes, Section 618.375, et seq.
Toxic Substances - Right to Know
Nevada Revised Statutes, Section 668.380.
Nevada Revised Statutes, Section 618.370.

{94.08} UNEMPLOYMENT COMPENSATION LAWS

Nevada Revised Statutes, Section 612.010, et seq.

{94.09} WORKERS COMPENSATION LAWS

Nevada Revised Statutes, Section 616.570, et seq.

{94.10} EMPLOYMENT-AT-WILL DEVELOPMENTS

Public Police Exception
Hansen v. Harrah's 675 P.2d 394 (Nev. S. Ct., 1984).
Implied Contract Exception
Southwest Gas Crop. v. Ahmad, 668 P.2d 261 (Nev. S. Ct., 1983).

NEW HAMPSHIRE

{95.01} LABOR RELATIONS LAWS

State Employees Bargaining Rights
New Hampshire Revised Statutes, Chapter 273-A:1, et seq.
Municipal Employees Bargaining Rights
New Hampshire Public Acts, Chapter 255 (L.1955).
Nonright-to-Work Policy
Section 14(b) of the labor management relations act
"Yellow-Dog" Contracts
New Hampshire Revised Statutes, Chapter 275:2.

{95.02} STRIKES, PICKETING, AND BOYCOTT LAWS

Unlawful Assembly
New Hampshire Revised Statutes, Chapter 644:1
Striker Replacements
New Hampshire Revised Statutes, Chapter 275-A:2.

Strikebreakers
New Hampshire Revised Statutes, Chapter 275-A:2.
Restrictions on Use of National Guard in Strikes.
New Hampshire Revised Statutes, Chapter 111:1.

{95:03} Mediation and Conciliation Laws

New Hampshire Revised Statutes, Chapter 210:12, et seq.
New Hampshire Revised Statutes, Chapter 542:1.

{95.04} Regulation of Union Activities

New Hampshire Revised Statutes, Chapter 664:1, et seq.
New Hampshire Revised Statutes, Chapter 207:1-7.

{95.05} Regulation of Employment Practices

Anti-Discrimination Laws
New Hampshire Revised Statutes, Chapter 354-A:1, et seq.
Employment of Aliens
New Hampshire Revised Statutes, Chapter 275-A:4-5.
Freedom of Expression (State Employees)
New Hampshire Revised Statutes, Chapter 98-E:2.
Protection of Military Personnel
New Hampshire Revised Statutes, Chapter 110-B:65.
Unlawful Procurement of Employees
New Hampshire Revised Statutes, Chapter 275:7.
Access to Personnel Records
New Hampshire Revised Statutes, Chapter 275:55.
Consumer Reporting Agency Requirements
New Hampshire Revised Statutes, Chapter 359-B:3.
Equal Pay
New Hampshire Revised Statutes, Chapter 275:36-41.

{95.06} Wage and Hour Laws

Child Labor
New Hampshire Revised Statutes, Chapter 276A:4.
Payment of Wags
New Hampshire Revised Statutes, Chapter 275:43.
Payment Upon Termination
New Hampshire Revised Statutes, Chapter 277:44(I).
New Hampshire Revised Statutes, Chapter 277:44(II).
Medical Examinations and Insurance Coverage Continuance
New Hampshire Revised Statutes, Chapter 275:3.
New Hampshire Revised Statutes, Chapter 500:3.

{95.07} Safety and Health Laws

New Hampshire Revised Statutes, Chapter 277:11.
  New Hampshire Revised Statutes, Chapter 277:12.
  Toxic Substances-Right to Know
  New Hampshire Revised Statutes, Chapter 277-A:1, et seq.

{95.08} Unemployment Compensation Laws

New Hampshire Revised Statutes, Chapter 282-A:1, et seq.

{95.09} Workers Compensation Laws

New Hampshire Revised Statutes, Chapter 281-A:1, et seq.

{95.10} Employment-at-Will Developments

Covenant of Good Faith and Fair Dealing Excepting
  Monge v. Beebe Rubber Co., 316 A.2d 549 (N.H., 1974).
  Public Policy Exception
  Cloutier v. Great Atlantic and Pacific Tea Co., 436 A.2d 1140 (N.H., 1980).
  Independent Consideration Exception
  Foley v. Community Oil Co., 64 F.R.D. 561 (D N.H., 1974).

NEW JERSEY

{96.01} Labor Relations Laws

Public Utility Labor Disputes Act
  New Jersey Statutes Annotated, Section 34:13B-13.
  New Jersey Statutes Annotated, Section 34:13B-1.
  State Employees' Bargaining Rights
  New Jersey Statutes Annotated, Section 34:13A-1
  New Jersey Statutes Annotated, Section 34:13A-5.4
  Nonright-to-Work Policy:
  New Jersey Statutes Annotated, Section.14 (b).
  "Yellow-Dog" Contracts
  New Jersey Statutes Annotated, Section 34: 12-2.

{96.02} Strikes, Picketing, and Boycott Laws

Anti-Injunction Laws
  New Jersey Statutes Annotated, Section 2A: 15-51, *et seq.*
  Unlawful Assembly
  New Jersey Statutes Annotated, Section 2A:126-4.
  Restriction of Railroad Picketing
  New Jersey Statutes Annotated, Section 48:12-164, *et seq.*

Striker Replacements
New Jersey Statutes Annotated, Section 30:8-40.
New Jersey Statutes Annotated, Section 34:8-25.

{96.03} MEDIATION AND CONCILIATION LAWS

New Jersey Statutes Annotated, Section 34:13-1 *et seq.*

{96.04} REGULATION OF UNION ACTIVITIES

New Jersey Statutes Annotated, Section 56:2-1, *et seq.*
New Jersey Public Acts, Chapter 246 (L. 1962, 1963).

{96.05} REGULATION OF EMPLOYMENT PRACTICES

Anti-Discrimination Laws
New Jersey Statutes Annotated, Section 10:5-1, *et seq.*
Protection of Political Freedom
New Jersey Statutes Annotated, Section 19:34-27.
Reemployment Rights of Military Personnel
New Jersey Statutes Annotated, Section 10:5-5 (g); 10: 5-12.
Polygraph Restrictions
New Jersey Statutes Annotated, Section 2C:40 A-1.
Jury Duty (Public Employees)
New Jersey Statutes Annotated, Section 2A:69-5.
Convictions
New Jersey Statutes Annotated, Section 2C:52-1, et seq.
Medical Coverage Continuance
New Jersey Statutes Annotated, Section 17B:27-51.12.
Authorization of State Employees' Union Dues Deduction
New Jersey Statutes Annotated, Section 52:14-15.9C.
Equal Pay
New Jersey Statutes Annotated, Section 34:11-56.2.

{96.06} WAGE AND HOUR LAWS

Child Labor
New Jersey Statutes Annotated, Section 34:2-3,8, 11 and 15.
Payment of Wages.
New Jersey Statutes Annotated, Section 34:11-4.2.
Payment Upon Termination
New Jersey Statutes Annotated, Section 34:11-4.3.
Garnishment
New Jersey Statutes Annotated, Section 2A:170-90.4

{96.07} SAFETY AND HEALTH LAWS

General Provisions
New Jersey Statutes Annotated, Section 34:6A-3.
Toxic Substances - Right to Know
New Jersey Statutes Annotated, Section 34:5A-1.

{96.08} UNEMPLOYMENT COMPENSATION LAWS

New Jersey Statutes Annotated, Section 43:21-1, et seq.

{96.09} WORKER' COMPENSATION LAWS

New Jersey Statutes Annotated, Section 34:15-1, et seq.

{96.10} EMPLOYMENT-AT-WILL DEVELOPMENT

Public Police Exception
Lalley v. Copygraphics, 428 A.2d 1317 (N.J., 1981).
Implied Contract Exception
Wooley v. Hoffman-LaRoche, Inc., Case No. A-98-82 (N.J. S. Ct., 1985).

NEW MEXICO

{97.01} LABOR RELATIONS LAWS

State Employees' Bargaining Rights:
New Mexico Labor-Management Relations Regulations, Section 3.
New Mexico Labor-Management Relations Regulations, Section 16.
New Mexico Labor-Management Relations Regulations, Section 1, et seq.
Nonright-to-Work Policy:
New Mexico Labor-Management Relations Act, Section 14(b).
"Yellow-Dog" Contracts:
New Mexico Public Acts, S.B. 402 (L., 1967).

{97.02} STRIKES, PICKETING AND BOYCOTT LAWS

Anti-Injunction Statute:
New Mexico statutes, Section 59-2-1, et seq.
Unlawful Assembly:
New Mexico statutes, Section 41-1210.
Interference with Ingress:
New Mexico statutes, Section 50-2-2(b).

{97.03} MEDIATION AND ARBITRATION LAWS:

New Mexico statutes, Section 44-7-1.

{97.04} REGULATION OF UNION ACTIVITIES:

New Mexico statutes, Section 52-201, et seq.
   New Mexico statutes, Section 50-2-3.

{97.05} REGULATION OF EMPLOYMENT PRACTICES:

Anti-Discrimination Laws:
   New Mexico statutes, Section 28-1-1, et seq.
   Protection of Political Freedom:
   New Mexico statutes, Section 3-10-11.
   Reemployment Rights of Military Personnel:
   New Mexico statutes, Section 28-15-1, et seq.
   Jury Duty:
   New Mexico statutes, Section 38-5-18.
   Blacklisting:
   New Mexico statutes, Section 30-13-3.
   Arrest Records (Public Employees):
   New Mexico statutes, Section 28-2-3(B).
   Credit Bureau Requirements:
   New Mexico statutes, Section 56-3-5.

{97.06} WAGE AND HOUR LAWS

Child Labor:
   New Mexico statutes, Section 50-6-2.
   Voting Time:
   New Mexico statutes, Section 1-12-42.
   Payment of Wages:
   New Mexico statutes, Section 50-4-2.
   Payment Upon Termination:
   New Mexico statutes, Section 50-4-4.
   New Mexico statutes, Section 50-4-5.

{97.07} SAFETY AND HEALTH LAWS

General Provisions:
   New Mexico statutes, Section 52-1-8. **Toxic Substance—Right to Know:**
   New Mexico statutes, Section 50-9-1, et seq.

{97.08} UNEMPLOYMENT COMPENSATION LAWS:

New Mexico statutes, Section 51-1-4B, et seq.

{97.09} Workers' Compensation Laws:

New Mexico statutes, Section 52-1-8, et seq.
New Mexico statutes, Section 52-1-9, et seq.

{97.10} Employment-at-Will Developments:

Public Policy Exception:
Vigil v. Arzola, 687 P.2d 1038. (N.M. S. Ct., 1984).
Implied Contract Exception:
Forrester v. Parker, 606 P.2d 191 (N.M. S. Ct., 1980).

NEW YORK

{98.01} Labor Relation Laws

New York State Labor Relations Act:
Consolidated Laws of New York, Labor Laws, Section 700, et seq.
General Right to Organize:
New York Constitution, Section 17.
Port Authority Employees' Benefits:
New York Public Acts, Chapter 1203 (L. 1971).
Public Employees' Bargaining Rights:
Consolidated Laws of New York, Civil Service Laws, Section 202. Consolidated Laws of New York, Civil Service Laws, Section 209.
Consolidated Laws of New York, Civil Service Laws, Section 200, et seq.
Labor and Management Improper Practices Act:
New York Labor and Management Improper Practices Act, Section 720, et seq.
Nonright-to-Work Policy:
New York Labor of Management Relations Acts, Section 14(b).
"Yellow-Dog" Contracts:
New York Public Acts, Chapter 11 (L. 1935).

{98.02} Strikes, Picketing, and Boycott Laws:

Anti-Injunction Statue: New York Anti-injunction Act, Section 807, et seq.
Interference with Employment:
Consolidated Laws of New York, Penal Code, Section 580.
Use of Detectives During Strikes:
Consolidated Laws of New York, General Business Law, Section 84.

{98.03} Mediation and Arbitration Laws:

State Civil Practice Law, Section 7501.
Consolidated Laws of New York, Labor Laws, Section 751, et seq.

General Municipal Law, Section 601, et seq.
Consolidated Laws of New York, Penal Code, Section 373.
Consolidated Laws of New York, Penal Code, Section 376 and 860.

{98.04} REGULATION OF UNION ACTIVITIES:

Consolidated Laws of New York, Labor Laws, Section 209.
Consolidated Laws of New York, Labor Laws, Section 209-a.
New York Labor and Management Improper Practices Act, Section 726.
New York Mitchell-Hollinger Law, Section 37, et seq.
Consolidated Laws of New York, Insurance and Banking Laws, Section 37, et seq.
Consolidated Laws of New York, Unconsolidated Laws, Section 9801, et seq.

{98.05} REGULATION OF EMPLOYMENT PRACTICES

Anti-Discrimination Laws:
Consolidated Laws of New York, Executive Laws, Section 291, et seq.
Employment Agency Requirements:
Consolidated Laws of New York, General Business laws, Section 187.
Psychogalvanic Stress Evaluation Exams:
Consolidated Laws of New York, Labor laws, Section 733, et seq.
Misrepresentation of Employment Opportunities:
Consolidated Laws of New York, General Business laws, Section 396-1.
Arrest and Conviction Record:
New York Executive Laws, Section 296(15) and (16).
Fingerprinting Limitations:
Consolidated Laws of New York, Labor Laws, Section 201-a.
Disclosure of Consumer Reports:
New York General Business laws, Section 380(a).
Jury and Witness Duty:
Consolidated Laws of New York, Judiciary laws, Section 519.
Consolidated Laws of New York, Penal Code, Section 215.11.
Importation of Migratory Farm Labor:
Consolidated Laws of New York, Labor laws, Section 212a.
Whistle-Blowing Statutes:
Consolidated Laws of New York, Labor laws, Section 740.
Protection of Railroad Employees:
New York Railroad Laws, Section 54-b.
Protection of Military Personnel:
New York Military Laws, Section 318.
Blacklisting:
Consolidated Laws of New York, Labor laws, Section 704(2).
Medical Examination Payment:
Consolidated Laws of New York, Labor laws, Section 210b.

Eavesdropping on Union Activities:
Consolidated Laws of New York, Labor laws, Section 704.
Equal Pay:
Consolidated Laws of New York, Labor laws, Section194.

{98.06} Wage and Hour Laws

Child Labor:
Consolidated Laws of New York, Labor laws, Section130.
Consolidated Laws of New York, Labor laws, Section 131(4).
Consolidated Laws of New York, Labor laws, Section 3215(4).
Voting Time:
Consolidated Laws of New York, election laws, Section 3.110.
Payment Upon Termination:
Consolidated Laws of New York, Labor laws, Section 191(3).
Garnishments:
New York Civil Practices Laws and Rules, Section 5252.
Medical Insurances Continuance:
Consolidated Laws of New York, insurance laws, Section 162(5)(a).

{98.07} Safety and Health Laws:

General Provision:
Consolidated Laws of New York, Labor laws, Section 28(2)(a).
Toxic Substances—Right to Know:
New York Toxic Substances laws, Section 875, et seq.

{98.08} Unemployment Compensation Laws:

Consolidated Laws of New York, Labor laws, Section 591, et seq.
See Consolidated Laws of New York, Labor laws, Section 591, et seq.

{98.09} Workers' Compensation:

Consolidated Laws of New York, Workers' Compensation laws, Section 1, et seq.
Consolidated Laws of New York, Workers' Compensation laws, Section 10 and 11.

{98.10} Employment-at-Will Developments:

Implied Contract Exception:
Weiner v. McGraw-Hill, 443 N.E.2d 441 (N.Y., 1982); as limited by certain requirement therein.
Promissory Estoppel Exception:
Myers v. Conradian Corp., 459 N.Y.S.2d 929 (1983).

NORTH CAROLINA

{99.01} Labor Regulation Laws

Ban Against Joining Unions (Public Employees):
General Statutes of North Caroline, Section 95-98.
Right-to-Work Statutes:
General Statutes of North Caroline, Section 97-78, et seq.

{99.02} Strikes, Picketing, and Boycott Laws:

Unlawful Assembly:
General Statutes of North Caroline, Section 15-30.
Possession of Weapons on Picket Lines:
General Statutes of North Caroline, Section 14-277.2.
Public Employee Strikes Prohibited:
General Statutes of North Caroline, Section 95-98.1.

{99.03} Mediation and Arbitration Laws:

General Statutes of North Caroline, Section 95-32, et seq.
General Statutes of North Caroline, Section 95-36.1, et seq.

{99.04} Regulation of Union Activities:

General Statutes of North Caroline, Section 95-101.2.
General Statutes of North Caroline, Section 80-8 and 80-9.

{99.05} Regulation of Employment Practices

Anti-Discrimination Laws:
General Statutes of North Caroline, Section 143-422.1.
General Statutes of North Caroline, Section 95-28.
Re-Employment Right of Military personnel:
General Statutes of North Caroline, Section 127A-201, et seq.
Blacklisting:
General Statutes of North Caroline, Section 14-355 and 14-356.
Unlawful Enticement:
General Statutes of North Caroline, Section 14-347.
General Statutes of North Caroline, Section 14-349.
Fraudulent Receipt of Wage Advancement:
General Statutes of North Caroline, Section 14-104.
Medical examination payment:
General Statutes of North Caroline, Section 14-357.

{99.06} Wage and Hour Laws

Child Labor:
General Statutes of North Caroline, Section 95-25.
General Statutes of North Caroline, Section 95-25.5(a) and (d).
Payment of Wages:
General Statutes of North Caroline, Section 95-25.6.
General Statutes of North Caroline, Section 95-98.
Payment Upon:
General Statutes of North Caroline, Section 95.25.7.

{99.07} Safety and Hour Laws

General Provisions:
General Statutes of North Caroline, Section 95-129(1).
General Statutes of North Caroline, Section 95-129(2).
Toxic Substance—Right to Know:
General Statutes of North Caroline, Section 95-143.

{99.08} Unemployment Compensation Laws:

General Statutes of North Caroline, Section 96-13, et seq.

{99.09} Workers' Compensation Laws:

General Statutes of North Caroline, Section 97-1 et seq.
General Statutes of North Caroline, Section 97-6.1.

{99.10} Employment-at-will Developments:

Brooks v. Carolina Tel. and Co., 290 S.E.2d 370 (N.C., 1982).
Roberts v. Mays Mills, Inc., 114 S.E. 530 (N.C., 1922).
Implied Contract Exception:
Still v. Lance 182 S.E.2d 403 (N.C. S. Ct., 1971); see also: Sides v. Duke Hospital, Case No. 83145C1308 (N.C. Ct., of App 1985).
Public Policy Exception:
Sides v. Duke Hospital, supra.

NORTH DAKOTA

{100.01} Labor Dakota Laws

North Dakota Labor Management Relation:
North Dakota Century Code, Section 34-12-01, et seq.

Teachers' Bargaining Rights:
North Dakota Century Code, Section 15-38.01-07.
Court Enforcement of Collective Bargaining Contracts:
North Dakota Century Code, Section 34-09-08.
Public Policy Regarding Bargaining Rights:
North Dakota Century Code, Section 34-09-01.
Right-to-Work Statute:
North Dakota Century Code, Section 34-01-14.
"Yellow-Dog" Contracts:
North Dakota Century Code, Section 34-08-04.

{100.02} Strikes, Picketing, and Boycott Laws

Anti-Injunction Statutes:
North Dakota Century Code, Section 34-08-03.
Stranger Picketing:
North Dakota Century Code, Section 34-09-12.
Secondary Boycotts:
North Dakota Century Code, Section 34-09-13.
Unlawful Assembly:
North Dakota Century Code, Section 34-19-06.
Striker Replacement Notices:
North Dakota public acts, chapter 255, Section 10(L. 1963).
Unlawful Interference with Employment:
North Dakota Century Code, Section 34-01-04, et seq.
Public Utility Strikes:
North Dakota Century Code, Section 37-01-06, et seq.

{100.03} Mediation and Arbitration Laws:

North Dakota Century Code, Section 34-11-01.
North Dakota Century Code, Section 34-11-01, et seq.
North Dakota Century Code, Section 34-11-03.
North Dakota Century Code, Section 34-29-01.

{100.04} Regulation of Union Activities:

North Dakota Century Code, Section 12-38-19.
North Dakota Century Code, Section 34-01-16.

{100.05} Regulation of Employment Practices

Anti-Discrimination Laws:
North Dakota Century Code, Section 14-02.4-03.
Rights of Military Personnel (Public Employees):

North Dakota Century Code, Section 37-01-25.1.
Backlisting:
North Dakota Century Code, Section 34-12-03.
Jury Duty:
North Dakota public acts, S.B, 2320 (L.1971).
Fraudulent Receipt of Wage Advancement:
North Dakota Century Code, Section 34-01-10.
Protection of Political Activities (Public Employees):
North Dakota Century Code, Section 34-01-10.
Medical Examination Payment:
North Dakota Century Code, Section 34-01-15.
Polygraph Requirements:
North Dakota Century Code, Section 41-31-03.
Equal Pay:
North Dakota Century Code, Section 34-06.1-03.

{100.06} Wage and Hour Laws

Child Labor:
North Dakota Century Code, Section 34-07-03, et seq.
Payment of Wage:
North Dakota Century Code, Section 34-14-02.
Payment Upon Termination:
North Dakota Century Code, Section 34-14-03(1).
North Dakota Century Code, Section 34-14-03(2).
Garnishments:
North Dakota Century Code, Section 32-09.1-18.

{100.07} Safety and Health Laws

North Dakota Century Code, Section 65-03-01.

{100.08} Unemployment Compensation:

North Dakota Century Code, Section 52-06-01, et seq.

{100.09} Workers' Compensation Laws:

North Dakota Century Code, Section 56-01-01, et seq.
North Dakota Century Code, Section 56-05-01, et seq.

{100.10} Employment-at-will Development:

Wood v. Buchanan, 5 N.W.2d 680 (N.D., 1942).
Aasmundstad v. Dickenson State College, 337 N.W.2d 792 (N.D., 1983).

OHIO

{101.01} Labor Relations Laws

Public Employment Bargaining Right
Ohio Statutes, Section 4117.03.
Ohio Statutes, Section 4117.11
Ohio Statutes, Section 4117.01, et seq.
Public Utility Bargaining
Ohio Statutes, Section 717.03.
Successor Employers Bargaining:
Ohio Statutes, Section 4113.30.
Nonright-to-Work Policy
Section 14(b) of the labor management relations act
"Yellow-Dog" Contract
Ohio Statutes, Section 4113.02.

{101.02} Strikes, Picketing, and Boycott Laws

Unlawful Assembly
Ohio Statutes, Section 3761.13.
Striker Replacements
Ohio Statutes, Section 4143.12.
Injury to Person or Property
Ohio Statutes, Section 2901.07.

{101.03} Mediation and Arbitration Laws

Ohio Statutes, Section 2711.01, et seq.
Ohio Statutes, Section 4129.02.
Ohio Statutes, Section 4129.03, et seq.

{101.04} Regulation of Unlon Activities

Ohio Statutes, Section 2911.27.

{101.05} Regulation of Employment Practices

Anti-Discrimination Laws.
Ohio Statutes, Section 4112.02.
Arrest Records
Ohio Statutes, Section 2953.42.
Conviction Records
Ohio Statutes, Section 2953.32.
Access to Medical Records
Ohio Statutes, Section 3113.23.

Jury and Witness Duty
Ohio Statutes, Section 2313.18.
Ohio Statutes, Section 2313.18.
Military Leave of Absence.
Ohio Statutes, Section 5903.061.
Use of Railroad "Spotters"
Ohio Statutes, Section 4999.17.
Protection of Political Activities
Ohio Statutes, Section 3599.06.
Blacklisting
Ohio Statutes, Section 1331.03.
Medical Examination Payment
Ohio Statutes, Section 4113.21.
Service Letter
Ohio Statutes, Section 4973.03.
Equal Pay
Ohio Statutes, Section 4111.17.

{101.06} WAGE AND HOUR LAWS

Child Labor
Ohio Statutes, Section 4109.01.
Ohio Statutes, Section 3331.01:4109.01.
Garnishments
Ohio Statutes, Section 2716.05.
Notice of Medical Insurance Continuance
Ohio Statutes, Section 1737.30.

{101.07} SAFETY AND HEALTH LAWS

Ohio Statutes, Section 4101.11.

{101.08} UNEMPLOYMENT COMPENSATION LAWS

Ohio Statutes, Section 4141.01, st seq.

{101.09} WORKERS COMPENSATION LAWS:

Ohio Statutes, Section 4121.01, et seq.
Ohio Statutes, Section 4123.90.
Ohio Statutes, Section 4123.54.

{101.10} EMPLOYMENT -AT-WILL DEVELOPMENTS

Henkel v. Educational Research Council of America, 334 N.E.2d 118 (Ohio, 1976).

Implied Contract Exception:
See, for example: Day v. Good Samaritan Hospital, Case No. 8062(2nd App. Dist. Of Ohio, 1983).
Promissory Estoppel Exception:
Jones v. East Center for Community Mental Health, Case No. L-83-280 (6th App. Dist. Of Ohio, 1984).
Public Policy Exception:
Merkel v. Scovill, Inc., 570 F. Supp. 133 (S.D. Ohio, 1983).

OKLAHOMA

{102.01} Labor Relations Laws

Collective Bargaining Laws.
Oklahoma statutes Annotated 11:51-101.
Oklahoma statutes Annotated 70:509.1, et seq.
Nonright-to-Work Police
Section 14(b) of the labor management relations act

{102.02} Strikes, Picketing, and Boycott Laws

Unlawful Assembly
Oklahoma statutes Annotated 21:1311, et seq.
Use of Prisoners During Strike
Title 57 Section 543.
Use of Detectives During Strike
Oklahoma statutes Annotated 40:169.
Strikebreakers
Title 40 Section 1991.1.
Strike Replacement
Oklahoma statutes Annotated 40:169.
Seizure of Property
Title 21 Section 1351.
Unlawful Interference with Employment
Oklahoma statutes Annotated 21:837 and 21:838.

{102.03} Mediation and Arbitration Laws

Oklahoma statutes Annotated 59:94 (c).
Oklahoma statutes Annotated 59:743 (c).

{102.04} Regulation of Unlon Activities

Oklahoma statutes Annotated 78:9, et seq.

{102.05} Regulation of Employment Practices

Anti-Discrimination Laws
Oklahoma statutes Annotated 25:1302.
Employment Under False Pretense
Oklahoma statutes Annotated Title 21 Section 1351.
Protection of Political Freedom
Oklahoma statutes Annotated 26:440.
Leaves of Absence for Political Activities
Oklahoma statutes Annotated Title 40 Section 184, et seq.
Jury Service
Oklahoma statutes Annotated 38:34.
National Guard Members
Oklahoma statutes Annotated Title 44 Section 208.
Freedom of Expression
See Oklahoma public acts, H.B.1128 (L.1981).
Service Letter
Oklahoma statutes Annotated Title 40 Section 171.
Backlisting
Oklahoma statutes Annotated 40:172.
Medical Examinations
Oklahoma statutes Annotated Title 40 Section 191, et seq.
Equal Pay
Oklahoma statutes Annotated 40:198.1.

{102.06} Wage and Hour Laws

Child Labor
Oklahoma statutes Annotated 40:71.
Oklahoma statutes Annotated 40:74 through 77.
Voting Time
Oklahoma statutes Annotated 26:7-101.
Payment of Wages
Oklahoma statutes Annotated Title 40 Section 165.
Payment Upon Termination
Oklahoma statutes Annotated 26:165.3.
Garnishments
Oklahoma statutes Annotated 14A:5-106.

{102.07} Safety and Health Laws

Oklahoma statutes Annotated Title 40 Section 403(1), et seq.

{102.08} Unemployment Compensation

Oklahoma statutes Annotated Title 40 Section 2-201, et seq.

{102.09} Workers Compensation Laws

Oklahoma statutes Annotated 85:1, et seq.

{102.10} Employment-at-will Developments

General Rule
Foster v. Atlas Life Ins., Co., 6 P.2d 428 (CA-10, 1984); Langdon v. Sage Corp., 569 P.2d 524 (Okla. App., 1976).
Implied Contract Exception
Vinyard v. King, 728 F.2d 428 (CA-10, 1984); Langdon v. Sage Corp., 569 P.2d 524 (Okla. App., 1976).
Hall v. Farmers Ins. Exchange, Case no.59584 (Okla. S. Ct., 1985).

OREGON

{103.01} Labor Relations Laws

Labor Peace Act
Oregon revised statutes, Section 663.005, et seq.
Nurses Bargaining Rights.
Oregon revised statutes, Section 662.705.
Public Employees Bargaining Rights
Oregon revised statutes, Section 243.662.
Oregon revised statutes, Section 243.672.
Oregon revised statutes, Section 243.650, et seq.
Nonright-to-Work Policy
Section 14(b) of the labor management relations act.
"Yellow-Dog" Contracts
Oregon revised statutes, Section 662.030.

{103.02} Strikes, Picketing, and Boycott Laws

Anti-injunction laws
Oregon revised statutes, Section 662.010 et seq.
Secondary Boycotts and Hot Cargo Clauses Forbidden
Oregon revised statutes, Section 663.210, et seq.
Unlawful Interference with Employment
Oregon revised statutes, Section 659.240.
Unlawful Assembly
Oregon revised statutes, Section.23-801.
Picketing of Farms
Oregon public Acts, Chapter 543 (L.1963).
Striker Replacements
Oregon revised statutes, Section 658.225.
Strikebreakers.
Oregon public Acts, Chapter 645 (L.1975).

{103.03} Mediation and Arbitration Laws

Oregon revised statutes, Section 662.405.

{103.04} Regulation of Unlon Activities

Oregon revised statutes, Section 661.210, et seq.

{103.05} Regulation of Employment Practices

Anti-Discrimination Laws.
Oregon revised statutes, Section 659.425.
Polygraph Restrictions
Oregon revised statutes, Section 659.227.
Jury Services
Oregon public Acts, Chapter 160 (L.1975).
Access to Personnel Records
Oregon revised statutes, Section 652.750.
Whistle-Blowing Statute
Oregon revised statutes, Section 240.3165.
Employment Under False Pretense
Oregon revised statutes, Section 659.260.
Fraudulent Receipt of Wage Advances.
Oregon revised statutes, Section 659.250.
Blacklisting
Oregon revised statutes, Section 659.330.
National Guard Duty
Oregon revised statutes, Section 408,210, et seq.
Anti-nepotism Discrimination
Oregon revised statutes, Section 659.340.
Medical Examinations
Oregon revised statutes, Section 659.330.
Prior Testimony
Oregon revised statutes, Section 659.270.
Juvenile Record
Oregon revised statutes, Section 659.030 (a).

{103.06} Wage and Hour Laws

Child Labor
Oregon Wage and hour commission Rules, OAR 21-215(1).
Payment of Wages
Oregon revised statutes, Section 652.120.
Payment Upon Termination
Oregon Revised Statutes, Section 652.140(1).
Garnishments

Oregon revised statutes, Section 23.185(5).
Medical Insurance Conversion
Oregon revised statutes, Section 743.850.

{103.07} SAFETY AND HEALTH LAWS

Oregon revised statutes, Section 654.010.

{103.08} UNEMPLOYMENT COMPENSATION LAWS

Oregon revised statutes, Section 656.001, et seq.

{103.10} EMPLOYMENT-AT -WILL DEVELOPMENTS

Implied Contract Exception
Fleming V. Kids and kin Head start, 693 P. 2d 1363 (Ore. S.ct., 1985).
Public Policy Exception
Nees v. Hocks, 536 p.2d 512(Ore., 1975).
Intentional Infliction of Emotional Distress Exception.
Smithson v. Nordstrom, Inc., 664 P.2p 1119(Ore Ct. of App., 1983).

PENNSYLVANIA

{104.01} LABOR RELATIONS LAWS

General Right to Organize
Pennsylvania statutes, Title 43, Section 191.
Pennsylvania Labor Relations Act
Pennsylvania statutes, Title 43, Section 211.1, et seq.
Public Employees Bargaining Rights
Pennsylvania Employee Relations Act, Section 401.
Pennsylvania Employee Relations Act, Section 101, et seq.
Public Transit Employees Bargaining Rights
Pennsylvania public laws Act, Section 288 (L.1967).
Firefighters and Police Officers Bargaining Rights
Pennsylvania public laws Act, Section 111 (L.1968).
Nonright-to-Work Policy
Section 14 (b) of the labor management relations.
"Yellow-Dog" Contracts
Pennsylvania statutes, Title 18, Section 4669.

{104.02} STRIKES PICKETING, AND BOYCOTT LAWS

Anti-Injunction Laws
Pennsylvania statutes, Title 43, Section 206a, et seq.

Strikebreakers Replacements
Pennsylvania statutes, Title 43, Section 23.
Pennsylvania public laws Act, Section 187 (L.1972).
Strikebreakers
Pennsylvania public laws Act, Section 111 (L.1968).
Right to Strike
Pennsylvania public laws Act, Section 187 (L.1972).
Interference with Railroads
Pennsylvania public laws Act, 872 (L.1939).
Pennsylvania statutes, Title 18, Section 4664, And Title 18, Section 4921.

{104.03} MEDIATION AND ARBITRATION LAWS

Pennsylvania statutes, Title 42, Section 7303.

{104.04} REGULATION OF UNLON ACTIVITIES

Pennsylvania statutes, Title 73, Section 105.
   Pennsylvania statutes, Title 25, Section 3225.

{104.05} ANTI-DISCRIMINATION LAWS

Pennsylvania statutes, Title 43, Section 955.
   Arrest Records
   Pennsylvania public laws, H.B.2095 (L.1978).
   Polygraph Restrictions
   Pennsylvania statutes, Title 18, Section 7321.
   Voice Stress Analyzers
   Pennsylvania statutes, Title 18, Section 7507.
   Employment Under False Pretenses
   Title 18, Section 4856, of the Pennsylvania.
   Interference with Employment
   Title 18, Section 4670, of the Pennsylvania.
   Protection of Political Freedom
   Pennsylvania statutes, Title 25, Section 3547.
   Jury Service
   Pennsylvania public laws Act, 17 (L.1978).
   Protection of Volunteer Firefighters
   Pennsylvania public laws Act, Section 83 (L.1977).
   Access to Personnel Records
   Pennsylvania public laws Act, 286 (L.1978).
   Medical Examination Payments
   Title 43, Section 1002, of the Pennsylvania.
   Equal Pay
   Pennsylvania public laws Act, 694 (L.1968).

{104.06} Wage and Hour Laws

Child Labor
Pennsylvania statutes, Title 24, Section 13-1391.
Payment of Wages
Pennsylvania public laws Act, 329 (L.1961).
Payment on Termination
Pennsylvania public laws Act, 329 (L.1961).
Medical Insurance Continuance
Title 40, Section 756.2, of the Pennsylvania.

{104.07} Health and Safety Laws

Title 43, Section 9, et seq. of the Pennsylvania.

{104.08} Unemployment Compensation Laws

Pennsylvania statutes, Title 43, Section 751, et seq.

{104.09} workers Compensation

Pennsylvania statutes, Title 77, Section 1, et seq.

{104.10} Public Policy Exception

McNulty v. Borden, Inc., 474 F.Supp. 1111 (E.D. Pa., 1979).
Independent Consideration Exception
Cory v. SmithKline Beckman Corp., 116 LRRM 3361 (E.D. Pa., 1984).
Intentional Infliction of Emotional Distress Exception
Shaffer v. National Can Corp., 565 F.Supp. 909 (E.D Pa., 1983)

RHODE ISLAND

{105.01} Labor Relations Laws

Rhode Island State Labor Relations Act
Section 28-7-1, et seq. of the Rhode Island General laws
Public Employees Bargaining Rights
Rhode Island General laws, Section 36-11-1, et seq.
Municipal Employees Bargaining Rights
Rhode Island General laws, Section 28-9.4-1, et seq.
Teachers Bargaining Rights
Rhode Island General laws, Section 28-9.3-9.
Firefighters and Police Officers Bargaining Rights
Rhode Island General laws, Section 28-9.1-2, et seq.
Rhode Island General laws, Section 28-9.2-2 et seq.

State Police Officers Bargaining Rights
Section 28-9. 5-1, et seq. of the Rhode Island General laws.
Nonright-to-Work Police
Section 14(b) of the labor management relations act
"Yellow-Dog" Contracts
Section 28-7-13, et seq. of the Rhode Island General laws

{105.02} STRIKES, PICKETING, AND BOYCOTT LAWS

Anti-Injunction Laws
Rhode Island General laws, Section 28-10-2 et seq.
Unlawful Assemble
Rhode Island General laws, Section 11-38-1.
Interference with Employment
Rhode Island General laws, Section 11-11-4.
Interference with Railroads
Rhode Island General laws, Section 11-36-3.
Use of Tear Gas Prohibited During Strikes
Rhode Island General laws, Section 28-10-7 and 28-10-8.
Strikebreakers and Replacement Notices
Rhode Island General laws, Section 28-10-10 et seq.
Rhode Island General laws, Section 28-10-13.

{105.03} MEDIATION AND ARBITRATION LAWS

Rhode Island General laws, Section 28-9-1.

{105.04} REGULATION OF UNION ACTIVITIES

Rhode Island General laws, Section 11-14-5.

{105.05} REGULATION OF EMPLOYMENT PRACTICES

Anti-Discrimination Laws
Rhode Island General laws, Section 28-5-7 et seq.
Polygraph Restrictions
Rhode Island General laws, Section 28-6.1-1.
Arrest Records
Rhode Island General laws, Section 28-5-7.
Medical Examinations Payment
Rhode Island General laws, Section 28-6.2-1.
Protection of Political Freedom
Rhode Island General laws, Section 17-23-5.
Confidentiality of Medical Information
Rhode Island General laws, Section 5-37.3-4(a).
Rhode Island public laws. Chapter 119 (L.1968).

Reemployment Rights of Military Personnel
Rhode Island General laws, Section 30-11-2 et seq.
Jury Duty
Rhode Island General laws, Section 9-9-28.
Equal Pay
Rhode Island General laws, Section 28-6-17.

{105.06} Wage Labor Hour Laws

Child Labor
Rhode Island General laws, Section 28-3-1 et seq.
Payment of Wages
Rhode Island General laws, Section 28-14-2.
Payment Upon Termination
Rhode Island General laws, Section 28-14-4.
Garnishments
Rhode Island General laws, Section 15-13-1.
Medical Insurance Continuance
Rhode Island General laws, Section 27-19.1-1.

{105.07} Health and Safety Laws

General Provisions
Rhode Island General laws, Section 28-20-8(a).
Toxic Substances-Right to Know
Rhode Island General laws, Section 28-21-1 et seq.

{105.08} Unemployment Compensation Laws

Rhode Island General laws, Section 28-44-1, et seq.

{105.09} Worker Compensation Laws

Rhode Island General laws, Section 28-33-1 et seq.

{105.10} Employment-at-will Developments

Lamoureax v. Burrillville Racing Ass'n., 161 A.2d 213 (R.I., 1960).

SOUTH CAROLINA

{106.01} Labor Relations Laws

Grievance Procedures
South Carolina public laws. H.B. 2626 (L.1982).
Code of laws of South Carolina. Section 8-17-110.

Right-to-Work Statute
Code of laws of South Carolina. Section 41-7-10.
"Yellow-Dog" Contracts
Code of laws of South Carolina. Section 41-7-30(2)

{106.02} Strikes, Picketing, and Boycott Laws

Unlawful Assembly Against Political Beliefs
Code of laws of South Carolina. Section 16-101.
Striker Replacement
Code of laws of South Carolina. Section 41-25-50(c).
Use of Detectives During Strikes
Article 8, Section 9, of the South Carolina Constitution.

{106.03} Mediation and Arbitration Laws

Code of laws of South Carolina. Section 41-17-10.
Article 6, Section 1, of the South Carolina Constitution.

{106.04} Regulation of Union Activities

Code of laws of South Carolina. Section 39-15-110.

{106.05} Regulation of Employment Practices

Anti-Discrimination Laws
Code of laws of South Carolina. Section 1-13-80 and 43-33-550.
Protection of Political Freedom
Code of laws of South Carolina. Section 16-17-560.
Reemployment Right of Military Personnel
Code of laws of South Carolina. Section 25-1-2310
Discrimination Against Union Members
Code of laws of South Carolina. Section 41-1-20.
Plant Closings
Code of laws of South Carolina. Section 41-1-40.
Voice Stress Analyzers
Code of laws of South Carolina. Section 40-53-40.

{106.06} Wage and Hours Laws

Child Labor
Code of laws of South Carolina. Section 41-13-110, et seq.
Payment on Termination
Code of laws of South Carolina. Section 41-11-170.
Garnishments
Code of laws of South Carolina. Section 37-5-106.

Medical Insurance Conversion
Code of laws of South Carolina. Section38-35-946.

{106.07} SAFETY AND HEALTH LAWS

General Provisions
Code of laws of South Carolina. Section 41-15-80.
Toxic Substances- Right to Know
Code of laws of South Carolina. Section 41-15-210.

{106.08} UNEMPLOYMENT COMPENSATION LAWS

Code of laws and govern of South Carolina. Section 41-27-10.

{106.09} WORKERS COMPENSATION LAWS

Code of laws of South Carolina. Section 42-1-10, et seq.

{106.10} EMPLOYMENT-AT-WILL DEVELOPMENTS

Todd v. South Caroline Farm Bureau Mut. Ins. Co., 278 S.E.2d 607 (S.C., 1981).
Tyler v. Macks Stores of South Caroline, Inc., 272 S.E.2d 633 (S.C. S. Ct., 1980).
Ludwick v. This Minute of Caroline, Inc., Case no. 22408 (S.C. S. Ct., 1985).

SOUTH DAKOTA

{107.01} LABOR RELATION LAWS

South Dakota Labor Relations Act
South Dakota Compiled Laws, 60-9A-1, et seq.
South Dakota Compiled Laws, 60-9A-7 and 12.
Public Employees Bargaining Rights
South Dakota Compiled Laws, Section 3-18-1, et seq.
Right-to-Work Statute
South Dakota Compiled Laws, Section 60-8-3, et seq.

{107.02} STRIKES, PICKETING, AND BOYCOTT LAWS

Unlawful Assembly
South Dakota Compiled Laws, Section 22-10-1, et seq.
Unlawful Interference with Employment
South Dakota Compiled Laws, Section 60-8-1.
Unlawful Picketing
South Dakota Compiled Laws, Section 60-10-9.
Strike Notice
South Dakota Compiled Laws, Section 60-6-19 and 20.

{107.03} Mediation and Arbitration Laws

South Dakota Compiled Laws, Section 60-10-1.

{107.04} Regulation of Union Activities

South Dakota Compiled Laws, Section 37-6-2.
   South Dakota Compiled Laws, Section 60-9-2.
   South Dakota Compiled Laws, Section 60-9-8.

{107.05} Regulation of Employment Practices

Anti-Discrimination Laws
   South Dakota Compiled Laws, Section 20-13-1, et seq.
   Protection of Political Freedom
   South Dakota Compiled Laws, Section 12-26-13.
   Jury Duty
   South Dakota Compiled Laws, Section 16-13-41.1
   Access to Personnel Records
   South Dakota Compiled Laws, Section 3-6A-31.
   Military Duty
   South Dakota Compiled Laws, Section 33-17-15.
   Medical Examination Payments
   South Dakota Compiled Laws, Section 60-11-2.
   Equal Pay
   South Dakota Compiled Laws, Section 60-12-15.

{107.06} Wage and Hour Laws

Child Labor
   South Dakota Compiled Laws, Section 60-12-2, et seq.
   South Dakota Compiled Laws, Section 60-12-4.
   Voting Time
   South Dakota Compiled Laws, Section 12-3-5.
   Payment of Wages
   South Dakota Compiled Laws, Section 60-11-9.
   Payment Upon Termination
   South Dakota Compiled Laws, Section 60-11-10.

{107.07} Safety and Health Laws

South Dakota Compiled Laws, Section 60-12-7, et seq.

{107.08} Unemployment Compensation Laws

South Dakota Compiled Laws, Section 61-6-20, et seq.

{107.09} Workers Compensation Laws

South Dakota Compiled Laws, Section 62-5-1, et seq.

{107.10} Employment-at-will Developments

Implied Contract Exception
Osterkamp v. Alkota Manufacturing, Inc., 332 N.W.2d 275 (S.D., 1983).
Presumption of Term Exception
South Dakota Public Laws, S.B. 263 (L., 1985).

TENNESSEE

{108.01} Labor Relation Laws

Professional Negotiations Act
Tennessee Code Annotated Section 49-5-601, et seq.
Public Transit Employees Bargaining Rights
Tennessee Code Annotated Section 7-56-102.
Collective Bargaining Sunshine Laws
Tennessee Code Annotated Section 8-44-201.
Right-to-Work Statute
Tennessee Code Annotated Section 50-1-201.

{108.02} Strikes, Picketing, and Boycott Laws

Use of Armed Guards During Strikes
Tennessee Code Annotated Section 50-1-102(d), (e).
"Sit-Down" Strikes
Tennessee Code Annotated Section 50-1-303.
Strike Replacement Notices
Tennessee Code Annotated Section 50-8-111.
Unlawful Inducement for Employment
Tennessee Code Annotated Section 47-1706.

{108-03} Mediation and Arbitration Laws

Tennessee Code Annotated Section 29-5-101.

{108.04} Regulation of Union Activities

Tennessee Code Annotated Section 47-25-407, et seq.

{108.05} Regulation of Employment Practices

Anti-Discrimination Laws

Tennessee Code Annotated Section 4-21-105, et seq.
Tennessee Code Annotated Section 8-50-103.
Freedom of Political Activities
Tennessee Code Annotated Section 2-19-34.
Jury Service
Tennessee Code Annotated Section 22-4-108.
Unlawful Enticement
Tennessee Code Annotated Section 50-1-101(a).
Selection of Physician
Tennessee Code Annotated Section 50-1-302(a).
Access to Personnel Records
Tennessee Code Annotated Section 8-50-108.
Tennessee Code Annotated Section 49-224.
Medical Examination Payments
Tennessee Code Annotated Section 50-1-302.
Equal Pay
Tennessee Code Annotated Section 50-2-202.

{108.06} WAGE AND HOUR LAWS

Child Labor
Tennessee Code Annotated Section 50-5-103, et seq.
Voting Time
Tennessee Code Annotated Section 2-1-108, et seq.
Payment of Wages
Tennessee Code Annotated Section 50-2-103(a).
Medical Coverage Conversion
Tennessee Code Annotated Section 56-7-1501.
Wage Assignments for Child Support
Tennessee Code Annotated Section 50-2-105

{108.07} HEALTH AND SAFETY LAWS

General Provisions
Tennessee Code Annotated Section 50-3-105.
Toxic Substances-Right to Know
Tennessee Public Laws, Ch. 417 (L. 1985).

{108.08} UNEMPLOYMENT COMPENSATION LAWS

Tennessee Code Annotated, Section 50-7-301, et seq.

{108.09} WORKERS COMPENSATION LAWS

Tennessee Code Annotated, Section 50-6-101, et seq.

{108.10} Employment-at-will Developments

General Rule
Whittaker v. care-More, Inc., 621 S.W.2d 395 (Tenn. App., 1981).
Public Policy Exception
Clanton v. Cain-Sloan Co., 117 LRRM 2789 (Tenn., 1984).
Implied Contract Exception
See, for example: Gee v. Express Corp., 710 F.2d 1181 (CA-6, 1983), applying Tennessee law.
Hamby v. Genesco, 627 S.W.2d 373 (Tenn. App., 1981).

TEXAS

{109.01} Labor Relations Laws

Fire and Police Employee Relations Act
Texas Statutes, Article 5154 (e) -1, Section 1, et seq.
General Right to Organize
Texas Public laws, Article 5152, (p.l.1899).
Right-to-Work Statute
Vernon's Texas statutes, Article 5207a, Section 2.

{109.02} Strikes, Picketing, and Boycott Laws

Secondary Boycotts
Section 1 of Article 5154F of the Texas Statutes.
Employment of Armed Detectives
Texas Statutes, Article 5207.
Public Employment Strikes
Section 3 of Article 5154c of the Texas Statutes.
Strikes Against Public Utilise
Texas Statutes, Article 1446a, Section 3.
Mass Picketing
Section 1 of Article 5154d of the Texas Statutes.
Interference with Employment
Texas Statutes, Section 2 of Article 5154d, Section 2.

{109.03} Mediation and Arbitration Laws

Texas Public Laws, Article 239 (L. 1895)

{109.04} Regulation of Union Activities

Texas Public Laws, Article 1061(L. 1895)
Texas Statues, Article 1690e.
Texas Statues, Article 5154a, Section 3.
Texas Statues, Article 5154a, Section 5.

Section 4b of Article 5154a of the Texas Statutes
Texas Statues, Article 5154b.

{109.05} REGULATION OF EMPLOYMENT PRACTICES

Anti-Discrimination Laws:
Texas Statues, Article 5221K, Section 1, et seq.
Texas Statues, Article 5547-300, Section 9.
Protection of Military:
Texas Statues, Article 5765, Section 7A.
Jury Service:
Texas Statues, Article 5207b.
Blacklisting:
Texas Statues, Article 5196, et seq.
Whistle-Blowing Statute (Public Employees):
Section 16(a) of Article 6252 of the Texas Statue.
Voice Stress Analyzers:
Section 4 of Article 4413 of the Texas Statue.
Political Activities:
Texas Education Code, Article 13.34a.
Service Letters:
Article 5196 of the Texas Statues.
Equal Pay (Public Employees):
Texas Statues, Section 6825.

{109.06} WAGE AND HOUR LAWS

Child Labor:
Texas Public Laws, Chapter 531 (L. 1981).
Voting Time:
Texas Election Code, Section 15.14 of Title 9.
Payment of Wages:
Texas Public Laws, H.B. 79 (L. 1983).
Payment Upon Termination:
Texas Statues, Article 5156, 5157, & 5158.
Texas Statues, Article 6431.
Wage Assignment:
West's Texas Family Code, Section 14.091(i).

{109.07} SAFETY HEALTH LAWS:

Texas Statues, Article 5182a, Section 10.23.

{109.08} UNEMPLOYMENT COMPENSATION LAWS:

Texas Statues, Article 5221b, Section 2, et seq.

{109.09} Workers' Compensation Laws:

Texas Statues, Article 8306, Section 1, et seq.
    Texas Statues, Article 8307c.

{109.10} Employment-at-will Developments

Public Policy Exception:
    Sabine Pilots, Inc. v. Hauck, 687 S.W.2d 733 (Tex. Ct. App., 1985).
    Implied Contract Exception:
    Reynolds Mfg. Co, Mendoza, 644 S.W.2d 536 (Tex. Ct. App., 1982).
    Johnson v. Ford Motor Co., 690 S.W.2d 90 (Tex. Ct. of App., 1985)

UTAH

{110.01} Labor Relations Laws

Utah Labor Relations Act
    Utah code Annotated, Section 34-20-7.
    Utah code Annotated, Section 34-20-8.
    Utah code Annotated, Section 34-20-1, et seq.
    Firefighters Bargaining Rights
    Utah code Annotated, Section 34-20a-1.
    Rights of Labor
    Utah Constitution, Article XVI, Section 1.
    "Yellow-Dog" Contracts
    Utah code Annotated, Section 34-1-24.

{110.02} Strikes, Picketing, and Boycott Laws

Anti-Injunction Statutes
    Utah code Annotated, Section 34-19-1.
    Unlawful Assembly
    Utah code Annotated, Section 76-9-101.
    Interference with Employment
    Utah code Annotated, Section 34-2-3.
    Sabotage
    Utah code Annotated, Section 76-8-802.
    Employment of Armed Guards
    Utah Constitution, Article XII, Section 16.
    Deputized Employees During Strikes
    Utah code Annotated, Section 34-19-12.

{110.03} Mediation and Arbitration Laws

Utah code Annotated, Section 78-31-1, et seq.
    Utah Public Laws, S.B. 133(L.1977).

{110.04} REGULATION OF UNION ACTIVITIES

Utah code Annotated, Section 76-10-1002.

{110.05} REGULATION OF EMPLOYMENT PRACTICES

Utah code Annotated, Section 35-35-6, et seq.
Protection of Political Freedom
Utah code Annotated, Section 20-13-6 and 20-13-7.
Polygraph Restrictions
Utah code Annotated, Section 34-37-16.
Blacklisting
Utah code Annotated, Section 34-24-1.
Access to Personnel Records
Utah code Annotated, Section 67-18-1, 63-2-66.
Military Duty
Utah code Annotated, Section 39-1-36.
Medical Examination Payments
Utah code Annotated, Section 34-33-1
Equal Pay
Utah code Annotated, Section 34-35-6.

{110.06} WAGE AND HOUR LAWS

Child Labor
Utah code Annotated, Section 34-23-1, et seq.
Voting Time
Utah code Annotated, Section 20-13-18.
Payment of Wages
Utah code Annotated, Section 34-28-3.
Payment Upon Termination
Utah code Annotated, Section 34-28-5(1).
Utah code Annotated, Section 34-28-5(2).
Garnishments
Utah code Annotated, Section 70B-5-106.

{110.07} SAFETY AND HEALTH LAWS

Utah Code Annotated, Section 35-9-5

{110.08} UNEMPLOYMENT COMPENSATION

Utah Code Annotated, Section 35-4-1, et seq.

{110.09} WORKERS' COMPENSATION LAWS

Utah Code Annotated, Section 35-1-1 et seq.

{110.10} Employment-at-will Developments

Bihlmaier v. Carson, 630 P.2d 790 (Utah, 1979).

VERMONT

{111.01} Labor Relations Laws

Vermont Labor Relations Law
  Vermont Statutes Annotated, Title 21, Section 1501, et seq.
  State Employees Bargaining Rights
  Vermont Statutes Annotated, Title 27, Section 901, et seq.
  Vermont Statutes Annotated, Title 27, Section 961 and 962.
  Teachers Bargaining Rights
  Vermont Public laws, Chapter 57(L.1969).
  Vermont Municipal Labor Relations Act
  Vermont Statutes Annotated, Title 21, Section 172, et seq.
  Nonright-to-Work Policy

{111.02} Strikes, Picketing, and Boycott Laws

Unlawful Assembly
  Vermont Statutes Annotated, Title 21, Section 521, et seq.
  Interference with Employment
  Vermont Statutes Annotated, Title 13, Section 931, et seq.
  "Sit-Down" Strikes
  Vermont Statutes Annotated, Title 13, Section 933.

{111.03} Mediation and Arbitration Laws

Vermont Statutes Annotated, Title 21, Section 521, et seq.

{111.04} Regulation of Unlon

Vermont Statutes, Ch. 337, Section 7759.

{111.05} Regulation of Employment

Anti-Discrimination Laws
  Vermont Statutes Annotated, Title 21, Section 495.
  Employment of Aliens
  Vermont public laws, Act 99 (L.1977).
  Jury or Witness Duty
  Vermont public laws, S.B. 98(L.1969).
  Military Duty
  Vermont Statutes Annotated, Title 21, Section 491, et seq.

Access to Personnel Records
Vermont Statutes Annotated, Title 1, Section 317 (b)(7).
Medical Examination Payments
Vermont Statutes Annotated, Title 21, Section 301.
Political Leaves of Absence
Vermont Statutes Annotated, Title 21, Section 496.
Equal Pay
Vermont Statutes Annotated, Title 21, Section 495.

{111.06} Wage and Hour Laws

Child Labor
Vermont Statutes Annotated, Title 21, Section 431, et seq.
Payment Upon Termination
Vermont Statutes Annotated, Title 21, Section 342 (c) (2).
Vermont Statutes Annotated, Title 21, Section 342 (c) (1).
Garnishments
Vermont Statutes Annotated, Title 12, Section 3172.

{111.07} Safety and Health Laws

Vermont Statutes Annotated, Title 21, Section 1301, et seq.

{111.08} Unemployment Compensation Laws

Vermont Statutes Annotated, Title 21, Section 1301, et seq.

{111.09} Workers Compensation Laws

Vermont Statutes Annotated, Title 21, Section 601, et seq.
Vermont Statutes Annotated, Title 21, Section 618, et seq.

{111.10} Employment-at-will-Developments

Brower v. Holmes Transp., Inc., 435 A.2d 952 (Vermont, 1981); Jones v. Keough, 409 A.2d 581 (Vermont, 1979).

VIRGINIA

{112.01} Labor Relations Laws

Right-to-Work Statute:
Code of Virginia, Section 40.1-60.
"Yellow-Dog" Contract:
Code of Virginia, Section 40.1-61.

{112.02} Strikes, Picketing, and Boycott Laws

Unlawful Assembly:
 Code of Virginia, Section 18.1-254.
 Interference with Employment:
 Code of Virginia, Section 40.1-53.
 Interference with Ingress or Egress:
 Code of Virginia, Section 40.1-53.
 Picketing of Residence or Dwelling:
 Virginia Public Laws, Chapter 711(L.1970).
 Public Employee Strikes:
 Code of Virginia, Section 40.1-55.
 Hospital Strikes:
 Code of Virginia, Section 40.1-54(1).
 See also Code of Virginia, Section 40.1-54(2). (However, this provision may well
be in contravention of the Federal Labor-Management Relation Act and, thereby
pre-empted by it.)
 Public Utilities Seizure Act:
 Code of Virginia, Section 56.1-509, et seq.
 Coal Industry Seizure Act:
 Code of Virginia, Section 45.1-145, et seq.

{112.03} Mediation and Arbitration Laws:

Code of Virginia, Section 8.01-577, et seq.
 Code of Virginia, Section 22.1-306, et seq.
 Code of Virginia, Section 2.1-114.5:1

{112.04} Regulation of union Activities

Code of Virginia, Section 40.1-76.
 Code of Virginia, Section 18.1-410.
 Code of Virginia, Section 40.1-54.

{112.05} Regulation of Employment Practice

Anti-Discrimination Laws (State Employee):
 Code of Virginia, Section 2.1-376.
 Employment of Aliens:
 Code of Virginia, Section 40.1-11.1.
 Polygraph Restrictions:
 Code of Virginia, Section 40.1-51.4:3.
 Blacklisting:
 Code of Virginia, Section 40.1-27.
 Medical Examination payments:
 Code of Virginia, Section 40.1-28.

Arrest Inquiries:
Code of Virginia, Section 19.2-392.
Jury Duty:
Virginia Public Laws (L. 1985, C. 436).
Military Duty:
Code of Virginia, Section 44-98.
Code of Virginia, Section 44-93
Equal Pay:
Code of Virginia, Section 40.1-28.

{112.06} WAGE AND HOUR LAWS

Child Labor:
Code of Virginia, Section 40.1-100, et seq.
Code of Virginia, Section 40.1-105, et seq.
Code of Virginia, Section 40.1-78, et seq.
Payment of Wages:
Code of Virginia, Section 40.1-29.
Payment Upon Termination:
Code of Virginia, Section 40.1-29(a).
Garnishments:
Code of Virginia, Section 34-29(f).
Medical Insurance Conversion:
Code of Virginia, Section 38.1-348.11.

{112.07} SAFETY AND HEALTH LAWS:

General Provision:
Code of Virginia, Section 40.1-51.
Toxic Substances—Compensation Laws:
Code of Virginia, Section 40.1-51.1(c).

{112.08} UNEMPLOYMENT COMPENSATION LAWS:

Code of Virginia, Section 60.1-1, et seq.

{112.09} WORKERS' COMPENSATION LAWS:

Code of Virginia, Section 65.1-1, et seq.
Code of Virginia, Section 65.1-40, et seq.

{112.10} EMPLOYMENT-AT-WILL DEVELOPMENT:

Public Policy Exception:
Bowman v. State Bank of Keysville, 331 SE2d 799 (Va. Ct. of App. 1985).
Implied Contract Exception:

Frazier v. Colonial Williamsburg Foundation, 574 F.Supp. 318(E.D. Va., 1983).
Presumption of Term Exception:
Hoffman Specially Co. v. 164 S.E. 397 (Va., 1932)

WASHINGTON

{113.01} LABOR RELATIONS LAWS

General Right to Organize
Revised Code of Washington, Section 49.36.010.
Public Employees' Bargaining Right:
Revised Code of Washington, Section 41.56.010.
Revised Code of Washington, Section 41.56.010, et seq.
Educational Employment Relation Act:
Revised Code of Washington, Section 41.59.010, et seq.
Academic Employees' Bargaining Rights:
Revised Code of Washington, Section 28.B.52.010, et seq.
Higher Education Collective Bargaining:
Revised Code of Washington, Section 28B.16.100, et seq.
Health-Care Collective Bargaining:
Revised Code of Washington, Section 49.66.010, et seq.
Marine Employees' Bargaining Rights:
Revised Code of Washington, Section 47.64.010, et seq.
Port District Employees' Bargaining Rights:
Revised Code of Washington, Section 53.18.010, et seq.
Public Utility Employees' Bargaining Rights:
Revised Code of Washington, Section 54.04.170, et seq.
Nonright-to-Work Policy:
Labor Management Relation, Section 14(b).
"Yellow-Dog" Contract:
Revised Code of Washington, Section 49.32.030.

{113.02} STRIKES, PICKETING, AND BOYCOTT LAWS

Anti-Injunction Statue:
Revised Code of Washington, Section 49.32.011.
Injury to Property:
Revised Code of Washington, Section 9.05.060.
Interference with Employment:
Revised Code of Washington, Section 9.22.010.
Unlawful Assembly:
Revised Code of Washington, Section 9.27.040.
Unlawful Breach of Contract:
Revised Code of Washington, Section 49.44.080.
"Sit-Down" Strikes:
Revised Code of Washington, Section 9.05.070.

Strikebreakers:
Revised Code of Washington, Section 49.44.100.

{113.03} MEDIATION AND ARBITRATION LAWS:

Revised Code of Washington, Section 7.04.010.
Revised Code of Washington, Section 49.08.010, et seq.

{113.04} REGULATION OF UNION ACTIVITIES:

Revised Code of Washington, Section 9.16.030.
Revised Code of Washington, Section 49.44.030

{113.05} REGULATION OF EMPLOYMENT PRACTICES

Anti-Discrimination Laws:
Revised Code of Washington, Section 49.60.010.
Military Duty:
Revised Code of Washington, Section 73.16.033.
Polygraph Restrictions
Revised Code of Washington, Section 49.44.120.
Employment Under False Pretenses
Revised Code of Washington, Section 49.44.040
Whistle- Blowing Statute
Washington Public Laws, Chapter 208 (L. 1982).
Service Letters
WAC, Section 296-126-050.
Blacklisting
Revised Code of Washington, Section 49.44.010.
Equal Pay
Revised Code of Washington, Section 49.12.175.

{113.06} WAGE AND HOUR LAWS

Child Labor
Revised Code of Washington, Section 26.28.060, et seq.
Revised Code of Washington, Section26.28.060 and 49.12.12.
Payment Upon Termination
Revised Code of Washington, Section 49.48.010.
Garnishments
Revised Code of Washington, Section 7.33.160.

{113.07} SAFETY AND HEALTH LAWS

General Provisions
Washington Public Laws, S.B. 2386 (L. 1973).

Toxic Substances -Right to Know
Washington Public Laws, S.B. 4831, Section 15 (L. 1984).

{113.08} UNEMPLOYMENT COMPENSATION LAWS

Revised Code of Washington, Section 50.20.001, et seq.

{113.09} WORKERS COMPENSATION LAWS

Revised Code of Washington, Section 50.04.010, et seq.

{113.10} EMPLOYMENT-AT-WILL DEVELOPMENTS

Public Policy Exception
Thompson v. St. Regis Paper Co., 685 P.2d 1081 (Wash., 1984).
Implied Contract Exception
Roberts v. Atlantic Richfield co., 568 P.2d 764 (Wash., 1977).
Intentional Infliction of Emotional Distress Exception
Contreras v. Crown Zellerbach Corp., 565 P.2d 1173 (Wash., 1977).

WEST VIRGINIA

{114.01} LABOR RELATION LAWS

West Virginia Labor Management Relation: West Virginia Code, Section 21-1A-1, et seq.
Nonright-to-Work Policy:
Labor Management Relation Act, Section 14(b).

{114.02} STRIKES, PICKETING, AND BOYCOTTS LAWS:

Unlawful: Assembly:
West Virginia Code, Section 61-6-6.
Use of Out-of-State Police:
West Virginia Code, Section 61-6-11.
Interference with Employment at Mines:
West Virginia Code, Section 22-2-77.

{114.03} MEDIATION AND ARBITRATION LAWS:

West Virginia Code, Section 55-10-1, et seq.
West Virginia Code, Section 21-1A-1.

{114.04} REGULATION OF UNION ACTIVITIES:

West Virginia Code, Section 47-2-3.

{114.05} REGULATION OF EMPLOYMENT PRACTICES:

Anti-Discrimination Laws:
West Virginia Code, Section 5-11-19, et seq.
Protection of Political Freedom:
West Virginia Code, Section 3-9-15.
Employment Under False Pretense:
West Virginia Code, Section 21-2-6.
Jury Duty:
West Virginia Code, Section 52-3-1.
Military Duty:
West Virginia Code, Section 15-1F-8
Polygraph Restrictions:
West Virginia Code, Section 21-5-5b
Medical Examination Payment:
West Virginia Code, Section 21-3-17.
Equal Pay:
West Virginia Code, Section 21-5B-3

{114.06} WAGE AND HOUR LAWS

Child Labor
West Virginia Code, Section 21-6-1, et seq.
Voting Time
West Virginia Code, Section 3-1-42.
Payment of Wages
West Virginia Code, Section 21-5-3.
Payment Upon Termination
West Virginia Code, Section 21-5-4(b).
West Virginia Code, Section 21-5-4(c).
Garnishments
West Virginia Code, Section 46A-2-131.
Medical Insurance Conversion
West Virginia Code, Section 33-16A-1.

{114.07} SAFETY AND HEALTH LAWS

General Provisions
West Virginia Code, Section 21-3-1.
Toxic Substances- Right to Know.
West Virginia Code, Section 21-3-18.

{114.08} UNEMPLOYMENT COMPENSATION LAWS

West Virginia Code, Section 21A-1-1, et seq.

{114.09} Workers Compensation Laws

West Virginia Code, Section 23-1-1, et seq.

{114.10} Employment-at-Will Developments

Public Police Exception
   Harless v. First Nat'l Bank in Fairmont 246 S.E.2d 270 (W.Va., 1978).
   Implied Contract Exception
   McMillion v. Appalachian Power Co., 701 F.2d 166 (CA-4, 1983).
   Intentional Infliction of Emotional Distress Exception
   Harless v. First Nat'l Bank in Fairmont, supra.

WISCONSIN

{115.01} Labor Relations Laws

Employment Peace Act
   Wisconsin Statutes, Section 111.01, et, seq.
   Municipal Employees Bargaining Rights
   Wisconsin Statutes, Section 111.70, et, seq.
   State Employees Bargaining Rights
   Wisconsin Statutes, Section 111.80, et seq.
   Police Officers and Firefighters Bargaining
   Wisconsin Statutes, Section 111.77, et seq.
   Nonright-to -Work Police
   Section 14(b) of the labor management relations act.
   "Yellow-Dog" Contracts
   Wisconsin Statutes, Section 101.52.

{115.02} Strikes, Picketing, and Boycott Laws

Anti-Injunction Statues
   Wisconsin Statutes, Section 103.56.
   Unlawful Assembly
   Wisconsin Statutes, Section 347.02.
   Interference with Employment
   Wisconsin Statutes, Section 343.683.
   Disorderly Conduct
   Wisconsin Statutes, Section 348.5.
   Mass Picketing
   Wisconsin Statutes, Section 111.06(2)(e).
   "Sit-Down" Strikes
   Wisconsin Statutes, Section 111.06(2)(b).
   Strikebreakers
   Wisconsin Statutes, Section 348.472.

Picketing of Resident or Dwelling
Wisconsin Statutes, Section 111.06(2)(a).
Secondary Boycotts
Wisconsin Statutes, Section 111.06(2)(g).

{115.03} MEDIATION AND ARBITRATION LAWS

Wisconsin Statutes, Section 298.01.
    Wisconsin Statutes, Section 111.50, et seq.

{115.04} REGULATION OF UNLON ACTIVITIES

Wisconsin Statutes, Section 132.19.
    Wisconsin Statutes, Section 211.01, et seq.
    Wisconsin Statutes, Section 111.08.

{115.05} REGULATION OF EMPLOYMENT PRACTICES

Anti-Discrimination Laws
    Wisconsin Statutes, Section 111.321, st seq.
Polygraph Restrictions
    Wisconsin Statutes, Section 111.37.
Protection of Political Freedom
    Wisconsin Statutes, Section 103.18.
Jury Duty
    Wisconsin Statutes, Section 756.25.
Arrest Records
    Wisconsin Statutes, Section 111.31, 111.335.
Access to Personnel Records
    Wisconsin Statutes, Section 103.13. et seq.
Backlisting
    Wisconsin Statutes, Section 343.682.
Plant Closure
    Wisconsin Statutes, Section 109.07.
Medical Examination Payments
    Wisconsin Statutes, Section 103.37.
While-Blowing Statute
    Wisconsin Statutes, Section 230.80, et seq.
Equal Pay
    Wisconsin Statutes, Section 111.36.

{115.06} WAGE AND HOUR LAWS

Child Labor
    Wisconsin Statutes, Section 103.66, et seq.
    Wisconsin Statutes, Section 103.78.

Voting Time
Wisconsin Statutes, Section 6.76.
Payment Upon Termination
Wisconsin Statutes, Section 109.03.
Garnishments
Wisconsin Statutes, Section 812.235.
Medical Insurance Conversion
Wisconsin Statutes, Section 632.897.

{115.07} SAFETY AND HEALTH LAWS

General Provision
Wisconsin Statutes, Section 101.11, et seq.
Toxic Substances-Right to Know
Wisconsin Statutes, Section 101,58, et seq.

{115.08} UNEMPLOYMENT COMPENSATION LAWS

Wisconsin Statutes, Section 108.01, et seq.

{115.09} WORKERS COMPENSATION LAWS

Wisconsin Statutes, Section 102.01, et seq.
Wisconsin Statutes, Section 102.01, et seq.

{115.10} EMPLOYMENT-AT-WILL DEVELOPMENTS

Implied Contract Exception
Ferrero v. Voelsch, 350 N.W.2d 735 (Wis. S. Ct., 1985),
Public Policy Exception
Ward v. Frito-Lay Inc., 290 N.W.2d 356 (Wisconsin Ct. of App., 1980).

WYOMING

{116.01} LABOR RELATIONS LAWS

General Right to Organize
Wyoming Statutes, Section 27-7-101.
Firefighters Bargaining Rights
Wyoming Statutes, Section 27-10-101, et seq.
Right-to-Work Statute
Wyoming Statutes, Section 27-7-108.
"Yellow-Dog" Contracts
Wyoming Statutes, Section 27-245.3.

{116.02} Strikes, Picketing, and Boycott Laws

Anti-Injunction Statute
Wyoming Statutes, Section 27-7-103.
Unlawful Assembly
Wyoming Statutes, Section 6-10-108.
Use of Police During Strikes
Wyoming constitution, article 19, Section 6.

{116.03} Mediation and Arbitration Laws

Wyoming Statutes, Section 1-36-103.

{116.04} Regulation of Union Activities

Wyoming Statutes, Section 27-7-245.

{116.05} Regulating of Employment Practices

Anti-Discrimination Laws
Wyoming Statutes, Section 27-9-105, et seq.
Protection of Political of Political Freedom
Wyoming Statutes, Section 22-341, et seq.
Jury Service
Wyoming Statutes, Section 1-11-401(a).
Military Duty
Wyoming Statutes, Section 19-3-105(e).
Access to Medical Records
Wyoming Statutes, Section 27-11-113.
Equal Pay
Wyoming Statutes, Section 27-4-301.

{116.06} Wage and Hour Laws

Child Labor
Wyoming Statutes, Section 27-6-107, et seq.
Voting Time
Wyoming Statutes, Section 22-2-111.
Payment on Termination
Wyoming Statutes, Section 27-7-104.
Garnishments
Wyoming Statutes, Section 40-14-506.

{116.07} SAFETY AND HEALTH LAWS

Wyoming Statutes, Section 27-11-105(a).

{116.08} UNEMPLOYMENT COMPENSATION LAWS

Wyoming Statutes, Section 27-3-101, et seq.

{116.09} WORKERS COMPENSATION LAWS

Wyoming Statutes, Section 27-12-101, et seq.
   Wyoming Statutes, Section 27-12-401, et seq.

Index

Note: Page numbers followed by "*n*" refer to notes.

Milton Keynes UK
Ingram Content Group UK Ltd.
UKHW031138141024
449569UK00024B/1231